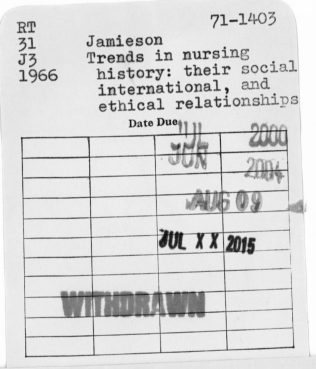
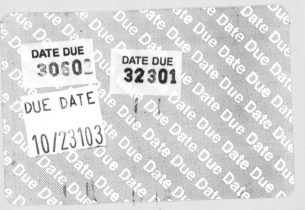

TRENDS IN NURSING HISTORY

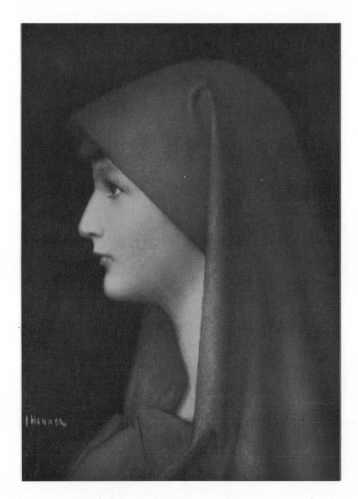

FABIOLA
An Early Christian Nurse

Sixth Edition

Illustrated

TRENDS IN NURSING HISTORY

THEIR SOCIAL, INTERNATIONAL, AND ETHICAL RELATIONSHIPS

ELIZABETH M. JAMIESON, R.N., B.A.
Late Director of Nursing,
Fabiola Hospital School of Nursing,
Oakland, California

MARY F. SEWALL, R.N., B.S.
Formerly Director of Nursing Education,
Methodist Hospital School of Nursing,
Los Angeles, California

ELEANOR B. SUHRIE, R.N., B.S., M. Litt.
Associate Professor of Nursing,
University of Pittsburgh,
Pittsburgh, Pennsylvania

W. B. SAUNDERS COMPANY · PHILADELPHIA · LONDON

Reprinted February, 1968 and March, 1969

Trends in Nursing History

Preface

In this sixth edition of *Trends in Nursing History* an introductory chapter on "International Relationships" tells of events of the 12th quadrennial Congress of the International Council of Nurses, held in Melbourne, Australia, in the spring of 1961. This corresponds with the method used in general education of beginning a course in history with events of the present in order to provide incentive for going back to discover the succeeding stages of development through which mankind has traveled to make such a setting possible. Opportunity is offered here also for bringing out the viewpoint that nursing transcends national boundaries and national cultures.

With the second printing of this edition changes have been made to show the recent restructuring of the American Nurses' Association, the National League for Nursing, and the U. S. Public Health Service, as well as the new headquarters of the International Council of Nurses and the Florence Nightingale International Foundation in Geneva, Switzerland. Emphasis continues to be placed upon the general trend of events rather than many details, the purpose of which is to provide a satisfactory foundation on which students may build through reading current journals and other literature.

As students of today prepare to take their places in a more closely associated and interdependent world than did those of yesterday, knowledge of nursing history, past and present, can induce confidence in assuming their roles as instruments of social progress. Boundless opportunities will present themselves for utilizing their special knowledge and skills in helping to build a democratic world in which each individual can be free from disease and find opportunity for his own growth and development. An understanding of the historical traditions, ideals of service, and Christian principles of those who have gone before them is the rightful inheritance of all nurses and will add dignity and meaning to their work.

Pacific Grove, California   MARY FRANKLIN SEWALL

Pittsburgh, Pennsylvania   ELEANOR BRADY SUHRIE

Contents

INTRODUCTION

Chapter 1

INTERNATIONAL RELATIONSHIPS 3

    Business Meetings 6
    Student Meetings 8
    Closing Sessions 10
    Suggestions for Study 11
    References 11

Part One. ANCIENT CIVILIZATIONS
               Circa 5000 B.C. to 500 A.D.

Chapter 2

BEGINNINGS OF CIVILIZATION: 5000 B.C. to 1 A.D. 15

    The Near East 18
        Egypt 18
        The Fertile Crescent 23
        Persia (Now Iran) 27
    The Far East 28
        India 28
        China 31
    The Americas 33
    Suggestions for Study 34
    References 37

Chapter 3

THE MEDITERRANEAN WORLD 39

    Greece 39
    The "Birth of Reason" 43
    Rome 46
    Suggestions for Study 51
    References 52

Chapter 4

EARLY CHRISTIAN ERA: 1–500 A.D. 53

    Saul of Tarsus 56
    Early Christian Orders of Women 58
        Deaconesses 58
        Widows and Virgins 59
    Persecution of Christians 60
    Influence of Constantine the Great 61
    Roman Matrons 61
    Diakonia and Xenodochia 63
    Status of Medicine and Nursing 65
    The Fall of Rome in 476 A.D. 68
    Suggestions for Study 70
    References 72

Part Two.   THE MIDDLE AGES
               Circa 500 to 1500 A.D.

Chapter 5

EARLY MIDDLE AGES: SOCIETY IN SMALL COOPERATIVE UNITS 77

    Christian Monasticism 78
        Rise of Benedictine Monasteries 79
        Women of Monasticism 81
    Feudalism 83
    Guilds 85
    Islam, a Rival of Christianity 86
    Medicine and Nursing, 500–1000 A.D. 91
    Suggestions for Study 92
    References 93

Chapter 6

LATE MIDDLE AGES: SOCIETY BECOMING MOBILE;
DETACHMENT OF INDIVIDUALS 94

Pilgrimages to Palestine 94
The Crusades (1096–1271) 95
    Orders of Military Nurses 97
    Medieval Social Problems 99
    Rise of Mendicant Orders 102
    Rise of Secular Orders 104
    Gains and Losses of the Crusaders 107
    Social Changes Associated with the Crusades 107
    Chivalry Influences the Position of Women 109
Great Plagues of the Fourteenth Century 110
Saint Catherine of Siena; Hospital Nurse and
    Visiting Nurse 111
Medicine During the Late Middle Ages 113
    Growth of Hospitals 117
    Nursing of the Late Middle Ages 120
Suggestions for Study 124
References 125

Part Three. **THE MODERN ERA OF SCIENTIFIC AND SOCIAL EVOLUTION**
Beginning Circa 1500 A.D.

Chapter 7

RENAISSANCE, REFORMATION, AND A DECLINE IN NURSING 129

The Renaissance 129
    The Classic Revival 130
    Political Revolution 131
    Industrial Revolution 132
The Reformation 133
Transfer of European Culture to America 134
Medicine of the Renaissance 137
    Medicine in America 139
Era of Sanitation 142
Women of the Renaissance 143
    Rise of Feminism 144
    Women of the Industrial Revolution 146
A Decline in Nursing 147
Suggestions for Study 151
References 152

Chapter 8

EARLY HOSPITALS OF THE AMERICAS 154

New Spain 154
New France 157
    Canada 158

Louisiana 165
New England 165
American Revolution (1775–1783) 170
    Philadelphia Dispensary 171
    Nurse Society of Philadelphia 171
    Growth of Hospitals 172
Suggestions for Study 173
References 174

Chapter 9

SOCIAL REFORM MOVEMENTS 175

Catholic Social Reform 175
    Social Service Established 175
    Order of Sisters of Charity Founded 176
Protestant Social Reform 178
    Prison Reform 180
    Reform in Care of the Mentally Ill 182
    Prevailing Nursing Methods Exposed 183
    Order of Modern Deaconesses Founded 184
Florence Nightingale: Reformer of Hospitals and
    Nursing 191
    Early Life 191
    First Position 195
    Crimean War Service 1854–1856 196
    Postwar Activities 203
Suggestions for Study 206
References 207

Chapter 10

DEVELOPMENT OF SOCIAL AGENCIES 208

Nonsectarian Nursing Reform 208
District Nursing Established 212
Workhouse Infirmary Reform 213
Birth of the Red Cross in 1863 214
The American Civil War (1861–65) 217
    Work of the Sanitary Commission 217
    Volunteer Nursing 219
    Organization of Army Nursing 221
American National Red Cross 222
Reform of Nursing in America 223
    Pre-Nightingale Reform 223
    Nightingale Reform 225
    First Preliminary Courses 233
    First Textbooks 233

Prevailing Methods 234
Adoption of Uniforms 235
Other Social Reforms 236
Salvation Army 237
Settlement Houses 237
Y.M.C.A. and Y.W.C.A. 238
Medical Missionaries 238
The New Nurse 239
Medicine Enters a Revolutionary Period 240
Suggestions for Study 244
References 245

Chapter 11

FIRST NURSING ORGANIZATIONS AND THREE WARS 247

Nursing Organizations of Great Britain 247
New World Organizations 248
International Council of Nurses 250
National Organizations of Canada 250
Wars of Late Nineteenth Century 253
Spanish American War 253
South African War 254
U.S. Army and Navy Nurse Corps 255
American Red Cross Nursing Service 255
Graduate Education for Nurses 256
Changes in Organization 259
World War I (1914–1918) 260
Royal College of Nursing 263
Postwar Reconstruction 265
Vocational Rehabilitation 265
League of Red Cross Societies 266
Postgraduate Courses at Bedford College 266
League of Nations 266
General Trends in Nursing 267
Broader Aims in Medicine 268
Suggestions for Study 271
References 273

Chapter 12

NATIONAL SURVEYS OF NURSING AND MEDICINE 274

Rockefeller Survey (1920–1923) 274
Grading of Nursing Schools (1926–1934) 277
Surveys in Canada and England 280
Revision of Nurse Practice Acts 281
Survey of Medical Practice (1927–1932) 282

Social Security Act of 1935 283
Florence Nightingale International Foundation 284
    FNIF Associated with the ICN 285
Suggestions for Study 286
References 288

Part Four. ACCELERATED SCIENTIFIC AND SOCIAL EVOLUTION

Chapter 13

WORLD WAR II AND POSTWAR DEVELOPMENTS 291

Postwar Problems 298
UNRRA 299
The United Nations 300
Postwar Developments 305
    Three Studies of Nursing 307
    School Data Survey of 1949 309
Hill-Burton Act 310
The President's Commission 310
U.S. Department of Health, Education, and
    Welfare; Public Health Service 311
Structure Changes in Organized Nursing 314
National Accreditation of Nursing Schools 316
National Accreditation of Hospitals 316
Rise of Psychiatry 318
Expansion of Rehabilitation Services 319
Suggestions for Study 320
References 321

Chapter 14

MODERN TRENDS IN NURSING 323

Structure Changes of 1966 and 1967 323
American Nurses' Association 324
National League for Nursing 330
National Student Nurses' Assocation 333
American Journal of Nursing Company 335
Canadian Nurses' Association 336
Expansion of Nursing Research Programs 339
    Associate Degree Research Programs 340
    ANA Research Programs 341
    American Nurses' Foundation for Research 344
    NLN Research Programs 346
    USPHS Nursing Research Programs 348
    Yale's Study of Studies 349

Report of the Surgeon General's Consultant Group 350
AMA Committee on Nursing 354
Suggestions for Study 354
References 356

Chapter 15

GRADUATE NURSING CAREERS 358

Career Opportunities 358
Government Services 366
Canadian Government Services 375
    Department of National Defense 375
    Department of Veterans Affairs 375
    Department of National Health and Welfare 376
    Victorian Order of Nurses for Canada 376
U.S. Exchange Visitor Program 378
Moral and Legal Responsibilities of Nurses 379
    Laws Regulating Nursing Practice 380
    Contracts of Employment 381
    Legal Status of Employed Persons 381
    Torts versus Crimes 382
Economic Security for Nurses 383
Educational Funds for Nurses 385
    Nurses' Educational Funds, Inc. 386
    USPHS Traineeship Awards 386
    U.S. Children's Bureau Awards 388
    Other Funds for Nurses 388
    WHO Fellowships for Foreign Study 389
    Fulbright Scholarships 390
Suggestions for Study 390
References 392

Chapter 16

NURSING IN MANY LANDS 394

Latin America 394
    Mexico 396
    El Salvador 398
    South American Republics 399
France 401
Germany 403
Belgium 405
Northern Europe 407
Italy 408
Israel 410

Africa 412
Republic of India 417
China 418
Formosa 418
Japan 419
Korea 420
References 424

INDEX 426

INTRODUCTION

Chapter 1

INTERNATIONAL RELATIONSHIPS

In April, 1961, more than twenty three hundred graduate nurses from forty four countries and two hundred student nurses from seven countries gathered in Melbourne, Australia, as guests of the Royal Australian Nursing Federation. For what special purpose had they come by train, ship, and plane, and what were their accomplishments? These present and future members of national nursing organizations, affiliated with the International Council of Nurses, were to attend the 12th quadrennial ICN Congress being held for the first time in the South Pacific. While it was spring in the Northern Hemisphere that many had left behind, flowers and shrubs gave evidence that it was fall in the land "down under."

An International atmosphere was everywhere present. National flags and banners of member associations decorated the balcony of the large Exhibition Building where meetings were held. The music of many nations was furnished by the Royal Australian Air Force Band, and a "Song of Welcome" by the choir of the Australian Christian Movement. The national dress of African and Oriental countries was worn by some of their nurses. Australian student nurses, in school uniforms, formed an honor guard at the auditorium entrance as officials of the Australian government, heads of churches and various services, and other distinguished guests arrived. Members of the lay press were present in order to report proceedings to their own country and to other parts of the world as well.

At the previous Congress, held in Rome, Italy, in 1957, the watchword, "Wisdom," had been given by the retiring president for the quadrennium to follow, and the theme of the Melbourne Congress was to be "Wisdom and Guidance through Professional Organization." Official

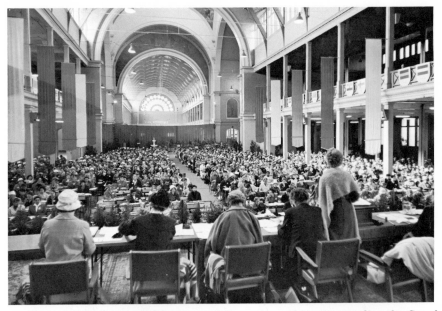

Figure 1. International Delegates and Congress participants attending the Grand Council of the International Council of Nurses in the Exhibition Building, Melbourne, 1961. (International Nursing Review, May/June, 1961. Courtesy of the Australian News and Information Bureau.)

proceedings were opened by the president, *Agnes Ohlson* of the United States, who spoke of today's emphasis on the welfare of the individual and of public awareness of need for adequate health care. She spoke also of the responsibility of governments for assisting with provision for health services and of nursing organizations for helping to solve problems of the nations and the world. *Daisy C. Bridges* of England, retiring general secretary of the ICN after 13 years of devoted service, stated that, "The International Council of Nurses with its world-wide membership and high professional ideals can be a powerful influence for the promotion of world health and for international understanding."[1]

Lyle Creelman of Canada, Chief of the Nursing Section of the World Health Organization, brought greetings from headquarters in the Palais des Nations of Geneva, Switzerland, and spoke of the value of close working relationships between the WHO, which is a specialized agency of the United Nations, and the International Council of Nurses. Through its status of official relationship with the World Health Organization, the ICN acts as expert adviser to the WHO on subjects relating to nursing education and service.

Marie Jahoda, social psychologist of England, gave the keynote address during which she stated that perhaps the most distinctive feature of a profession is that its "members possess specialized knowledge which is acquired through formal education beyond the schooling that is

---

[1]American Journal of Nursing, July, 1961, p. 62.

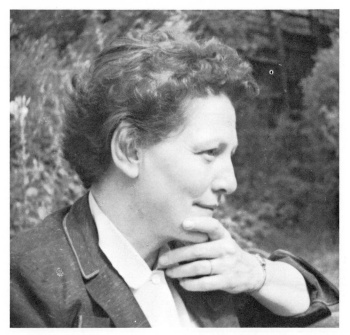

Figure 2. Marie Jahoda, Social Psychologist. (International Nursing Review, Aug., 1960.)

common to all members of a nation as prescribed by the law of the land." She then went on to say that "a profession implies that the quality of work done by its members is of greater importance in their own eyes and in the eyes of society than the economic rewards they earn."[2] She also warned of a possible danger in the inclination to talk as if problems of every culture and country could be solved under the tremendous good will of the International Council of Nurses.

Alice Girard, past president of the Canadian Nurses' Association, included the following in her address: "We represent professional nurses from all parts of the world. We work under every existing condition— political, economic, geographical, and climatic. We are deeply integrated into the fabric of our countries and these countries vary in terms of national aspirations. Notwithstanding the possibilities of division inherent in the variety of backgrounds that make up our profession, we are all united in a common purpose and a common goal. In this unanimity of purpose we are indeed fortunate since, in a world full of conflict, it provides a broad international basis for mutual effort, interest and understanding."[3]

The speaker then went on to say that three forces at work in the world today are constantly bringing about social changes of which the

---

[2]International Nursing Review, May/June, 1961, p. 11.
[3]INR, May/June, 1961, p. 22.

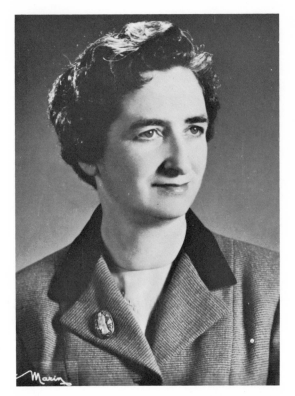

Figure 3. Alice Girard,
ICN President, 1965–1969.

nursing profession must have knowledge and understanding. These are a revolution in science and technology profoundly affecting the practice of medicine and nursing; increasing anxieties among the people due to opening up of wider horizons through educational and scientific advances; and a rising level of education with more and more rapid means of communication and transportation.

BUSINESS MEETINGS

In addition to plenary sessions, special business meetings were held by the two ICN governing bodies, the *Board of Directors* and the *Grand Council,* the former made up of ICN officers and the presidents of member associations, and the latter, which is the voting body, consisting of the same group together with four official delegates from each member association. The Board of Directors met in Wellington, New Zealand, a week before the Congress opened, as guests of the New Zealand Registered Nurses' Association. The Grand Council held five meetings to which all other registrants were invited. The Board of Directors meets every two years but the Grand Council convenes only during the quadrennial Congresses.

Reports and recommendations of the *Nursing Service Division* and the *Florence Nightingale Education Division* were received and acted upon, and a new *Social and Economic Welfare Division* was brought into being. *Frances Beck* of England, director of the Nursing Service Division, spoke on "The Responsibility of a Professional Nurses' Association for the Improvement of Nursing Service." She stressed the necessity for unity of purpose while representing the interests of nurse educators, administrators, and other specialists, and for the development of communication skills by all nurses. She spoke also of the responsibility of national nursing associations for sound ethical practices, for participating in international work through the ICN, and for representing nursing to governmental and non-governmental organizations. She urged acceptance of individual and collective responsibility for future improvement of all nursing services.

Ellen Broe of Denmark, director of the Florence Nightingale Education Division, said that "The nurse of the future must be prepared to move freely between hospital and home; she would have to be familiar with work in day hospitals, outpatient centers, clinics, and rehabilitation units. She might have the responsibility for the health of a group of families. For these reasons it is essential for the nurse to learn to work with people and to cooperate with a variety of colleagues."[4]

The Florence Nightingale Education Division of the ICN was originally an entirely separate organization under the name of *Florence Nightingale International Foundation,* which was established in 1934 as a living, educational memorial to Florence Nightingale. In 1949 the FNIF was brought into association with the ICN and now functions as its Education Division while retaining its original identity as a separate organization.

The objective of the new Social and Economic Welfare Division was defined as that of advising and assisting national nursing organizations to improve employment practices, while regarding problems of shorter hours, higher salaries, and desirable working conditions as contributing factors to solution of that greater problem of improving their social service. In line with this aim of encouraging high standards of nursing practice, the Nursing Service Division carries on research directed toward this end, and a booklet, "ICN Basic Principles of Nursing Care," has been prepared under the guidance of *Virginia Henderson* of the United States and is being used extensively throughout the world.

An interesting measure agreed upon by the Grand Council was for the preparation of a booklet on *Nursing Ethics* which would embrace the *International Code of Ethics* now available from ICN headquarters, 35–37 rue de Vermont, 1200 Geneva, Switzerland. There was

---

[4]California Nurses' Association Bulletin, Sept., 1961, p. 140

agreement, too, on a measure for future consideration of the advisability of preparing a pledge, based on the International Code of Ethics, that would be suitable for taking at graduation exercises all over the world.

In addition to messages from the ICN Divisions, others were received from the *Publications and Public Relations Department* and the *Information on Professional Qualifications Department,* the former of which spreads knowledge of developments in nursing on a world-wide basis through bi-monthly publication of the *International Nursing Review* and other literature; while the latter evaluates the credentials of nurses who are seeking opportunities for study or employment outside of their own countries under the ICN *Exchange of Privileges for Nurses Program.*

Statistics presented to the Grand Council by the Information on Professional Qualifications Department showed that hundreds of nurses, many of them refugees, have been working for stipulated periods, studying, or observing nursing methods outside of their own countries, and the number has been increasing in recent years. Arrangements for this experience are made by some nurses through their own national associations in cooperation with the ICN and by others through individual channels. An ICN file of available opportunities is maintained as well as a clearing house through which exchanges of nurses are arranged and policies relating to them defined.

STUDENT MEETINGS

Nursing students at the Melbourne Congress represented schools of Australia, Canada, Great Britain, Korea, Malaya, New Zealand, and the United States. They attended all sessions including the official ICN banquet, and their earnestness and enthusiasm were everywhere

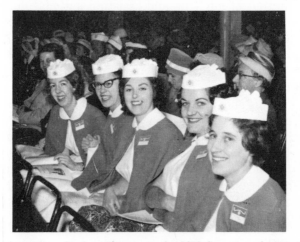

Figure 4. Australian Student Nurses at the ICN Congress of 1961. (International Nursing Review, May/June, 1961.)

in evidence. They also held meetings of their own during which correspondence that had been received since the last Congress was reviewed. This brought out the fact that an effort had been made to get in touch with as many national student nurses' associations as possible and that information had been acquired about Florence Nightingale, the International Council of Nurses, exchange visits among nursing students, research in relation to writing term papers, and the uniforms worn by students and nurses in various parts of the world. A few pen friends in foreign countries had been acquired.

The International Student Nurses' Unit of the ICN, formed at the 1957 Congress in Rome, was discussed and the problems associated with possibilities for its continuance due to changing populations of nursing schools between quadrennial meetings. The feeling was expressed that they wanted all students to attend their meetings regardless of whether or not their national nurses' associations had been admitted to ICN membership. The final decision was to hold in abeyance all resolutions in regard to the ISN Unit until some future time.

Special teas for students were held at several nursing schools in Melbourne, to all of which they were transported by taxi or bus. On the way, they saw stuffed kangaroos and Koala bears displayed in many places and purchased them in large numbers. On the last day of the Congress they were dinner guests of Australian students at the Royal

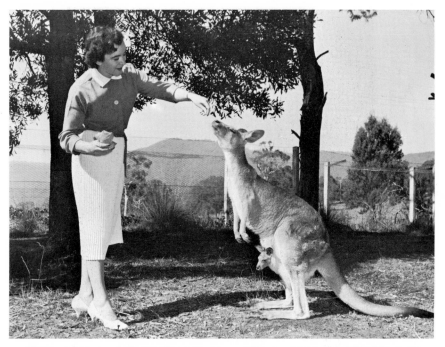

Figure 5.   Young Lady Feeding a Kangaroo. (Nursing Times, Dec. 25, 1959. Courtesy of the International Council of Nurses.)

Children's Orthopedic Hospital in Frankston, a distance of twenty miles from Melbourne. Dinner was followed by singing of familiar songs and autographing of programs and a tendency to delay the moment of departure as long as possible.

CLOSING SESSIONS

As the Congress was coming to a close, a colorful ceremony admitted to membership the national nursing associations of thirteen countries, bringing to fifty nine the number affiliated with the ICN. The new associations were those of Burma, British Guiana, Egypt, Ghana, Jordan, Kenya, Mexico, Nigeria, Poland, Republic of China, Singapore, Thailand, and Venezuela. As the name of each nation was called, a representative of its association accompanied by a member of a sponsoring association and preceded by an Australian student carrying that nation's flag, marched down the long center aisle of the auditorium to the stage where they were received by Agnes Ohlson, ICN president, amid music of the Royal Australian Air Force Band and great applause. Another flag was then added to those decorating the balcony.

Officers were elected making *Alice Clamageran* of France the new ICN president for the ensuing quadrennium. Mlle Clamageran is

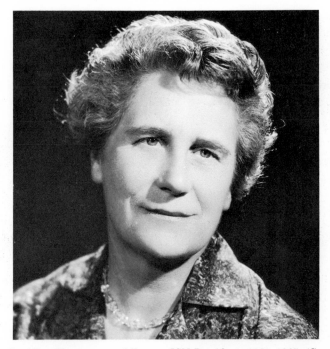

Figure 6. Alice Clamageran of France, ICN President, 1961–1965. (Courtesy of the International Council of Nurses.)

director of the School of Nursing and Social Work at the Hôtel Dieu, Rouen, and at that time president of the National Association of the Trained Nurses of France. Invitations for their countries to be the meeting place for the next Congress were extended by the presidents of the national associations of Canada, the United Kingdom, and Germany, but it was *Ruth Elster,* president of the German Nurses' Federation, who persuaded the delegates to cast their ballots in favor of Frankfort, Germany, for 1965. The watchword, "Inquiry," was given by Agnes Ohlson, retiring president, for the intervening four years, who went on to say that "Inquiry is the spirit of research, the curiosity of mind that must be ours."[5]

Suggestion for Study

What do you consider to have been the accomplishments of the 12th quadrennial ICN Congress, held in Melbourne, Australia, in 1961?

References

INTERNATIONAL NURSING REVIEW

1899-1959 Jubilee Issue. July, 1959. ICN Chronology, p. 3
"ILO Report – Employment and Conditions of Work of Nurses," August, 1960, p. 26
"The Importance of Professional Organization – National and International," Jan./Feb., 1961, p. 5
"International Congress, Melbourne," May/June, 1961, p. 3
"The Story of the Florence Nightingale International Foundation," – Killby. Nov./Dec., 1963, p. 25
"News from ICN House," Jan./Feb., 1964, p. 3
"International Summer Schools," Sept./Oct., 1964, p. 17

AMERICAN JOURNAL OF NURSING

"The ICN, the ANA, and the UN," Jan., 1959, p. 83
"With the ICN in Australia," July, 1961, p. 60
"Students at the ICN Congress," July, 1961, p. 92
"Consider the ICN Congress," – Schutt. Nov., 1964, p. 77

NURSING OUTLOOK

"Nursing is International!" – Bridges. April, 1961, p. 238
"12th International Congress of Nursing," June, 1961, p. 372

---

[5]International Nursing Review, July/Aug., 1961, p. 4

Part One

ANCIENT CIVILIZATIONS

Circa 5000 B.C. to 500 A.D.

Chapter 2

BEGINNINGS OF CIVILIZATION
5000 B.C. to 1 A.D.

Primitive man was a hunter and a nomad until he learned to select a suitable place to till the soil and provide a permanent abode for himself and his family. He lived in caves and wandered from place to place in search of food in the form of animals, birds, and fish as well as fruits, berries, and nuts. The stone was discovered to be a useful implement and, in the beginning, any detached piece of rock was thrown in its original state, but in time its shape was adapted to many purposes and this first manufactured implement is known as a "fist hatchet," and is often unearthed today. It was used with such skill that this earliest period of human habitation of the earth is known as the *Old Stone Age* or *Age of Hunters,* and is the longest period of human history, extending back several thousand years.

Primitive man continues to survive, very much in his original state, in isolated parts of Australia and Africa, and remnants may be seen in some of the Indian tribes of North and South America. Available records of his life, discovered in cave pictures, carvings, and excavations, show that there was early division into small, well defined groups built up around the nucleus of family relationship, with mutual protection in a difficult world as a basic reason for development. Each individual was expected to serve, to his utmost capacity, the common welfare and failure to be useful was sometimes cause for his elimination. Scarcity of food or imminent danger might lead to extermination of all dependents, and the aged and the sick were either destroyed or abandoned.

Customs or *mores,* peculiar to each tribe, constituted a chief means

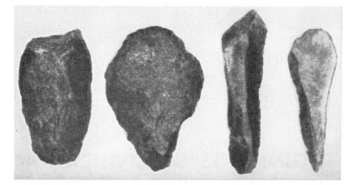

Figure 7. Rough stone implements of primitive man. (Courtesy of the Metropolitan Museum of Art.)

of perpetuating it, and habits of action that had proved expedient were looked upon as the only right way of doing things. Children brought up in the mores of one group accepted them or, if an individual now and then rebelled against what experience had proved desirable for the good of the tribe, he was destroyed or sent out to meet hostile nature alone. This strong tendency to adhere to established customs gave to some of them the fixity of law.

Animism. In the roving existence which was man's, constantly changing experiences were met. All about were myriad forms of life toward knowledge of which he had no science to guide him, but information gradually was acquired which enabled him to distinguish the harmful from the useful, and food and medicinal values in plants were learned empirically. At the same time it was natural for him to ascribe to all forms of nature, with which he was so closely associated, the same qualities as those of which he became conscious in himself. His rivers, trees, and sky, his rocks, plants, animals, birds and fish were believed to possess an inner reality and to make responses similar to his own. This *animism,* as we call it, opened up to man a still greater world, that of his imagination.

Eventually man found himself surrounded by a veil of superstition which he has not so far been able to destroy completely. While it brought added beauty into his life, it brought also fear and unnecessary ugliness. Spirits came to be considered as either *good* or *evil,* and to their influence were assigned the catastrophes as well as the benefits of everyday life. While some happenings brought happiness, added strength, or new life to the little bands of human wanderers, others brought sadness, weakness, or death. Disasters like storms, earthquakes, drought, flood, lightning, fires, or illness were explained by the presence of evil spirits, or even of good spirits that needed to be appeased.

In learning protection from the ravages of disease, the comforting effects of applying water externally were experienced in river bathing. It is possible that this knowledge was first obtained from observation of animals, for these cleanse their wounds by licking, and have been known to keep them submerged in water until inflammation subsided. Experience of emesis or catharsis, following the use of certain plants for food, doubtless underlay discrimination in choice. It is possible that some of this knowledge also was obtained from creatures of the animal kingdom, for examples of animal instinct in selection of plant remedies are known. His own wonderful invention of fire making by means of friction acquainted man with the comforting value of heat. In his use of heated stones lies the origin of later methods of searing and counter-irritation.

Medicine Men and Priest Physicians.   Some individuals became more expert than others in divining symptoms and applying special remedies and were known as "medicine men." Modern science now credits them with amazing knowledge of some valuable drugs, the use of which along with baths, manipulations, and much unconscious psychotherapy doubt-less brought about many cures. Each of these men was accepted as an outstanding figure in his tribe and in order to maintain this prestige it was necessary for him not only to be wise in medical lore but also to assume an intimacy with the good and evil spirits which men learned to either blame or exhort in attempts to solve the mystery surrounding cause and effect in disease.

As time went on the imagination of the medicine man often exceeded his wisdom and he adopted strange disguises to inspire fear in the super-natural. Attired in combinations of skins of animals, horns, feathers, grasses, snakes or toads, he struck awe into the hearts of those who beheld him and convinced them of his ability to frighten off evil spirits as he danced, made loud noises, and indulged in strange antics before them. However, he also must demonstrate power to invoke the help of good spirits in driving off the evil ones as well as the power to bring disaster on all enemies. It was necessary for him to learn the art of *white magic* for kindly, helpful purposes and of *black magic* for hostile and destructive aims.

The cure of disease gradually took on the quality of ritualistic religious ceremony and the medicine man was set apart from other men as a functionary of holiness. Ceremonial rites gave an added support in the presence of misfortune of any kind and, eventually, medicine men were succeeded by *priest physicians* to whom was passed over a strange mixture of fact and superstition.

Meanwhile the nomadic manner of life followed by primitive man brought constant changes in location of tribes and they tended to move toward the south where warm temperatures and luxuriant vegetation made it possible to live with less effort than was possible in northerly sections. This movement, it is now generally believed, radiated from the interior of Europe and Asia toward the warm shores of the Mediterranean Sea, India, and China. A lesser migration led toward western Europe and the British Isles, and travel and settlement usually followed the shores of great rivers. Regions bordering on the Mediterranean Sea came to form the greater part of the known world and this body of water was believed to occupy the center of the earth, as its name implies. All areas to the east of it were known as *Eastern,* those to the west as *Western.*

THE NEAR EAST

EGYPT

The long, narrow fertile strip, lying on either side of the Nile River and fringed by deserts, constitutes what came to be known as Egypt. The people who settled in this green valley were destined to go through the same stages of development as other regions, but at an earlier period. By 5000 B.C. they had added to man's early invention of stone implements, other inventions which brought radical changes into their manner of living. The grindstone enabled them to give tools a sharpness and smoothness that facilitated the work for which they were intended. Some ingenious person added a handle to the fist-hatchet and the axe was invented, which gave mastery over the forest and opened up opportunity to build a new type of home to replace the ancient cave dwelling, and to build ships and engage in commerce.

From observation of germination of seeds dropped inadvertently, man learned to control his supply of edible plants and grains, and he arrived at the *New Stone Age* or *Age of Farmers.* No longer compelled to wander constantly in search of means for subsistence, his energies were turned into new channels, and inventions increased in number. The wheel and cart were among the earliest, and by 4000 B.C., the observations and calculations of Egyptians had produced a calendar consisting of twelve months of thirty days each, with five extra days to celebrate the birthdays of their gods.

By 3000 B.C., writing had been introduced, at first in the form of pictures and later as signs or hieroglyphics, the earliest of which were cut in stone but later were written in ink on papyrus. The invention of writing was one of tremendous importance in the life of Egypt. It gave impetus to trade and the rewards of trade enabled those pioneers of civilization to express themselves in many ways. Buildings assumed the dignity of architecture and palaces, temples, and tombs arose over the land, and sculpture was produced to adorn them.

Religion and Medicine. By this time men had arrived at a stage in their beliefs where they were building up a world inhabited by gods whose wisdom and strength far exceeded theirs. Mythology was displacing animism, and a trinity of gods ultimately came into control of bodily and spiritual affairs. *Isis,* Mother Earth, gave help to the sick, most frequently through the medium of dreams. *Osiris,* her husband, was god of light or sun-god, and sat in judgment on the souls of the dead, for man had now arrived at belief in immortality and Egyptians were the first to make happiness in an after life dependent upon character. *Horus,* son of Isis and Osiris, from whom the Pharaohs believed themselves descended, learned medical lore from his mother.

As time went on the first temples increased in size and beauty and today their ruins bespeak to us the grandeur which they finally attained. Priests presided over them, and among those who sought their help were many who came because of illness. The temple thus assumed the dual aspect of church and hospital, and the priest became a *priest-physician,* thus strengthening the bond already existing between medicine and religion. From all priest-physicians of ancient Egypt, history singles out *Imhotep* as the greatest. So successful was he in healing the sick and so strikingly generous and kindly in personality that, after his death, Egyptian belief in Imhotep led the people to erect statues and temples in his honor, and worshipers addressed prayers to their wise and beloved physician.

The significance of the temple as a moulding influence in all early civilizations cannot be overestimated. Beginning as a meager shelter of crudest form to protect the image of a god from the eroding effects of weather, the temple arose to a magnitude and attained a magnificence that was in towering contrast to the early simplicity of human existence. The temples of Karnak and Luxor, near Gizeh, are today points of especial interest for every tourist. Nearly two thousand years of effort are said to have been spent on the Temple of Karnak alone, and the walls of its front gate are forty nine feet thick.

Temples became centers of community and national life, and when

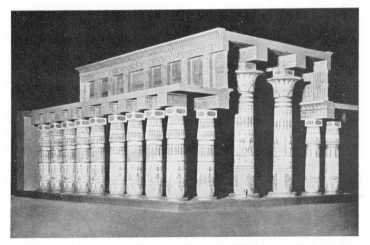

Figure 8. Reconstruction of the great Hypostyle Hall in the Temple of Karnak at Thebes, Egypt. (Courtesy of the Metropolitan Museum of Art, New York City.)

frequented by those in search of health, priest-physicians shared their task with a group of *temple women* who were often of high social position and held the rank of *priestess*. They are believed to have performed some nursing duties, especially for those who remained over night to seek priestly intercession with the gods, but history fails to make this point clear. It is probable that nursing care in ancient Egypt, as well as other countries of that time, was chiefly the responsibility of the mother or daughter in the home. The mother occupied a position of authority, and the level of woman's place in Egyptian society was relatively high.

The priests determined all ethical standards and gradually collected in written form their religious and other precepts and such mores as time had fixed into law. Included with the forty two Sacred Books eventually completed were six in which were gathered much of that medical lore tested out by primitive mothers, medicine men, and priest-physicians which has come down to us on rolls of papyrus. Of these first medical books, the one purchased in 1874 by Dr. Ebers of Germany and known as the "Ebers' Papyrus," is considered the best. It contains a classification and description of diseases and many complex prescriptions, one of which contains 35 ingredients.

Great wisdom was ascribed to Egyptian gods and any deviation from their teachings was a crime, punishable by law. The finality of thus placing all decisions in their hands took away from man all initiative. His life was ordered for him. All experimentation in medicine was discouraged. Dissection was not permitted. If a patient died following treatment varying from that prescribed in the Sacred Books, the priest-physician paid with his life. All further advance in medicine was checked.

Belief in Immortality. Egyptian belief in immortality, which was dependent upon preservation of the body, led men to devise permanent homes for the latter. An elaborate process of embalming was developed, the techniques of which were so elaborate that mummified bodies can be seen today. These give knowledge of some diseases existing at that time and of the art of bandaging. As many as a thousand yards of linen of various widths were sometimes used on one mummy and moistened with a gluey substance which hardened to form an impervious case for an aseptically cleansed body from which the internal organs had been removed. Should the mummified body be destroyed, a statue as nearly identical as possible could take its place in the afterlife, according to Egyptian teachings.

Assured of the preservation of body and soul for all time, tombs were erected to provide a safe repository for them, and food and other property necessary for comfort in life were buried with them. The pyramid type of tomb was the choice of Pharaohs and the pyramids erected for mummies of those rulers and their families still stand in the vicinity of Gizeh, near Cairo. The Cheops Pyramid, covering thirteen acres

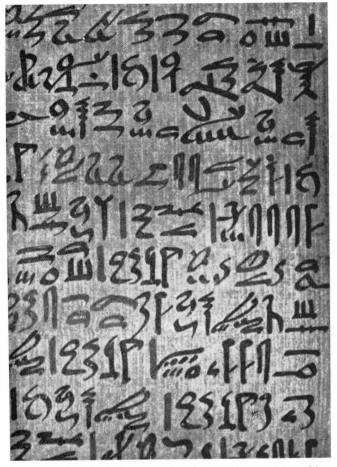

Figure 9. Babylonian medical prescription in cuneiform writing. (Museum of the University of Leipzig.)

at its base and nearly five hundred feet in height, stands as a memorial to a civilization then at the height of its grandeur. It is estimated to have required twenty years to build for the Pharaoh Cheops, and to have consumed the labor of 120,000 slaves.

In 330 B.C., came invasion and conquest by *Alexander the Great,* king of Macedonia and former pupil of Aristotle's. As a fortunate aftermath of this disaster, a new and great city grew and flourished on the Nile delta. Alexandria was, in time, to be celebrated as the home of *Cleopatra,* Queen of Egypt, but the real fame of the new city rested on a library of ancient manuscripts which attracted scholars of the world. A museum which was, in reality, a university drew teachers of eminence and became renowned among students. Distinguished physicians from many countries were among them and scientific medicine was studied, for the culture introduced by Alexander the Great was Greek, and the methods of Hippocrates were used in the school which he founded. The museum achieved honor throughout the world for its work in medicine, mathematics, geography, and astronomy.

The glory of the Alexandrian Empire was not to last. A greater Empire was already on the horizon of world affairs and in 30 B.C., the Romans came to Egypt, led by *Octavius,* successor to Julius Caesar. Cleopatra, its queen, found herself at the head of a country too weak to withstand him. Roman organization and Roman tyranny succeeded the culture of Greece along the banks of the Nile, and continued for nearly seven centuries.

Control of Egyptian territory was wrested from the Romans about 650 A.D., when great hordes of Moslem zealots from Arabia swept over their country on horseback in a westerly direction to spread Mohammed's teachings around the Mediterranean Sea and claim the land and its inhabitants for a great new Moslem Empire to be ruled by one of their caliphs. Theirs was a lasting influence and, even though a mixture of blood flows through their veins, today the Egyptians regard themselves as Arabs and are adherents of the Moslem religion.

Progress in the form of ensuring sufficient food for millions of their people is now taking place by construction of a new high dam to replace the present smaller one near the city of Aswan on the Nubian Desert. This undertaking will control the flow of the Nile River and form a vast lake 300 miles long to be used for irrigation purposes, but it also is making it necessary for Nubian Desert dwellers to abandon their long-established homes and lead a new type of life in hastily constructed villages between Aswan and Luxor. The Nubians have been greatly admired by many tourists for their integrity, gentleness, cleanliness, and wit, and they are said to be a people without crime.

The Aswan Dam, when completed about 1975, is destined to cover up for all time, and disintegrate, a multitude of irreplaceable archeological remains, including ancient temples and tombs and sculpture as well as rock carvings and cave paintings. Nearby granite quarries supplied the rock for early Egyptian genius to create monuments which, in this land of little rain, have been maintained in an excellent state of preservation. They are being unearthed and studied by archeologists, and secrets of the first colonists of the Nile Valley are being revealed. Authentic historical information is being acquired, not only of ancient Egyptians but of the beginnings of the human race as well.

To prevent an impending catastrophe, the United Arab Republic and the Republic of Sudan requested the assistance of the United Nations Educational, Scientific, and Cultural Organization (UNESCO), a responsibility of which is to safeguard our cultural and scientific heritages, and they have offered to surrender to contributing nations at least one half of all future excavation discoveries in the threatened area. A worldwide UNESCO appeal has been launched to raise sufficient funds with

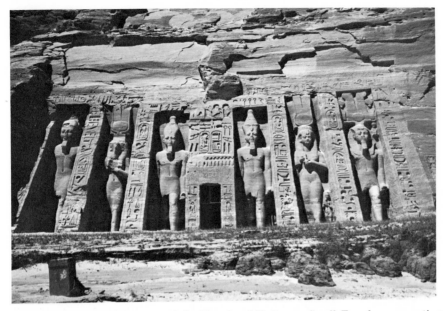

Figure 10. Six Colossuses of the Temple of Hathor or Small Temple representing Rameses II (1290–1223 B.C.) and his Wife Queen Nefertari (in danger of being submerged by the Aswan High Dam). (UNESCO/Laurenza.)

which to remove as many treasures as possible and save them for posterity. As they find their way to museums around the world, all will have the privilege of seeing them and contemplating upon the infancy of human race and the general direction in which mankind is moving.

THE FERTILE CRESCENT

The three ancient countries of Babylonia, Assyria, and Palestine formed a crescent-shaped strip of land extending from the Persian Gulf in the east to the Mediterranean Sea in the west, which because of the presence of three great rivers and good soil became known as the "Fertile Crescent." *Babylonia,* now Iraq, formed the eastern portion in the valleys of the lower Tigris and Euphrates Rivers and was originally called, "Mesopotamia," or the land between the Rivers. Here, as in Egypt, archeologists have been active during the last fifty years, and it has been determined that the beginnings of civilization appeared as early as 4000 to 3000 B.C. with so rich a development of morals, learning, and the arts that it has been called by some, "the cradle of all culture."

By 2100 B.C. Babylonians had attained a status of such importance that their lands were known as the Babylonian Empire. Their king, *Hammurabi,* substituted for long continued policies of warfare a constructive program that was distinctive in its originality. A very religious man, he built temples for his people. He also developed systems of irrigation. His fame, however, rests chiefly on his collection of all the older laws and customs of business, legal, and social life, and his systematic arrangement of these into a comprehensive Code of Law. This he had engraved on a great shaft of stone in one of the temples of Babylon, their capital city. Today it is the oldest preserved code of ancient law, and the sense of justice it displays is regarded as surprising, as well as the consideration shown for the poor and defenseless classes.

Medicine in Babylonia. \Hammurabi's Code of Law also provided for regulation of the arts of medicine and surgery, and differentiated between fees for operation on a "gentleman" and those chargeable to a freedman or a slave. Severe penalties fell upon the surgeon whose work was not successful. In case of failure to cure a gentleman, the operator's hands were to be cut off; in the case of an uncured servant, he must pay the owner the current price of a slave. Both these and the punishments inflicted upon criminals and those guilty of minor delinquencies seem harsh, but account must be taken of the fact that religion at that time did little to soften men's hearts, and that the value placed on life was inestimably less than that which followed the advent of Christianity.

The practice of medicine was considered of utmost importance at this early date of Babylonian history. Surgery was in advance of internal medicine, which concerned itself mainly with magical formulas to banish demons, the general belief being that gods of evil spirits avenge themselves upon erring human beings by visiting disease upon them. Their surgeons understood cataract removal, blood letting, and the use of facial applications in cases of erysipelas. Bodies of sacrificed animals supplied the only opportunity for anatomical research. Babylonian priests ascribed the source of epidemics to inauspicious astral influence. They diagnosed human ailments by examining the livers of dead animals. Indeed, their system of medicine placed noteworthy reliance on *divination,* or ascertaining, which was attempted by many means. Communion with the dead, crystal-gazing, palmistry, card-reading, omens, falling of meteors—even the instinctive acts of birds or animals—were all used as its medium.

Women were never held in high regard in Babylonia. Their opportunities were strictly domestic and polygamy was practiced. The upper classes of women enjoyed less freedom of action than was accorded those of the middle and lower groups of society.

The little country of *Assyria* arose in the middle portion of the Fertile Crescent and constituted the upper valleys of the Tigris and Euphrates Rivers. As Assyrians acquired culture, Nineveh, their capital city, became the center of art and culture of the East. Here lived their king in dazzling splendor, surrounded by a throng of officials who assisted him in administrative duties. They were a warlike race who built up the Assyrian Empire, the greatest that the world had yet known.

A custom of Assyrians was writing on tablets of soft clay which were then baked in the sun or in ovens, and a library of clay tablets recently unearthed reveals them as superstitious people believing in the influence of lunar changes and using charms and amulets. Sickness represented punishment for sin, and was curable by repentance, while medical practice otherwise confined itself to magic and empiricism. So much time was occupied with war that little was left for anything but military tactics. Education was restricted to the priesthood. Needless to say, Assyrian womanhood did not achieve a high position.

While members of Semitic tribes were drifting into the regions of Babylonia and Assyria from the arid parts of Arabia, other members of the same tribes were making their way into the region of *Palestine* at the western end of the Fertile Crescent. The natives whom they overran gave them the name of "Hebrews," or the "people from beyond." In time they migrated to Egypt, where they were taken into captivity and remained as slaves for more than four hundred years. They escaped under the leadership of Moses in the fifteenth century, B.C., and after forty years of wandering re-entered Palestine, and the country was divided up among their twelve tribes.

Religion was to constitute the chief contribution of the Hebrews to the betterment of a world that had come to have sore need of it. During centuries of confusing uncertainty they had held with considerable loyalty to the one Father, God, who had emerged supreme from an early polytheism. In his organization of a code of laws in harmony with the needs of his times, Moses developed the Mosaic Law around the worship of this one ethical Father God who demanded obedience from his children. The debt of mankind to the Hebrews came not through the adoption of any new ritual, but through the acceptance of this idea of one God, Jehovah, Maker of all things, a beneficent Being from whom all good can be expected to come, and with whom men may use their intelligence in individual communion through the spirit of prayer. By 1 A.D. this religion had been recorded in what we know as the Old Testament. It was written by many authors and, mainly, in the Hebrew language.

In an age in which people had inherited so many gods that religious worship was fast becoming a mechanical and meaningless official routine which knew not at all the significance of a life of the spirit, the Hebrew emphasis on the *brotherhood of man* made all men equally eligible to the favor of a strict but kindly Father. Its teaching of charity toward others and the dignity with which it clothed human life softened human attitudes and broadened human outlook. Indeed, the Old Testament of the Hebrews combined with the New Testament, written in the early Christian era, have proved the greatest forces in the development of modern civilization.

Rising empires seized Palestine, each in its turn, and by 1 A.D. the country was under the rule of Rome. In that day, Hebrew religion shared, in common with other religions of the time, a nullifying burden of routine ceremonial and the low invasion of idolatry had become very apparent. Prophets had long since foretold the coming of a Christ or Messiah. During captivity and wanderings the Hebrews had seen the good as well as the evil in human beings and had learned to conceive of a sphere, the bounds of which were not set by any one nation. This was the kingdom of God.

Medicine in Palestine.   From a medical standpoint, the Hebrews have a wonderful record of achievement in the practice of hygiene and sanitation and systematic prevention of disease, much of which undoubtedly was learned during captivity in Egypt. The laws ascribed to Moses, who undertook the responsibility of their leadership on the post-exilic journey from Egypt to Palestine, were designed to cover the camp life of more than two million people who had to find subsistence along the way. Inspection of food, regulation of diet, slaughtering of animals for food, diagnosis and reporting of communicable disease, isolation and quarantine — all were regulated. Circumcision as a religious practice was ensured as a sanitary measure. Priest-physicians took on the function of health inspectors and reporting of disease was made compulsory. Orders for treatment and isolation, if warranted, were received from the priest, who also saw to the disinfection of body, clothing, and habitation. Persons excluded from the camp because of disease were compelled to secure permission from the priest before re-entering it.

Women of Palestine.   Biblical stories in which women appear portray impartially all types common to feminine human nature. *Ruth* exemplifies loyal friendship; *Jezebel* has been called the prototype of Lady Macbeth; *Huldah* was a prophetess; *Deborah,* a judge and a Joan of Arc; *Delilah,* utterly treacherous; and *Vashti* defied a royal husband's command, thereby raising alarm among his courtiers lest all women might follow her example and become difficult to manage. Her action, indeed, led to an ordinance declaring men to be rulers in their homes. The sweetness of all romance, however, enters into the story of *Rebekah,* a heroine of decision and action. In the twenty-fourth chapter of Genesis we see her setting out by camel train with her nurse, another Deborah, to meet Isaac, who was to become her husband. Although Deborah was a child's nurse and a companion, no doubt at times she was called upon to perform some nursing duties and, therefore, represents the first nurse to have her name come down to us in history.

Hebrew women, like all others, held a relatively better position in the early days of tribal clans than in later times. Divorce and polygamy brought various restrictions upon them. At times they were sold into captivity. However, the home atmosphere, as interpreted in general, was an exemplary one. The family bond was strong. Children were taught to honor both parents, as shown in one of the Ten Commandments of Moses which reads, "Honor thy father and thy mother; that thy days may be long upon the land which the Lord thy God giveth thee." Parents shared responsibility for children's education. Morality, health, habits which affected physical or mental welfare, and manners were taught with the assistance of Biblical tradition and precept. Fathers must teach trades to sons, mothers must make daughters good housekeepers and homemakers. The virtues of that mother whose children will "arise up, and call her blessed" show her to be wise, kindly, capable, and businesslike.

The equality which their religion gave to Hebrews, as children sharing in common the gifts of a merciful Father, was a stimulus to charity in their dealings with one another. Continual reminders are given by their leaders, of their past condition of servitude in Egypt and of the many experiences of lack of kindness among people of that country. The stranger, the fatherless, the widow, and the poor are not allowed to be forgotten. The borrower who is unable to redeem his pawned clothing before night must have it returned that he may use it as a sleeping garment (Deuteronomy 24:12, 13). The hired servant is not to be oppressed whether he be Hebrew or of alien birth. He is also to receive his pay promptly, "for he is poor and setteth his heart upon it."[1] Owners of vineyards must leave some fruit on the vines, those who have olive orchards must refrain from beating down the olives more than once, corners of grainfields must be left unreaped, and forgotten sheaves or gleanings are not to be gathered from the open fields. The way is thus opened to the poor who followed harvesters (Deuteronomy 24:19–22). Consideration is urged even for an enemy, "if thou meet thine enemy's ox or his ass going astray, thou shalt surely bring it back to him."[2]

A system of tithing gave into the hands of the church, for clerical support and distribution to the poor, one-tenth of each property owner's profit after the second year and one-tenth of his harvest annually. Support for the *xenodochia* or lodging houses provided for strangers depended on this tithing system. These institutions later developed, as an accessory to their service, the care of the sick and in this way became predecessors of the modern hospital.

PERSIA (Now Iran)

To the east of *Babylonia,* and running between the Persian Gulf and the Caspian Sea, lay the Plateau of Iran occupied in ancient times by peoples known respectively as Medes and Persians. By the fifth century B.C. the Persians had not only conquered their neighbors, the Medes, and carried the boundary of Persia eastward to the Indus River in India, but had extended their rule westward in the greatest empire then known to mankind.

Into religion the Persians brought belief in a god of goodness and a

---

[1]Deuteronomy 24:15.
[2]Exodus 23:4.

god of evil. The Zendavesta or sacred books of Persia owe their authorship, in the main, to one *Zoroaster* who lived about 600 B.C. The world,
according to the Zendavesta, is ruled by two Creators, one making light
and good, the other darkness and evil. Good and evil are at constant war
for mastery, and good is always triumphant. Fire, earth and water are
sacred elements, and of these fire is purest. The principal virtues are
those of veracity, virility, and hard work.

It has been said that Persians and Hebrews contributed more than
any other ancient peoples to the elevation of standards of human morality. The resemblance between their religious ideals will be seen readily.
Both make *good* their guiding star. Both reward good living in an after
life. Both essay to control physical health by religious law and practice.
To medicine, Persia contributed little in comparison with Palestine. Like
the religion of the Hebrews, Zoroastrianism sank into ritualistic routine,
but the dignity with which it endowed labor in an age of slavery is important. The god of good was as busy as he expected those to be who
worshiped him. His work was to shape the universe and his industry
sanctified all work. His followers, like him, worked and fought.

THE FAR EAST

INDIA

India, in the form of a triangular peninsula with two great rivers,
the Indus and Ganges, lies in the southern part of the Far Eastern
continent. Like the valleys of the Nile, Tigris, and Euphrates, that of
the Indus River has been yielding secrets of the past to archeological
exploration.

Aryan tribes migrating from central Asia in ancient times filtered
through the mountain passes on the north and found in India a race of
people darker in color than themselves, enjoying a warmer climate and
a richer vegetation than they had known. In time these northern Aryans
took the country away from its Dravidian inhabitants by conquest. In her
social development, India shows the influence of this early mixture of
races which merged old and new without assimilation. Her caste system
with its characteristic acceptance of inequality in birth and uneven division of wealth originated in these early days.

Hinduism.　Pre-eminent in influence on the outlook of the people of
India is Hinduism, known as the "mother of all religions." The teachings
of Hinduism were gathered together by its ancient priests and preserved
for posterity in two collections of about one hundred sacred books known
as the "Vedas" and the "Upanishads." These are written in beautiful
Sanskrit language. They contain philosophic and metaphysical specula-
tions of the highest order in relation to the Spirit of the Universe, which

they know as *Brahman*. Rules of conduct are given for everyday living as well as priestly ceremonials and hymns for special occasions.

For students of medicine and nursing, there is special significance in the fact that, in the Vedas, man is pictured as free from sin and disease at birth. One book in particular, known as the *Ayur Veda,* or the Veda of Longevity, is medical in viewpoint and content and stresses hygiene and prevention of sickness. It teaches man to preserve a perfect body by his own determination to practice precepts that have been culled from general experience. Inoculation against smallpox is mentioned. Curative practice in medicine, surgery, and pediatrics is discussed. Materia medica and psychiatry are included.

Rise of Buddhism. About 500 B.C. there was born in India a Hindu child of the princely caste who was to become the founder of another gentle and peaceful religion which, in time, would spread over a large portion of Asia and to other parts of the world as well. Gautama, who was to be known as *Buddha* or the "Enlightened One," was not entirely satisfied with the Hindu religion which accentuated caste differences and induced fear of a lower caste after death. While still a young man he stoically abandoned his wife, his child, and a life of ease to become a mendicant monk, aspiring to bring contentment to all men. After meditating forty-nine days under a Bo tree, he received enlightenment as to the meaning of life, and the religion which he finally offered required no sacrifices to the gods and completely disregarded caste.

REINCARNATION. It was natural that Buddhism should retain many of the precepts of Hinduism. Like it, Buddhism embodies the basic ethical concept of an endless cycle of rebirths and reincarnations until, through self-discipline, lives of good works and discovery of the truth, release from the "Wheel of Karma" is attained. Karma, operating as the law of moral cause and effect through successive lifetimes, determines the desirable or undesirable pattern of each life. Inevitably, everyone builds up for himself either a good or a bad karma. This agrees with the Christian parable of the sower, "Whatsoever a man soweth, that shall he also reap."[3]

By disregarding caste Buddhism made possible for everyone the practice of a system of self-education which would bring freedom from worldly evils and entrance into a mystical state of perfect peace or *Nirvana.* Complete renunciation of self with charity toward all men was further expression of a kindly religion to which India turned eagerly. Images of Buddha do not represent a god but are a symbol of that perfection of character which is attainable, through work, by the devout Buddhist.

Reign of Good King Asoka. About 250 B.C., in the very beginning of a long reign which was to make him one of the foremost rulers in his-

---

[3]Galatians 6:7.

tory, *King Asoka* of India became a convert to Buddhism. Reared in the tradition of war, he had entered upon a campaign of invasion with the aim of acquiring territory, but his remorse for the human suffering that he caused was so real that he refused to fight again. Instead, he introduced methods of arbitration that brought him fame among potential enemies. War, he told men, should be a spiritual conquest. "It is in the conquests of religion that the gods take pleasure."[4] As a Buddhist, peaceful penetration became his aim in the future, and the influence of his gentle spirit was felt far beyond his realm.

In proclamations inscribed upon rocks, King Asoka urged his people to study the new religion. He exhorted them to show kindness to slaves and to give alms to the poor. In a world which set little value upon life he succeeded in organizing what amounted to a national society for the prevention of cruelty to animals. By his own example, as well as by precept, he persuaded the people of India that all living things are worthy of respect.

The wise rule of "Good King Asoka" brought prosperity. Improved buildings were provided for the use of travelers in India. These compare with the hotel and garage of today, for they gave shelter to animals as well as to their owners. Hospitals were founded. Buddhist monasteries of great magnificence were built for the men and women who wished to retire from the work-a-day world to pass lives of purity in study and contemplation. Buddha had founded similar religious communities during his lifetime, and they were now a source of help to King Asoka, whose chief desire was to give to all the world the doctrines of peace and love inherent in Buddhism.

Medicine in Early India. India set high moral standards for those who chose care of the sick as a life work. Her exaction of a king's permission for right to practice medicine was akin to our license system. Prevention of disease was a matter of first importance, and care of the body a religious duty. Compulsory hygienic measures were adopted. Bathing twice a day was a regulation that must have been readily enforced in a climate of distressing heat. Trustworthiness and skill were demanded of midwives who, in common with doctors, were admonished to have short fingernails. Operations were preceded by religious ceremony and prayer. By 1 A.D., the methods prescribed by magic had already been altered to conform with more up-to-date practice, although the priest-physician still controlled the field of medicine, and retarded it considerably by his refusal to come into contact with blood or pathological tissues. As in Egypt, dissection of the human body was forbidden.

Position of Women. Socially the women of India in the period preceding 1 A.D. held a relatively high position. Monogamy was the general rule, although polygamy was practiced. King Asoka had shown interest

---

[4]Steel, F. A.: India Through the Ages. New York, E. P. Dutton & Co.

in the education of women, and their status presents a sharp contrast to that to which they were to be reduced in later times. Woman's activities were, in the main, those connected with management of her home. Doubtless she performed the duties of a nurse when sickness befell a member of her family. In institutions these duties were entrusted to old women and to men.

CHINA

Ancient China lay across the great range of the Himalaya Mountains, far to the northeast of India. Like India it was cut off from the Mediterranean world and lacked the stimulation of ideas which accompanies a freer intercourse among peoples. The Chinese are thought to have come from central Asia about 3000 B.C. No record has been found of their Stone Age, but they developed another of the great civilizations that record man's progress beyond the primitive. Just as in the Near East and in India, there developed among the people of Eastern Asia a mythology. Sacred books also were written which compare with the ancient Papyri of Egypt and the Vedas and Upanishads of India.

Confucianism. About 500 B.C., while the teachings of Buddha were changing the outlook of men in India, *Confucius* entered the life of China. As a child, he studied sacred books and learned to revere their teachings. As a man, he turned to them for the inspiration that was to make him one of the greatest reformers and teachers the world has known.

Born into a period of political disturbance and unhappiness that had been induced by corruption in the governing group, Confucius sought means of relieving oppression in his country by going back to ancient customs for the basis of a governmental ideal. He hoped to solve the problems of government by demanding fair and kind dealing on the part of a ruler in exchange for the respect and veneration of his people. The empire would be an ideal family in which the emperor took the place of both father and mother and guided the destiny of subjects bound together by ties of brotherly love.

The patriarchal rule, which China had developed in common with other peoples, appealed to Confucius as a fundamental factor in the attainment of a good life for all. The sacred books held record of this system, still in force but greatly weakened. He revived it. The family became the unit of society and the father assumed responsibility for its welfare. Owner of all property, and endowed with supreme authority, he was expected to rule with wisdom and kindliness. On the foundation of such family units — all subject to the rule of an emperor, also wise and kind — Confucius, the reformer, hoped to build up a contented, peaceful empire.

Ancestor Worship. Ancestor worship has been a phase of religious growth among all human beings, and in China the descent was traceable through fathers of families only. No worship was accorded to female ancestors, for the mother's share in the honors of descent was ignored. Through the efforts of Confucius ancestor worship attained great strength in China, a strength which resisted the passage of time much longer than elsewhere.

The philosophy passed down to us by disciples of Confucius is composed of precepts and rules of etiquette. Great emphasis was placed on the value of knowledge in solving life's problems. Faithfulness and sincerity were chief among virtues. Confucius urged men to think good thoughts and to treat each other as brothers, doing nothing to others that they would not have others do to them. The Confucian formulary made its strongest appeal to men of his own aristocratic and more enlightened class.

On the whole, and especially through its glorification of the past, the influence of Confucian teaching on Chinese development was arresting. It failed to stimulate ambition for better things. Nevertheless, it was the Chinese who invented the mariner's compass and discovered how to make gunpowder. They made use of bronze money as early as 1100 B.C. European missionaries of a later era were surprised to find that the Chinese not only had collected great libraries, but were able to demonstrate, in addition to paper making, the art of printing on paper with wood blocks. From this has developed the indispensable art of modern printing.

By 200 B.C., or after about three centuries of Confucianism, another ideal of life was brought into China from India. Buddhism became the religion of the populace. With its advent monasteries in charge of monks or nuns arose, and the Buddhist influence continues to be a strong one in China today.

Position of Women.   Although records have been found which would indicate a different status for women in China as early as 2000 B.C., their position, as ultimately defined by custom and quite definitely by Confucius, was inferior to that of men. A woman was expected to become a fruitful and submissive wife. The education of her daughters, it is true, was in her hands but marriage automatically transferred them to membership of subordinate character in the families of husbands.

Medicine in Early China.   China's medical knowledge dates far back in her history. Before 2000 B.C. dissection was permitted. Studies of the circulation were made and great stress placed on behavior of the pulse. Systematic methods of physical diagnosis were used, and four words were set as final guides for the physician, "Look, Listen, Ask, Feel." In common with other peoples, the Chinese had their system of massage, and they are said to have been willing to assign this form of treatment to operators who were blind. The bath was used for reduction of fever, and blood letting resorted to as a means of helping an evil spirit to escape from the prison of the body.

THE AMERICAS

Empires of the Near East, the Far East, and the Mediterranean World had risen and disappeared before their builders became aware that, far to the west, across what seemed an endless expanse of sea, lay riches far greater than any of those which they had spent centuries in wresting one from the other. Here there was being developed another civilization that might outshine any civilization thus far achieved. The earliest inhabitants of the unknown continent that was to be America are believed to have come from Central Asia and to have crossed the relatively narrow and island-strewn strait of Bering into the state that we know as Alaska.

These Indians, as *Columbus* named their descendants, filtered over the land, principally in easterly and southerly directions. Waterways were the natural lead, and traces of very early Indian occupation are found as far east as the Atlantic coast. Eventually they abandoned hunting and, as time went on, drifted into agriculture and established a more settled mode of life. Scientists differ in setting a period for the habitation of this area. Some place it as far back as ten, or even twenty thousand years ago, and some dare to say that men reached civilization in the Americas earlier than they did in Egypt. In any case, it is thought that American Indians, as we now speak of them, progressed culturally very much as men had done elsewhere, from the Stone Age onward, slowly, and under the influence of varied climatic conditions.

Among these groups of pioneers from another continent, several attained a high degree of civilization. Some were still in the Stone Age in 1492 A.D. The *Toltecs,* the *Aztecs,* the *Mayas* and the *Incas,* occupying the land from Mexico to Peru, not only acquired wealth, but left behind them monuments of man's achievement in the building of temples and palaces which challenge the art of the Egyptian. The Incas also built great highways and are said to have been gifted beyond the others. Writing was known, and some of the finest temples produced by early America originated between 1000 B.C. and 1 A.D.

As we have found is customary among primitive people, the offices of religion, medicine, nursing, and pharmacy were combined in one individual who was set apart from other men. Medicine men, and later priests, essayed to conquer Indian ills of body or mind. Little has been carried down to us except as folklore, for it is believed that sacred books were destroyed by Spanish invaders. With the stimulus of modern interest in archeological study of these people, it is probable that we shall learn to value our inheritance from them proportionately. We owe to them the origin of various processes of commercial value. Their baskets still defy our skill and patience. They learned to utilize wood ashes as a cleaning powder, to tan leather with oak bark and to develop a glue from fish. They were the next people to be reached in the enlarging circle of acquaintanceship around the globe.

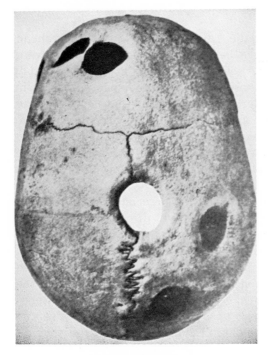

Figure 11. Prehistoric skull showing trephine openings made during life. "The rounded edges of the openings show that the bone has grown after the wound was made. Thus we know they were made while the owner was living. Excavated in Peru." (Clendening, Logan: Behind the Doctor. Alfred A. Knopf, New York.)

Among Indians in the tribal state, the position of the Indian woman was, in some respects, unusually good. While she obeyed certain restrictions set by tribal practice as masculine rights, the Indian woman retained complete authority over her home. The children were in her charge until admitted to tribal membership and, in at least one group, a woman's council took part in discussion of all affairs affecting the welfare of the tribe.

Suggestions for Study

1. Show the advantages to primitive man of placing great emphasis upon family relationships, and of building up mores to control habits of action.
2. What is animism?
3. (a) How did primitive man explain the benefits and catastrophes of everyday living? (b) How did this affect his attitude toward disease?
4. What were some of the first methods used to offset the ravages of disease, and from what source are some of these believed to have been learned?
5. (a) Differentiate between a medicine man and a priest physician. (b) Between white and black magic.
6. In what region is man believed to have originated, and in what general directions did he migrate?

7. How did the Mediterranean Sea get its name?
8. Show how care of the sick came to be a responsibility of women.
9. From what sources is knowledge of the prehistoric period obtained?
10. Show why this earliest period is known as the Old Stone Age or the Age of Hunters.

EGYPT

1. How does the period of development of Egypt compare with that of other ancient civilizations?
2. What invention attributed to the Egyptians brought about a gradual change from the Old Stone Age or Age of Hunters to the New Stone Age or Age of Farmers?
3. Give the names and attributes of the trinity of gods that ultimately was believed to control the welfare of Egyptians?
4. Tell something of the priest physicians of ancient Egypt, and the one who stands out as greatest of these men.
5. (a) Of what significance were the early temples?
   (b) What were the duties of temple women?
6. Into what books did the priests of Egypt collect their religious precepts, and in which one is the medical world especially interested?
7. Name two circumstances which prevented progress in medical knowledge of the Egyptians?
8. Egyptian belief in immortality led to what practices, evidence of which are still in existence?
9. Tell what you know of the ancient city of Alexandria, and how its influence was terminated.
10. What brought about an end of Roman rule, and when did it occur?
11. What is the significance of the great new Aswan Dam from an historical viewpoint?

THE FERTILE CRESCENT

1. Give the geographic location of Babylonia, Assyria, and Palestine, naming their principal rivers.
2. Justify the statement that Hammurabi exerted a great social influence.
3. For what great achievement is Hammurabi best known today?
4. Name several drawbacks to the practice of Babylonian medicine and surgery.
5. What was the general position of Babylonian women?
6. Tell what you know of the Assyrians.
7. What was the chief contribution of the Hebrews toward world betterment?

8. Show how teachings of the Hebrews far excelled those of others around them.
9. (a) Why are the Hebrews credited with great advances in the practice of hygiene and sanitation? (b) Why is Moses known as a "great sanitarian" and also as "the law-giver"?
10. What laws did Moses give to the Hebrew people, and in what book of the Bible are they recorded?
11. Show how the virtues emphasized by the Hebrew religion led to provision for institutional care of the sick.
12. How were Hebrew women affected by practices of this early period?

PERSIA (Iran)

1. Give the location of ancient Persia and the name by which it is known today.
2. What was the sacred book of the Persians, and who was its principal author?
3. How were problems of the universe accounted for in the Zendavesta?
4. What elements were sacred according to Persian teachings, and what were the principal virtues?
5. What two ancient peoples are considered to have made the greatest contributions to standards of morality?
6. What circumstances prevented these same two peoples from continuing to exert a high moral influence?

INDIA

1. Name the two large rivers of India, show their historical importance and state the bodies of water into which they flow.
2. What is the origin of the caste system of India?
3. Why is Hinduism sometimes called the "mother of all religions"?
4. Tell what you know of the Vedas and Upanishads of India and their authors.
5. In which Veda is medicine and nursing particularly interested, and why?
6. (a) In what important way did the religion offered by a great man of India differ from that of Hinduism? (b) What was the teaching of both in regard to the "Wheel of Karma"?
7. (a) Why is Buddhism regarded as having characteristics in common with Christianity? (b) What do statues of Buddha represent?
8. In what ways did Good King Asoka exert an uplifting social influence?
9. What procedure comparable to licensing was required of a physician before being permitted to practice in India?
10. What practices were required of doctors and midwives for the protection of their patients?

11. What circumstances affected the position of women of India during this early period?

CHINA

1. Name several circumstances which tended to retard the development of ancient China.
2. Give causes for unhappiness among the people of China, and show how Confucius attempted to relieve them.
3. Name several inventions of ancient China.
4. What new type of religious influence was brought into China about 200 B.C., and what is its status today?
5. Tell what you know of the position of women during this early period.
6. How did the practice of medicine in China compare with that of other peoples?
7. Make a list of the great men who lived about 500 B.C., with contributions of each.

THE AMERICAS

1. (a) The earliest inhabitants of North and South America are believed to have come from what region? (b) What probably caused them to migrate? (c) What line of travel are they believed to have followed?
2. (a) What Indian tribes attained the highest degree of culture? (b) Where did they locate? (c) Name some of their accomplishments.
3. What evidence is there that the position of women was exceptionally good in some tribes?
4. Which group of women of the various regions studied demonstrated a remarkable spirit of independence?
5. What is known of the nursing of this early period?
6. (a) What was the general condition of the known world at the beginning of the Christian Era? (b) Give reasons for the fact that contentment was not possible for the average man or woman.

References

Austin, Anne L.: History of Nursing Source Book. New York, G. P. Putnam's Sons, 1957. Chapter I.
Breasted, J. H.: The Conquest of Civilization. New York, Literary Guild of America, 1938.
Brown, Lewis: The World's Great Scriptures. New York, The Macmillan Co., 1946.
Ceram, C. W.: Gods, Graves and Scholars. The Story of Archeology. New York, Alfred A. Knopf, 1956.

Durant, Will: Our Oriental Heritage. New York, Simon and Schuster, 1935.

Editorial Staff of *Life:* The World's Great Religions. (Special edition for young readers.) New York, Golden Press, 1958.

Old Testament of the Bible:
  Exodus 20:3-17 inc., The Ten Commandments.
  Book of Ruth (love story of Ruth).
  I Kings, Ch. 18, 19, 20 (Jezebel).
  II Kings, Ch. 9 (Jezebel).
  II Kings, Ch. 22, 14-20 (Huldah).
  Judges, Ch. 4 and 5 (Deborah).
  Judges, Ch. 16 (Delilah).
  Esther, Ch. I (Vashti).
  Genesis, Ch. 24 (Rebekah).

Chapter 3

THE MEDITERRANEAN WORLD

GREECE

Jutting out into the Mediterranean Sea from the southeastern part of Europe is a peninsula that we know as Greece, but the tiny kingdom of the twentieth century is but a remnant of an ancient Greece. For their history, the mixture of peoples who later came to be known as Greek learned to rely on the writings of *Homer* who recorded the deeds of ancient heroes in his poems, "The Iliad" and "The Odyssey." Written about 1100 B.C., these became the sacred books of Greece, and are believed to have been the beginning of a moral revolution. Through mythology the Greeks traced their origin to *Chiron,* strongest of a race of Centaurs, or men whose bodies were half human and half horse.

Apollo, god of the sun, was also god of health — and of medicine, the supporter of health. Apollo's son, *Asklepios,* was known as "The Blameless Physician." Representation showed him holding the staff of the traveler, entwined with the serpents of wisdom — emblems still used by the medical profession in the caduceus. Asklepios' wife shared his work, for she was revered as "The Soothing One." One son was the possessor of hands which were an asset in surgical work. Another gave his attention to internal medicine. Of their daughters, *Hygeia* served as goddess of health, while *Panacea* presided over the administration of medicine and was known as the healer of all ills.

The loveliness of their surroundings made a deep impression on the responsive Greek people. They enjoyed the opportunity given them for outdoor life. In meeting the exigencies of war, poverty, and disease they exhibited a practical bent. Hospitality was to them a virtue and a religious duty, the demands of which they met by providing organized

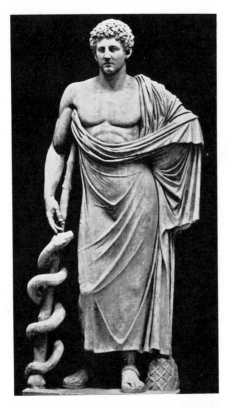

Figure 12. Aesculapius, Greek marble in the Vatican Museum.

charity and care for those who were poor or sick. To be sure, they denied this care to incurable cases and to women in confinement, but it must be remembered that they were not alone in considering both death and birth sources of pollution. The chief interest of the Greek people was not held by sickness and misery in which lie neither beauty nor perfection. They looked and worked for the positive states of health and happiness.

Institutional Care of the Sick. Care for the sick was provided by the *xenodochion* which was similar in function to the xenodochium of the Hebrews. After Christianity had awakened men to the extent of human misery and their responsibility for doing something about it, this type of institution was to be copied wherever the religion of brotherhood was preached. It became the hospice of the early church. Originally the xenodochion was built for the purpose of providing lodging and refreshment for the strangers whose number increased with the development of travel and commerce. Sickness among these wayfarers was inevitable and, in all likelihood, the provision of medical and nursing care was soon added. The work of the xenodochion, carried on under municipal management, might be considered a forerunner of the modern city or county hospital.

The *iatrion* was another civic undertaking of the Greeks. The work done in it would correspond most closely with that of the out-patient department or clinic of a hospital. Medical advice could be obtained at the iatrion by the ambulatory sick, operations were performed if necessary, and prescriptions were compounded and issued. No provision was made at the iatrion for hospitalization of those who needed care in bed.

Temples. The appreciative people of Greece found in the topography of their country opportunity for selection of lofty sites of unusual beauty for their temples. The artistic genius of architects and sculptors was not restrained. Neither money nor toil was spared in bringing to successful completion such conceptions as those of the Parthenon in Athens which is still regarded as the most perfect building ever conceived by the mind

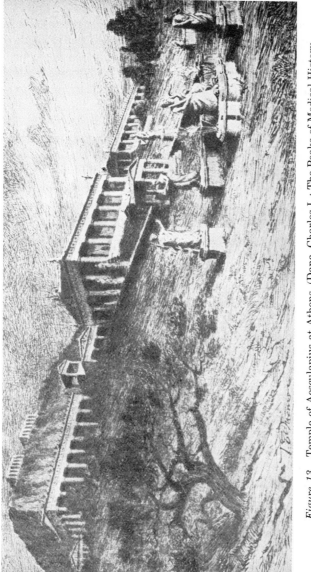

Figure 13. Temple of Aesculapius at Athens. (Dana, Charles L.: The Peaks of Medical History. Paul B. Hoeber, Inc., New York.)

or built by the hand of man. The *Temple of Epidauros,* in its beautiful
mountain setting near Athens, bears especial interest for us because
of the part that it has played in medical history.

But the temple was more than a building, crude or beautiful as it
might be. It was the pulse of national life. Its records are national history.
Rulers made use of it for broadcasting information or laws. Its priests
comforted, healed, exhorted, or swayed the public in this common gathering place. In the absence of microphones or radios, nature frequently
supplied echoes, or exaggerated sound waves traveling through caverns,
to amplify the human voice. Many functions besides that of worship
occupied men in or near the temple. They made it a bank, a market, a
social welfare society, a community recreation center, sometimes a
school, always an object of lavish adoration and best creative effort. It is
not surprising, therefore, that high on mountain tops, on plains or
deserts, in cities, even buried under ruins of former civilizations, we find
these memorials which men intended to last forever. They were the
centers from which radiated religion, education, medicine, and nursing.

Temples of Asklepios.   Temples devoted to the worship of Asklepios
(Æsculapius, as he was called later by the Romans) were the main centers of medical work in Greece. *They illustrate the best development of
the constant association between religion, medicine, and nursing that
existed in early times.* They also represent a national effort to bring about
physical and moral health among the people. Greek reverence for physical perfection retarded medical advancement when it prohibited marring
the body by dissection. At the same time, it brought about development
of a group of priests who attained skill in the care of the sick who came
with the well to join in prayers to Asklepios. Their success caused them
to be set apart in a group known as the *Asklepiades.* They shared their
wisdom with selected students and as early as the eighth century B.C.
had originated a form of medical school in Greece. By 500 B.C. they were
practicing in the xenodochion, the iatrion, and in certain temples of
Asklepios which had been given over to them.

EPIDAUROS, A TEMPLE OF ASKLEPIOS.   Some temples of the Asklepiades assumed the character of health centers in which the core of activities was the Greek ideal of health as a balanced state of well-being
in mind, body, and soul. The most celebrated of these was at Epidauros,
a few miles from Athens. On a scenic site amid groves of trees, Epidauros
offered places of worship, hotels, libraries, gymnasia, a stadium with
a capacity for twelve thousand spectators, a theater, and a hospital.
Sixteen thousand people could be accommodated in the theater, which
was one of the most beautiful of the outdoor theaters of the Greeks.
Like all the other buildings of Epidauros, it was of white marble.

To the hospital men thronged in response to reports of miraculous
cures performed by priest-physicians who interpreted treatment prescribed by Asklepios. We are told that, upon entrance, the patient met

the same efforts to induce confidence that characterize the reception of patients in our hospitals today. Until the time of Hippocrates it was not customary to make any physical examination, but priests endeavored to inspire hope by assurance of the super-human skill of Asklepios. The patient was bathed and clad in white garments. Clean, relaxed, and quite tired out by a journey, probably made on foot, and by the excitement of being admitted to the haven for which he had longed, he was assigned to a bed in a building or on a porch provided for the sick. Evening worship was conducted, and after that he went to sleep. A message purporting to come from Asklepios was delivered to him during the night. It has been suggested that the priest-physicians made rounds when all was quiet and talked to patients drowsy with sleep or drugs. No record verifies this. Treatments defined by the dream oracle took the form of warm baths, massage, inunctions, catharsis or blood-letting, with diet regulation and other hygienic measures. The aid of the sacred serpent might also be invoked. Snakes of nonpoisonous variety moved at will among the patients and by licking wounds gave cleansing treatment which often helped them to heal.

The routine of care was largely hygienic and took full advantage of the sunlight and fresh air available in rural surroundings. Ample provision was made for instruction, exercise, bathing, and entertainment. The worship of the god Asklepios, revered for his character as well as for his wisdom in matters pertaining to health, lifted patients above themselves and increased their faith. The aura of magic which surrounded all the work of the Asklepiades may have been a concession to the times, but it met with popular approval.

THE "BIRTH OF REASON"

Greek civilization continued to progress and many changes took place. Slavery increased, as did poverty. Nevertheless, the intellectual and artistic prestige of Athens gave inspiration to the Greek people. To *Aristotle,* whose insatiable desire for knowledge of the meaning of life led him to dissect animals, men owe the foundation of the science of biology as well as the study of comparative anatomy. *Hippocrates* laid the foundation of scientific medicine; *Socrates* and *Plato,* those of philosophy and government. By the work of these and many other men of genius and scholarship Greece was able to broadcast culture throughout a waiting world. Greek influence meant not only a change from empiric to scientific methods; it made apparent, forever after, a distinction between the sound and the unsound. Indubitably, it affected the work of the nurse as well as that of the physician.

Hippocrates. *Hippocrates* was the son of a priest-physician and one of the Asklepiades. He was born on the island of Cos in 460 B.C. Here was a school of medicine already well known, and we may suppose that

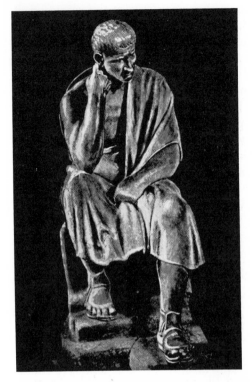

Figure 14. Aristotle.

the youth grew up in the traditions surrounding the sacred cult of his father. Destiny pointed to him as the man who would dispel the mists of magic and expose to the light of knowledge all those superstitions which served to obscure the whole question of how to keep health in the human body. Hippocrates, who forced the transition from magic to science, is said to have spent much time in observing symptoms and to have gleaned considerable knowledge regarding the ills of those who sought treatment. He found groups of symptoms shared in common by groups of people. When such was the case, he reasoned, there must be a common cause. Present-day medicine dates its beginning from the work of Hippocrates, which made it possible for scientific medicine to supersede the empiric. He is still known as the "Father of Scientific Medicine."

The new viewpoint which Hippocrates offered to physicians made necessary a searching inquiry into each patient's history and symptoms. Treatment must be individual and dependent upon the diagnosis reached. While no writings ascribed to Hippocrates were made public for fifty years after his death, the course to be taken in medical investigation and treatment for ages to come after him were, in their scientific trend, the work of this great scholar. The medical profession found a solid foundation in his ideals of ethical conduct and practice. Portions of the oath required of his students are still used in an oath taken by students graduating from medical schools today.

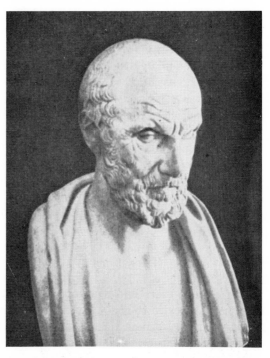

Figure 15. Hippocrates.

Strangely enough, the enviable place in history gained by this country of scholarly wisdom was reached in spite of, and actually through, political subjugation. In 338 B.C. Philip of Macedonia conquered Greece. The education of his son, Alexander, he placed in the hands of a Greek scholar and when this young man succeeded his father, he possessed an appreciation of Greek civilization so sincere that he included in his ambition to conquer the world a determination to endow it with the culture of Greece. His success was acknowledged when he became known as "Alexander the Great." Cities that he took from Greece became greater; cities that he built were Grecian in character. The city of Alexandria in Egypt, which was named after him, became the gathering place of scholars from all over the world. In Alexandria medical science received the encouragement of permissible dissection, which it had failed to receive in Greece. Greeks carried all that their country stood for in the way of scholarship or art to this and other foreign centers. It was indeed, a historic period of cultural flowering. It made the thinker a leader.

Some discontent was doubtless due to the insecurity of Greece's political position. Alexander, who had elevated her so suddenly to a position of world fame, did not live long enough to stabilize the government. Without Alexander's leadership it fell quickly to pieces, for a new power was rising in the west. After a series of disheartening attempts to maintain her prestige, Greece fell into the hands of her grasping neighbor, Rome, by 146 B.C.

The period about 500 B.C. marked more than a Golden Age for Greece.

The Birth of Reason which brought her fame was bringing about changes in far-off India and China. Her philosophies had counterparts in other lands. In India Buddhism was offering its hope of peace to discontented and suffering men. In China Confucius was making his appeal to the intellectual class in the hope of working out a scheme of living which might systematize and render more agreeable the lives of all. When his teachings failed to reach all men, Buddhism became the solace of the poor of China. Everywhere there was evidence of a striving to understand the meaning of life and death. Blind worship of old gods did not fill man's need. Worry, ambition, poverty, cruelty and pain seemed to be taking an ever greater place in life. Nobody was satisfied, and many were thinking. The world was preparing for 1 A.D.

Greek Women.   To this Birth of Reason which so stimulated thought and education some have traced a decline in the status of women. They were not included by the Greeks in its benefits. The mores of the time kept women strictly confined to home duties. When men turned to mental interests, study and public life altered their attitude toward the home. Work became more and more specialized, ambitions changed, and there was born a desire to rise above the demands of a purely physical existence, to have freedom for contemplation, to use creatively the mental power of which men were now conscious.

The girl baby did not meet with a hearty welcome in Greece. When she came to marry she was not free to choose her husband. She had a dower value. The higher her social position, the less free was she to mingle with other people. Her only alternative to the protection of marriage was slavery or prostitution. During her whole life she was, legally, a minor. She was not even permitted to act as hostess to her husband's friends, but withdrew to a separate part of the house after she had seen that preparations for their entertainment were complete. The duties which fell to her lot confined her strictly to the family circle and, probably, nursing was often an arduous task for the housewife who was responsible for the care of her men so often called upon to be soldiers, for her children, and for varying numbers of slaves.

ROME

While Greece was developing into a world renowned home of art and reason, there lived on a long peninsula beside her an agricultural people whom we know as Latins. These people were preparing to wield tremendous influence of a different nature over the future of mankind. The peninsula was Italy, separated from Greece by only a narrow sea, and divided down the middle by a chain of mountains. Level plains on the western side had been chosen by the Latins for their home.

In due time a civilization grew up, with a capital city located near the mouth of the Tiber. Legend places the birth date of this city of Rome at 753 B.C., and enwraps the event with the uncertainty of a variety of mythological interpretations. Its site on seven hills appears to have been the choice of twin brothers, Romulus and Remus, themselves indebted for life to the nourishment and care given them by a kindly wolf who found them on a mountain top, abandoned by a goddess mother.

By 500 B.C., when Greece was entering upon her Golden Age, and the influence of Buddha and Confucius was dawning upon an unhappy India and an intellectual minority in China, the city of Rome had struggled into the status of a *republic* with a ruler chosen by election. Its citizens were still, in the main, farmers, and theirs was an honored occupation. The civilization of the world beyond had not touched the Latin state deeply. Even the temple, so characteristic a feature of other infant cultures, was not essential to the religion of the early Roman. Gods were borrowed and temples built for worship later, but his deities were few and their functions highly practical. Small images of them were used for worship, which could be carried on at home. *Jupiter* was charged with the welfare of the city, *Juno* was a woman's patroness, *Mars* was god of war and *Janus* was the god of openings or beginnings who guarded the archway gate through which the soldiers marched to war. This arch, later replaced by the temple of Janus, remained open for the duration of a war. Its closing announced peace.

Contacts with Greece gave Roman citizens some appreciation of its famous culture and, by 146 B.C., this country was under their control. Greek scholars were made Roman slaves and became teachers of men, women, and children in what was to be the Imperial City of the World. Greek physicians of the Hippocratic school, who were also slaves, introduced their ideas on the practice of medicine. Rome not only proceeded to take the place of Alexander the Great in the eastern world, but she was on the way to subjugating a large part of Europe as well. Time would thoroughly Romanize Italy, Spain, and France. Roman territory would spread from Britain to the Black Sea and would encircle the Mediterranean. Meanwhile, the gates of Janus seldom closed. By the time Julius Caesar came to power in the first century B.C. men acknowledged her triumph by admitting that "All roads lead to Rome." The eyes of the world were turned her way.

History has accepted *Julius Caesar* (100–44 B.C.) as a brilliant example of the Roman warrior statesman. Bent on conquest, swiftly decisive in thought and action, constructive in his attitude toward the conquered, ever alert to his own advancement as well as to his country's glory, Caesar has handed down to us a record of his work in the Commentaries on his wars. This "Father of his Country," as Romans came to know him, subjugated and introduced to civilization, western Europe and Britain, while he rose to the position of dictator in what was now the Roman Empire. His person was declared sacred. His office was considered

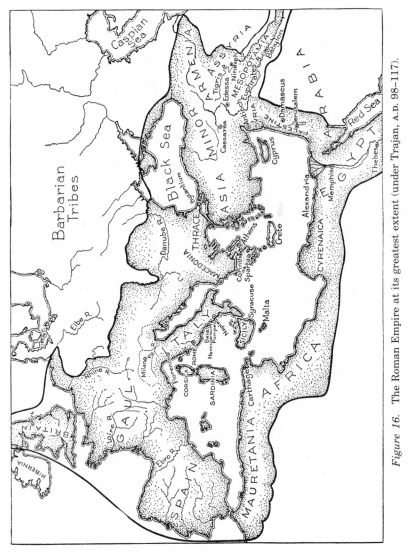

Figure 16. The Roman Empire at its greatest extent (under Trajan, A.D. 98–117).

divine. This did not prevent his assassination by close associates, who explained it as a "sacrifice" for the good of a state just emerging from its experiment in republican government and giving itself over reluctantly to one-man rule.

Julius Caesar was not allowed to finish all the social reforms that he planned, but he had proved himself well fitted for the difficult task of being the pioneer of Roman monarchy, and his succession in 29 B.C. by a grand-nephew to be known as *Augustus Caesar* brought a peace within the City of Seven Hills which was to last for two centuries.

Before the dawn of the Christian era, Rome was excessively rich. Her trade had become enormous. She was attaining a degree of culture. *Virgil* wrote the history of her ancestors in the Aeneid, *Horace* gave her a name

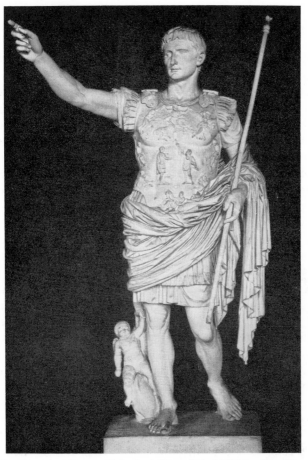

Figure 17. Augustus Caesar (Octavian). From "World History" by Hayes, Moon and Wayland, 1955. By permission of The Macmillan Company, New York.

in poetry, *Livy* and *Cicero* wrote her prose, while the latter also exemplified her best achievement in oratory. As slaves were brought home from conquered countries, those of her people who were wealthy also became idle. The custom of bringing home art as well as treasure from dispossessed peoples put beauty into their hands. The transition from the rugged life of the pioneer to a life of ease had been abnormally rapid. Old domestic virtues were being undermined. Divorce was common.

Roman Medicine. In medical advancement Rome fell far short of Greece. She appreciated hygiene as a foundation for the fighting strength that she could not do without. Her health work in the way of sanitation was marvelous. Sewers and drains, and paving on the streets, made cities clean. Great aqueducts brought pure drinking water into them and supplied the citizens of Rome with bathing facilities. Baths with heated water appeared in the homes. It has been said that public health practices began in Rome. Notwithstanding what would seem to have been

a high degree of civic and individual cleanliness, the city was the prey
of frequent epidemics of disease, much of which was brought in with
conquests. Moreover, the marshes surrounding the city persisted, in
spite of drainage, and fostered the malaria to which history has ascribed
Rome's ultimate downfall.

For help when sickness came, the Romans clung to their gods, to
herbs or to superstition, which might even include the keeping of snakes
in their houses. Although Greek physicians were allowed to do most of
the medical work after 200 B.C., Hippocratic medicine failed to make
much headway. No great physicians arose among Roman scholars themselves before the first century. Army hospitals were conducted well and
Roman soldiers received good care wherever they might be. The dispensaries provided for the care of the public were badly managed.
Weakness won contempt rather than pity.

Roman Women.   Turning to the women of Rome, we find them of a
caliber to match that of the men. Indeed, Romans are said to have conquered all people save their own women. Coarser in grain, stronger in
personality, the Roman woman quite lacked the retiring submissiveness
that characterized the typical Greek woman. Both were minors in the
eyes of the law, but that was a resemblance which custom failed to up-
hold. The Roman woman got around the law. She succeeded in making
hers a better position and actually acquired the right to hold property in
her own name and to appear in court to give testimony. She was companion worker with a busy husband, of enduring physical and moral
strength, a capable, resourceful housekeeper and a good mother. Stoically
she sacrificed her sons to her country's growth.

When wars ceased Roman women proceeded to enjoy with the men
the fruits of conquest. They appeared in public, went to theaters, sports,
and banquets. Their independence developed to such strength during the
frequent absence of their husbands that it was a problem to subdue them
in time of peace. They did work that would continue to be traditionally
woman's work for centuries to come, but before the first century they were
equipped beyond their predecessors in civilization with an independence
of spirit that would enable them to emerge into other spheres at the first
opportunity.

In her own home the Roman woman held acknowledged sway. Subordinate to her husband outside of it, she was addressed by him as
"domina" in its privacy. She could come and go as she pleased under the
protection of her "stola matronalis," a garment worn over her tunic on
the street and donned when she married. She entertained guests and sat
with them at table. She could nurse ill members of her household or turn
that work over to Greek slaves if she had them. She could dally with
philosophy if she chose to do so. When riches came, she might go in for
"society," which frivolous institution she is credited with originating.
But, as in all ages, there must have been great numbers of Roman women

who did traditional work and represented traditional virtues in their "constantly changing world."

Suggestions for Study

GREECE

1. (*a*) Give a description of the location and climate of Greece. (*b*) Where is the island of Crete? (*c*) Of Cos?
2. Give the author, names and date of writing of the sacred books of Greece.
3. Make a list of Greek gods that influenced the practice of medicine, naming an outstanding characteristic of each.
4. Describe the people of Greece and their attitudes toward illness and birth and death.
5. Compare the functions of the xenodochion and the iatrion.
6. (*a*) Show how the temples of Asklepios illustrate the close association between religion, medicine, and nursing. (*b*) Describe the temple of Epidauros.
7. Account for the statement that scientific medicine and ethical principles of the present day had their beginnings in ancient Greece.
8. Make a chart of the great men of all ancient civilizations who lived about 500 B.C., during the period known as the "Birth of Reason."
9. Show the effects of building of the Alexandrian Empire on the spread of Greek culture.
10. Tell what you know of Greek women before 1 A.D.
11. What do you think of the implications of the Greek ideal of "moderation in all things"?

ROME

1. Compare Greece and Rome in regard to geographical location, climate, and people.
2. (*a*) How does the time of the founding of Rome compare with that of other ancient civilizations? (*b*) What is the legend in regard to it?
3. What gods were revered in ancient Rome?
4. (*a*) Name several sanitary practices of the ancient Romans. (*b*) Do they justify the statement that public health began here?
5. The development of Roman hospitals and medicine was directed toward what purpose?
6. How did Roman women compare with those of Greece?
7. Who was Emperor of Rome at the time of the birth of Jesus of Nazareth?

References

Austin, Anne L.: History of Nursing Source Book. New York, G. P. Putnam's Sons, 1957, Chap. 1.

Bury, J. B.: A History of Greece. New York, The Modern Library, 1902.

Carcopino, Jerome: Daily Life in Ancient Rome. New Haven, Yale University Press, 1940.

Durant, Will: Life of Greece, New York, Simon & Schuster, 1935.

Gibbon, Edward: The Decline and Fall of the Roman Empire. New York, The Modern Library.

Toynbee, Arnold J.: Hellenism. The History of a Civilization. New York, Oxford University Press, 1959.

Chapter 4

EARLY CHRISTIAN ERA
1–500 A.D.

The history of mankind now divides itself into two periods, one leading up to 1 A.D., the other following that date. Superficially, we would say that a new calendar was initiated at this time, but reasons far deeper than measure of time underlay what were revolutionary changes. Discerning minds of men like the Hebrew prophets, like Confucius, Buddha, Zoroaster and the philosophers of Greece had seen the futility of life if it could not yield a measure of satisfaction to all men, but in spite of prophecy, religions, and philosophy, the predominant ideal of humanity remained that of subjugation of the weak by the strong. The Roman Empire represented the epitome of this ideal, and Rome was now supreme over nearly all the peoples of the known world. Although nominally a republic, her emperor, Caesar Augustus (majestic), was an absolute ruler whose acts were believed to be authorized by the gods.

In many respects conditions in this greatest empire duplicated those experienced by its predecessors. Hardy virtues of earlier times were disappearing. Taxation was oppressive. Religion had come to represent formal duties imposed upon disinterested worshipers. Everywhere lands had passed into the possession of a few. A great chasm separated rich and poor, and slavery had lessened the value of life. The majority of people in the world knew that they could get nowhere. The minority, wherever it was possible, set examples of wasteful extravagance, callousness of heart, idleness. In Rome so many slaves now did all kinds of work that work seemed to her citizens the occupation of a slave class, and they chose idleness in preference to work. While there was more wealth in the world than had yet been known, the need of distributing it fairly enough to maintain human dignity was not yet seen.   **53**

The questioning of idealists who had been seeking the good life for several centuries was answered by a Child of Destiny who was born about this time in Bethlehem, a town of Palestine. Life was preparing this *Redeemer of Mankind* to understand hardship. He grew to manhood among people accustomed to both poverty and toil. His native land was a crossroads of trade which gave opportunity for observation of many kinds of people and for learning about those who dwelt in far countries. The greater part of humanity appeared to be in the grip of misery, the cause of which seemed to Him to lie in greed and injustice. Men overvalued power and put too much emphasis on the acquisition of wealth. Something could be done to make life worthwhile to the masses if higher ideals could be put before them and before those who, perhaps unwittingly, oppressed them. Life would be better if class barriers were done away with, if cruelty were changed into kindliness, if peace and service replaced war and servitude.

The new Redeemer began to show the possiblity of a world ruled by love, to advocate the responsibility of each individual for the general welfare, to urge a common faith in one Father God. By thus awakening in men the sense of their brotherhood as children of one family, He sought to do away with distinctions of race, position, and creed which raised walls of misunderstanding among them. Hatred of enemies, long looked upon as a virtue, He wished to transform into brotherly love. He hoped to send forth, even to the farthest corners of the great world, teachers whom He himself would prepare to influence all humanity toward a unity which it had never known. Among His teachings, the following contained seeds of social revolution:

1. "Whosoever shall do the will of my Father who is in heaven, he is my brother and sister and mother." Matthew 12:50. (Distinctions of race, creed and social status which had been built by men were without foundation.)
2. "Thou shalt love thy neighbor as thyself." Matthew 19:19. (Selfish interests should cease to dominate men.)
3. "Love your enemies, do good to them that hate you." Luke 6:27. (Hating was a virtue cultivated when men spent the greater part of the time at war with one another.)
4. "Blessed are the peacemakers, for they shall be called the children of God." Matthew 5:9. (War had come to be man's chief occupation. Its results had been proved evil. Peace would bring good.)
5. "If thou wouldst be perfect, go sell that which thou hast, and give to the poor, and thou shalt have treasure in heaven." Matthew 19:21. (This teaching, in many instances, was followed by early Christians.)
6. "Whatsoever ye would that men should do unto you, do ye even so unto them." Matthew 7:12. (The Golden Rule.)
7. "Inasmuch as ye have done it unto one of the least of these, my brethren, ye have done it unto me." Matthew 25:40. (Pity was not a common characteristic of men in ancient times. They worshipped strength. This new outlook helped women, children, the poor and the sick.)
8. "Even as the Son of man came not to be ministered unto, but to minister, and to give his life as ransom for many." Matthew 20:28. (Dignity in work, beauty in service.)

9. "For I was hungry, and ye gave me to eat; I was thirsty, and ye gave me to drink; I was a stranger, and ye took me in; naked, and ye clothed me; I was sick and ye visited me; I was in prison, and ye came unto me." Matthew 25:35, 36. (Stimulus to charity, medicine, nursing, and work among prisoners.)

The story of the Good Samaritan was one which turned particular attention toward the sick poor, and by so doing also affected nursing, medicine, and charity. It was a plea for sympathy, individual effort, and generosity in providing shelter and care.

"A certain man was going down from Jerusalem to Jericho; and he fell among robbers, who both stripped him and beat him, and departed, leaving him half dead. And by chance a certain priest was going down that way: and when he saw him, he passed by on the other side. And in like manner a Levite also, when he came to the place, and saw him, passed by on the other side. But a certain Samaritan, as he journeyed, came where he was: and when he saw him, he was moved to compassion, and came to him, and bound up his wounds, pouring on them oil and wine; and he set him on his own beast, and brought him to an inn, and took care of him. And on the morrow he took out two shillings, and gave them to the host, and said, 'Take care of him; and whatsoever thou spendest more, I, when I come back again, will repay thee.' Which of these three, thinkest thou, proved neighbor unto him that fell among the robbers?"[1]

Jesus himself worked first among the poor who readily became adherents of One who brought to them a comfort that they needed sorely. They felt themselves rescued from an isolation which had enveloped them gradually, and their self-respect rose. Their enthusiasm and honest effort to live according to the principles that He explained to them so affected the social life about them that men and women of wealth and education were attracted to the group.

For a long time Christians had no meeting places but the homes of fellow Christians. From the beginning of His work, their Leader made use of group discussion in planning for effective organization of a living temple to replace the too formalized temple of the time. The new temple was to be the center of a movement for the people and by the people. It was to demonstrate all over the world the good life through everyday practice by individual believers of principles for which it stood. Its policy was to be a democratic one of participation by the membership in all activities, even to preaching.

The work of Jesus was confined to Palestine. In order to ensure its continued advance, He selected twelve leaders from the early disciples, or followers, and these He instructed in methods of procedure to be followed in organization of churches and in teaching. They were known as "apostles," and freedom to devote themselves wholly to the work and to

---

[1]St. Luke 10:30–36.

travel as new fields opened up was a requisite of their appointment. As time went on, the number of apostles increased to meet the need. Men from many walks of life were to be found among them—teachers, physicians, lawyers, and others of means and education. They carried the message of Christianity east and west through the known world, they recorded the history of the movement, and they gave clarity and permanence to its principles by setting them down in writing.

SAUL OF TARSUS

In the group which eventually became apostles of Christianity, one stands out among great men of all time. A contemporary of Jesus, and almost the same age, *Paul,* or *Saul* as he was also known, was a Jewish rabbi born in Tarsus, a town on the Asiatic coast of the Mediterranean, not far from the city of Antioch in Syria which early became a center of Christian activity. So deeply did Paul resent the intrusion of Christianity into the life of Palestine, that he secured permission to travel to Damascus for the purpose of preventing its further spread by imprisoning all who embraced it there. On the way he encountered a vision which appeared to him in such blazing light that he was blinded and completed his journey with difficulty.

Report of the presence in their city of a man reputed to have been harsh in his persecution of their brethren in Jerusalem spread rapidly among Christians of Damascus. One of them was divinely prompted to visit him. As they talked together, Paul's sight was fully restored and he hastened to become a Christian, too. From that time until his death about 62 A.D., he was able to make use of many talents and a rich enthusiasm which were invaluable to a young organization struggling to maintain a foothold. He worked amid a confusion of beliefs in a discontented world, and always in opposition to those who resisted change. An excellent education under Greek influence had prepared him for his task of teaching ever-changing groups. His management of an extensive field proved to be able and systematic, and his powerful preaching showed him qualified to catch and transmit the spirit of the Master.

St. Paul was especially well fitted for the work of a missionary in foreign fields. His energy was great, and travel apparently delighted him. Danger he could meet with calm strength, his personal comfort he could overlook. Undaunted by imprisonment or persecution, he taught in Palestine and Asia Minor, in the principal cities of Greece and, finally, in Rome. His journeys took him through the islands of the Mediterranean and adjacent seas, and it was his hope that he might carry the work into Spain.

St. Paul has been recognized as the chief exponent of progressive Christianity. He went back and forth among people of many nations, revisiting churches when necessary, collecting and transmitting to the parent church funds for its maintenance and for alms. It was his wish that Christians set aside on the first day of every week what they could spare for the church. In addition to searching out new opportunities for preaching, strengthening weak groups, and starting new ones, St. Paul was a prolific writer. Many books of the New Testament owe their authorship to him. In the Acts of the Apostles, a book credited to a companion worker, *St. Luke,* "the beloved physician," the adventures and trials of St. Paul are recorded. In the Epistles, written by Paul to his bishops or to churches under his supervision, he plans church organization, sets forth ideals of living, admonishes, exhorts, or praises, as the need may be.

St. Paul's Attitude Toward Women. This great preacher is said to have had an indirect influence in lowering the status of woman. Although St. Paul helped her by deprecating divorce and upholding monogamy, it must be admitted that he looked upon woman with the ancient belief in her power as a temptress of man. He may have been fearful, too, of misunderstandings incident upon her undertaking of work side by side with men when tradition outside of Rome confined her so exclusively to the home. He took his own work with extreme seriousness, and he desired the same attitude on the part of others.

We find St. Paul demanding that women be silent in church, that they wear veils, that their dress be of studied plainness. At the same time, he did not fail to speak highly of *Phoebe* who, as a deaconess in Greece, had been, as he says, "a helper of many, and of myself also."[2] To Phoebe, who preceded him to Rome on legal business of her own, he entrusted his letter to the Romans. This was a precious missive, containing as it did the presentment of his gospel and his intention of carrying it to the Gentiles. Much work and thought had gone into the preparation of his message, for it might be met with antagonism. The proud and callous city admitted his right to teach there if he wished to do so, but it was in Rome that he met martyrdom. However, before this time he was able to accomplish two years of fruitful work in the heart of that empire which controlled practically all the nations he hoped to reach.

Church Organization. Systematic organization and able leadership enabled the Christian movement to survive the early loss of its Founder, and the decimation of its ranks through long succeeding periods of persecution. Each little church of Christ emerged, ultimately, under supervision of a priest, presbyter, or elder. Bishops were placed in charge of designated groups of churches. A general council was in control, and met at stated intervals in different places. The Apostle, *Peter,* who later became first Bishop of Rome, carried on notably successful work in the city of Jerusalem where his own compelling influence had been

---

[2]Romans 16:1–2.

augmented by the astounding ability of his preacher assistants in the use of language. As the number of converts rose rapidly to five thousand souls, the difficulty of rendering necessary aid to many poor people increased. Seven men were appointed to assist the apostles. The name "deacon" was given them because it meant "a servant." No duty was too menial for deacons to undertake. One of their chief concerns became that of distributing among the needy the property handed over to the apostles in the early days of the church by those who literally "gave up all" to follow the Christ.

EARLY CHRISTIAN ORDERS OF WOMEN

DEACONESSES

Women had been active in the democratic mission of Christianity since its inception and it was to be expected that they would find work which they alone could do. The *deaconess* came into being and devoted herself to the needs of women converts. The church required her to be unmarried or a widow but once. Like the deacon, she was *ordained to service* and worked on an equal basis with him as a church official. Friendliness to all expressed the ideal of both deacons and deaconesses. The majority of early Christians were poor and, in response to a sympathy to which they were not accustomed, confided many needs. As the diaconate developed its own system and the work increased, an outlet was provided for supervised, effective charity on the part of rich and well-to-do persons who desired to share in Christian activities.

The beginning of concerted private effort in the cause of charity owes its inception to the social work and nursing done by these servants of the early church. Deacons and deaconesses carried the church into the home in a very practical way. They prayed with some, gave food and money to others, and coped as best they could with sickness and those other social ills arising from poverty. Doubtless, their nursing was but a carrying over of that mixture of magic, empiric remedies, and home treatments which women of the time used for their families. We know of no new methods in nursing introduced over a long, long period, but the functions of organized visiting nursing and social service were interpreted by these men and women who accepted the office of servant in the Christian church.

Phoebe, a Greek lady of influence and bearer of St. Paul's Epistle to the Romans, is first mentioned among the women selected for deaconess service. Because of this and her work in nursing the sick poor in their homes, she has been awarded the dual honor of being known as *the world's first deaconess and first visiting nurse*. Visiting nursing soon became a major part of the work of deaconesses, who assumed responsibility for it throughout the eastern, as well as the western, world. The

Christian church had made possible the care of many more people than had ever before received medical or nursing care. A nursing service was brought to the home which has continued ever since. An occupation was opened to women, especially to those who, being widows or unmarried, had held no definite place in society.

WIDOWS AND VIRGINS

Two other formal organizations of women, known respectively as *Widows* and *Virgins,* were developed. Women had held a place in the religion of most countries as priestesses of the temple. It was, therefore, not without precedent that they should occupy positions in the organization of the Christian church. Indeed, their loyal interest made them welcome. They provided lodging, food, and encouragement for the earliest leaders of Christianity. Their homes were the first church meeting places. They offered themselves for service with enthusiasm for the performance of all manner of tasks arising from the Christian assumption of work among the poor.

The Order of Widows was formed very early. Members had not been married, necessarily. The title "Widow" was sometimes used as designation of respect for age. If the widow had been married, it was required that she be the widow of one husband only, and must vow her intention of not marrying again. St. Paul, in the fifth chapter of his First Epistle to Timothy, has explained the qualifications which made widows acceptable. Piety and a character above reproach are first essentials. Freedom from home responsibilities which would interfere with service is another. The age requirement he sets at sixty, although it is said to have been reduced later to forty, and, later still, to an even lower level. "She that giveth herself to pleasure," he says, "is dead while she liveth."[3] This zealous missionary, who seems to have had his work made difficult by many of the failings so often imputed to youth in social or health work today, asks his church to refuse younger widows. Too anxious to marry are they, and inclined to idle also. Besides, they indulge in gossip, carrying tales from one house to another, and they talk too much! Paul recommends that, in their case, marriage be encouraged.

In spite of restrictions Widows allied themselves with the church in considerable numbers. They did a great deal of work of the same nature as that done by Deaconesses, but they were not ordained. An Order of Virgins was created when Christians began to interpret virginity as essential to purity of life. Women were consecrated to service in this, its third group of workers, to which men also are said to have belonged for a time. Virgins ranked in equality with the clergy, next to whom they sat in church gatherings. Ascetics as they were, society in the

---

[3]First Epistle of Paul to Timothy 5:6.

Christian groups of their time set them apart, and awarded them great honor for austerity of life—that crown of good works which they had chosen as an offering to God. Their chief duty seems to have been to assist with distribution of alms.

The three Orders of women which have just been discussed shared certain characteristics in common. All were enrolled for church service. Marriage automatically separated all from their groups. In the beginning, all wore the customary dress of women of the time, although distinctive garb is thought to have been adopted later. All lived in their own homes. If they needed it, all were entitled to receive an allowance from the church for, in its earliest days when converts literally gave up all to follow the Christ, they disposed of their property among the needy or handed it over to the church for distribution.

Under conditions which permitted the use of their own initiative, women were likely to make greater progress. The eagerness with which they entered the social and religious activities of the church probably, in part, bespoke a need. A warring world made many widows, while it kept thin the ranks of marriageable men. There had been times, too, when popularity of bachelorhood had given concern to imperial authorities. The dependent woman could not but know that she was an unwelcome expense, and she was denied self-expression. Eventually, entire Orders of Widows and Virgins were absorbed into community life and became nuns (non nuptae, not married). The number of deaconesses greatly declined. If she was religious, the nunnery offered the woman of this era a measure of independence and the supervision of a woman helped to avoid criticism of conduct.

Throughout the development of the primitive Christian church, women, as we have seen, took an active part. The qualities of character which Jesus upheld were qualities which men associated with mothers, wives, and sisters, and women discovered in Christianity opportunities for strengthening themselves in new activities. We can well imagine the enthusiasm with which they applied themselves to these when we remember that, up to this time, the majority of women had known none but home duties. They gave their sons to be preachers, they sewed for the poor, they unceasingly shared their hospitality with Christian travelers, and they served the church as Deaconesses, Widows, or Virgins, and later as nuns.

PERSECUTION OF CHRISTIANS

Christianity grew within an old pagan religion, and for some time the Christian churches were allowed to develop without interference. Romans were tolerant of people who helped with the vexing problem of caring for the poor. Rome itself had residents of many religions and bore a cosmopolitan atmosphere. Followers of the new religion were accepted with mild indulgence and some curiosity, but when attention was drawn to their refusal to admit the divinity of the emperor, or to sacrifice to any but one God, persecution began. As time went on Christians were stoned, beaten, imprisoned, tortured, or put to death. The church finally was crushed into secrecy, but the misery of Christians only intensified the virtues of pity, gentleness, and charity which they upheld. Men began to note the sincere piety and fine characters of many Christian wives and mothers. Writers of the time extolled the need of virtues such as theirs. Husbands followed wives into the church.

INFLUENCE OF CONSTANTINE THE GREAT

The unquenchable spirit of the Christian martyrs attracted the attention of many a pagan, but the attitude of the Roman government did not change until the early part of the fourth century when it had become apparent to Romans that these persistent Christians, wherever they dwelt, promoted peace and unity. Suddenly, after the worst of many persecutions, the empire under *Constantine the Great* discarded its efforts to uproot a faith which might prove to be a useful agent, and Christianity was adopted as the official religion of the Roman State in 324 A.D.

Constantine, who had been converted a few years previously, not only became the first Christian emperor of Rome, but also relinquished claim to authority of divine origin. By that time Christianity had penetrated the upper or patrician class of society throughout the Roman Empire. The basis of equality on which all were admitted to its privileges and shared in its work was a manifestation of Christian democracy which gave evidence of a nascent social order. In it were gathering the seeds of modern nursing. Monasticism was destined to provide shelter for the young plants and to nurture them as they grew.

ROMAN MATRONS

Strange to say, it is the gay and licentious city of Rome itself that has handed down to us the greatest number of illustrious names among patrician Christian women of the fourth and early fifth centuries. This is not surprising when we recall how well fitted was the Roman woman of the upper classes, by social life and traditional freedom of action, for the use of her initiative. Roman women had been interested in public affairs and had participated in them. Those who managed the houses of wealthy husbands successfully were of proven executive ability and social poise. In their affiliation with the cause of Christianity, they encountered the prejudice of friends and lived, often, in families which remained pagan. We owe considerable progress in organization of charity and care of the sick to the fact that they did not falter in their work.

Marcella. Three of the great names among Christian matrons of patrician Rome are those of *Marcella, Fabiola,* and *Paula.* All were members of a group of women meeting at Marcella's home on the Aventine Hill, which soon became a center of Christian study for her friends. Much inspiration came to them through a great friend and teacher, *St. Jerome,* translator of the Bible from its original Hebrew and Greek into Latin. His version is known as the "Vulgate" version, from the fact that he made use of that form of Latin in common use among the people. Jerome's influence in broadcasting the teachings of Christianity and making it a world religion was next to that of St. Paul. With Marcella and Paula, especially, he read and discussed much of this work. Both were able to render intelligent assistance, and Paula was endowed with mental gifts of an unusually high order.

In time Marcella made her luxurious home into a monastery for women and throughout the remainder of her life devoted herself to their instruction, to charitable work, and to prayer. Her companions, like herself, were sufficiently well educated to become good students of Hebrew and Greek, and the intellectual attainments of her group attracted admiration. This woman who had thus become head of *the first Christian monastery in Rome* was regarded as an authority when questions arose on scriptural passages which were difficult to understand. She had also assisted St. Jerome in his translation of the Hebrew prophets. Her work ended when, in 410 A.D., she was brutally attacked by invaders of the city who, expecting to find valuable plunder in her house, took revenge on her in their disappointment. She is said to have taken refuge in a nearby church where she soon died.

Fabiola. Fabiola, a young woman of storied beauty that caught the imagination of Henner, a famous French artist, was the idolized daughter of a great Roman family. Eagerly she had entered into the gay social life of the Empire, but disappointment awaited her. Marriage united her to a worthless husband whom she found it necessary to divorce. She married a second husband no better than the first, and, on becoming a Christian, realized that in accordance with her new beliefs a marriage following divorce made her guilty of sin. After publicly acknowledging her wrongdoing, Fabiola renounced the world and threw herself wholeheartedly into charitable work. Her charm and enthusiasm distinguished her among fellowworkers.

The *first Christian hospital in Rome* was founded by Fabiola in her own palace. She is said to have sought out the poor and the sick in the streets and byways of her native city and to have cared for them herself. We are further told that she had great fortitude when it was necessary to dress ugly wounds and sores. Toward the end of her life, Fabiola is reputed to have gathered together what was left of her fortune and to have joined with the son-in-law of Paula in building a great hospice for strangers at Ostia, a seaport of Rome. She died beloved of Rome and left behind her a lasting tradition of beauty, youth, and social opportunity given willingly as sacrifice to the expression of a selfless love for human beings. Thousands of young women, equally endowed, have followed her example through the ages since.

Paula. Paula had a daughter, Eustochium, who joined her mother in adopting Christianity and expressing its ideals through charitable work. Together they studied with Marcella. Paula was descended from famous lines and the possessor of a great fortune. Brokenhearted by the death of her husband, she prepared to devote herself to the care of the poor and the sick. Taking with her Eustochium, she set out for Palestine with the intention of living there for the remainder of her life. In the course of their pilgrimage they visited many places connected with the history of the early church and, ultimately, settled in Bethlehem where Paula organized a monastery. She built hospitals for the sick and hospices for pilgrims. In all of these the design and construction of buildings were of the plainest type, for a practical foresight made her determine to save all the money possible for the work to be done in them.

For twenty years Paula managed the institutions that she built and, following her death in 404 A.D., Eustochium conducted the monastery for fifteen years longer. A life story of Paula owes its authorship to her friend and co-worker, St. Jerome. He expresses appreciation of her wisdom and charity and comments on the number of poor who attended her funeral.

DIAKONIA AND XENODOCHIA

The responsibility of nursing care of the sick poor in private homes was so closely associated with activities of the Deaconess Order that the name popularly applied to these institutions was "diakonia." While their use was continued for centuries, another type of institution was developing in the house of the bishop of the church who was expected to make his home a place of welcome for all who needed help. Rooms for the sick or homeless were added to his house, or a separate building was erected nearby. Already the purposes of the ancient xenodochium had been fulfilled, and its well-known name was borrowed by Christians for an institution that soon gave promise of permanency.

By the third century the Christian xenodochium was on the way to becoming the center of a well-rounded system of relief. The hospital took its place within it as one of many departments. Orders of Deaconesses, Widows, and Virgins supplied it with nursing staffs. A considerable number of bishops and priests, who had been drawn from the ranks of physicians, became directors of institutions caring for the sick.

As time went on, the democratic ideal of Christianity brought about a better understanding of social conditions. It became clear that much more than shelter, spiritual consolation, or care during illness would be necessary if poverty was to be alleviated. Work had to be dignified, and work also had to be found. The ideal of brotherly love prompted the rich to free their slaves, many of whom thus became homeless and unable to support themselves. Epidemics of disease which carried off millions left behind numerous orphans.

Society had created beggary by accepting alms as the remedy for dependence. The church followed this tradition in its distribution of the money which came to it in steadily increasing volume. Charity was not yet very wise, but experience gradually made it plain that for many people, housing, funds, education, and a trade would be essential to general well-being. Concentration of charitable activities would be necessary. The xenodochium became the best possible source of expansion in function and concentration of effort and resources.

The magnitude of many Christian xenodochia is made clear by the statement that Constantinople, in 347 A.D., had a daily bread line of three thousand persons dependent on the charity of Christians. Besides food, it is logical to suppose that alms, with medical and nursing care, were included in this work of relief. The church also undertook to assuage the distress of prisoners, a function which it had carried out through the whole period of martyrdom when Christians so often endured this form of punishment. Prison work had become an expression of the Christian spirit identified with the visit of the deaconess.

Xenodochium of St. Basil. The extent to which Christianity succeeded in this task of giving protection and help to all who were poor, afflicted, or distressed is best understood by a study of one of its early accomplishments. About the middle of the fourth century, *St. Basil,* a Greek Bishop of Caesarea in Asia Minor, began to build up what was to be *the most famous of Christian xenodochia.* In its physical organization the institution, when completed, resembled a city. It was developed on the edge of town and its many buildings included the traditional hospice or inn for travelers, clinical facilities for ambulatory patients, a hospital for those who needed bed care, houses for the aged, for the crippled, for orphans, infants, and foundlings. There were buildings in which lepers and those suffering from communicable diseases were segregated. Living quarters were provided for full housekeeping and industrial staffs, and there was accommodation also for a staff of "ductores" or guides who were sent out to find patients and bring or lead them to the hospital.

In addition to housing facilities, it was necessary for a xenodochium of that period to provide for almost complete self-maintenance of the group within it. All among inmates who could perform any kind of labor were put to work. Factories did not exist which could supply the multitude of human needs for everyday living alone. These, and all articles of specialized uses had to be made on the premises. St. Basil's xeno-dochium contained work rooms, refectories, shoe and clothing shops, blacksmith shops, foundry, laundry, dairy, and all other facilities necessary to supply a small city with its needs.

Through the triumph of St. Basil, the hospital found a place as an institution within another institution which it held for many centuries. In the stress of those centuries, and under the uncertain influence of stagnant medical advance, such protection as the xenodochium offered was not only of extreme importance to development of hospitals and charity, but was a factor in disease control.

One of the most widespread plagues of early times occurred about the middle of the third century and "raged without interruption in every province, every city, and almost every family, of the Roman Empire. During some time five thousand persons died daily in Rome; and many towns that had escaped the hands of barbarians were entirely depopulated."[4]

STATUS OF MEDICINE AND NURSING

We have seen that a great increase in the number of people who received nursing care had been brought about by Christianity. Much of this care was given them in their own homes or in homes of Christians who wished to express their charity by giving refuge to the sick poor. At the same time, there was a considerable increase in the number of institutions provided for hospitalization of those who needed it. Strangely enough, there occurred little or no corresponding advance in medicine. The dominant western civilization, which had acquired all the traditions of Hippocratic medicine, neither assimilated much of them itself nor took the trouble to send them elsewhere. No Roman successor of greater wisdom than the "Father of Scientific Medicine" appeared.

All peoples were suffering the strain of exhaustion resulting from many wars, and Rome, in particular, was called upon to cope with communicable diseases introduced by foreign slaves and by soldiers and traders. The mosquitoes of the Tiber marshes infected Romans with malaria, which drained the vitality of citizens of the capital. Everywhere indifferent morals, idleness, and an impoverished populace served to weaken further a world that was growing old while still young.

Indirectly conducive to the failure to disseminate and advance Hippocratic teaching was the prevailing opportunity to have all work done by a slave class. This stigmatized work, and Greek physicians, the bearers of Hippocrates' message, were reduced to the position of slaves

---

[4]Gibbon, Edward: Decline and Fall of the Roman Empire. New York, The Modern Library, Vol. I, p. 244.

to their Roman conquerors and were forced to practice without social recognition. The status of medicine was lowered. Perhaps the real basis of an approaching medical stagnation, however, lay in a primitive tendency of the Roman to place reliance on a form of magic which related all troubles to omens and portents. Quackery flourished among a people who honored success in fighting above intellectual attainment. It was to the surgeon who attended injured gladiators and to the army surgeon that Rome offered the best experience in practice.

As the centuries passed, an ever-increasing influence against adequate care of the body came from the Christian church, which was making a virtue of lack of emphasis on physical things. The spiritual side of man and his future life were becoming all-important, with a tendency to belittle the value of medical care. Carelessness in regard to personal hygiene was pronounced in the eastern part of the Empire, whereas, in the west, Rome's interest in cleanliness and her provisions for its maintenance opposed neglect which might induce disease. This attitude deferred Roman understanding of Christian disregard for the body and hindered medicine.

Soranus of Ephesus.   In spite of obstructions which tended to slow down to stagnation the stream of medical progress, here and there throughout the Empire some man, usually a Greek or a student from the great school of Alexandria, would pour into it his contribution of new ideas to stimulate the current. One of these, *Soranus of Ephesus,* won fame as an obstetrician, pediatrician, and gynecologist and was the author of many practical medical treatises. One helped little children by exposing the stupefying mental results of whippings received from their school masters. Two names, however, stand out above all others during the first five centuries of the Christian era for their influence on the future course of medicine, those of *Celsus* and *Galen.*

Celsus.   Celsus was a Roman patrician of the first century who is best known for his writings, which included medical works. His great achievement was the rescue and preservation of knowledge of other men. The clarity of his descriptions and the usefulness of his material have been admitted by the surgeon of modern times. The intricacies of procedure in amputation, surgery of plastic nature, hernias, venesection, cataract, and other operations are among the valuable contents of his collection, which consists of eight books on subjects concerned with medicine— the group entitled "De Re Medicina" (The Subject of Medicine). In Celsus' own time the compilation did not attract great attention but, in a later time, men honored the author when they found an answer to a great need. During the Revival of Learning in the sixteenth century, these books of Celsus were among the first to be printed.

Galen.   Galen lived in the second century. Born at Pergamum in Asia Minor, he enjoyed the privilege of a good education which included work at the famous University of Alexandria. The knowledge of medicine

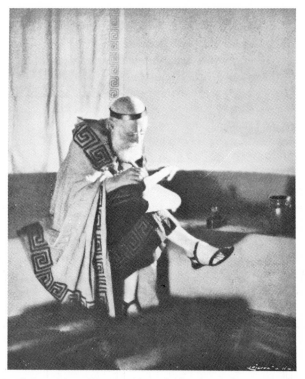

Figure 18. Celsus (*circa* 25 B.C. — 40 A.D.). A present-day conception. (Courtesy of Davis & Geck, Inc.)

which he acquired there and through much travel was supplemented by independent investigation by means of dissection. As dissection of human bodies had again become illegal, Galen was forced to work principally on animals, but he is known as the "Founder of Experimental Physiology." He was also a popular teacher of anatomy. His work was done in the scientific spirit, and he restored Hippocratic medicine which had been hidden under a scum of pedantry.

Ultimately settling down in the city of Rome, he became physician to the gladiators. In this capacity his experience with emergency and plastic surgery appears to have been extensive. His professional literary contributions accumulated greatly and so popular were his works that, as late as the sixteenth century, they were still consulted as the chief medical authority. Through these interpretations of Hippocratic medicine and the restoration of interest in scientific method which they brought about, Hippocrates and Galen, fortunately, gave direction to what medical thought and procedure continued throughout the Middle Ages.

The brief study which we have made of the nursing done during the first four centuries after the birth of Jesus shows that it was largely in the hands of intelligent, educated, wealthy women of noble birth. The emphasis which Christianity placed on pity gave prominence to the weak and suffering among mankind. It pointed to preservation of all, rather than to the maximum development of the fit. Infanticide was condemned, and because of the lessening of this common practice more children needed care and more women survived among the population. Service to all in need took the place of military glory as an aim of life. Self-sacrifice on the part of the rich was idealized, and poverty looked to them for its alleviation.

THE FALL OF ROME IN 476 A.D.

In spite of many dissensions Christian influence on the Roman Empire may be looked upon as steadily constructive. Other influences doomed to destruction whatever political integrity had been attained. The reign of Augustus Caesar (29 B.C.–14 A.D.) was the beginning of a considerable period during which Rome knew more peace, prosperity, and luxury than at any other time in her history. Romans were worn out by war, and they were satisfied with the decision of the new emperor to cease imperial expansion. Augustus confined Roman power within the following natural boundaries: The Danube and the Rhine rivers on the north, the Black Sea, the Euphrates River, and the Arabian Desert on the east, the Sahara Desert on the south, and the Atlantic Ocean on the west.

As happens during all periods of peace, some people took advantage of the opportunity to extend their culture. The majority tended in another direction. A fashionable license and coarseness among the wealthy minority made the prevailing status of morals low, for lower classes were encouraged to follow their example. Disease made its inroads on physical vitality. Persistent malaria in the city of Rome kept citizens under par and probably accounted, in some degree, for an increase in her vices. Recurring pestilence here and throughout the Empire reduced the general population by millions.

The worst menace, however, came from other sources. The constituent elements of the vast Empire felt no common interest in its successful administration. Protection of over two thousand miles of boundary proved to be very difficult. On the other side of it lived people still in the tribal state—Jutes, Angles, Saxons, Alemans, Burgundians, Franks, Vandals, Sueves, Lombards, Visigoths, and Ostrogoths. Huns and Alans, savage enemies of all, were straining forward from Asia toward southeastern Europe. The force of the general movement southward and westward made itself felt.

These people from the north were known as "barbarians" or "outsiders" to the Greeks and Romans. They were nature worshipers, and skins of wild beasts furnished their clothing in a rigid climate. They lived in fixed habitations, and the chief occupation of the men was fighting and hunting. Women performed the manual work and were subject to the rule of harsh husbands. None among these semisavage people could read or write. They made use of the cart and must have known something of farming, for they repeatedly stole Roman tools. Some of the earlier arrivals were assimilated as they replaced Roman farm laborers who left the country for the city. Many of them were marauders, who plundered property and carried off captives whose fate was slavery if not redeemed by ransom. Romans themselves engaged in slave trade with these neighbors, and some Romans married barbarian wives, while a good many barbarians became Roman citizens. On the whole, there seems to have been in progress, for several hundred years, a comparatively peaceful penetration of foreign peoples.

By the fifth century whole tribes began to settle on Roman lands. They coveted the wealth of those who had attained civilization and were ready to fight for it. They were also pushed over the border by enemies behind them. Invasion followed invasion in such rapid succession that it was as if a flood had been let loose. Roman armies were unable to control the sudden influx. Greece was plundered, Gaul devastated, and the capital city of Rome was sacked, all about the same time. In 476 A.D. Rome fell, and within a year wild tribes controlled the whole western division of the Empire. Some Romans were able to migrate to an eastern capital hastily set up in Constantinople. The majority had to stay where they were and submit to barbarian domination.

If the work of man for many centuries was not to be lost, there must be some force in civilization which would prove sufficiently strong to induce the invading hordes to discard barbarism. As we shall see, that force was in Christianity, and in the missionary and teaching spirit of its preachers lay the means of utilizing it. The world pays tribute to the men and women who so shaped the affairs of monasteries that they could perform this service for mankind. They had to deal with unlettered, half-savage people of many gods and languages. They had to teach them to read and to write, to desire and to learn all the practical arts as well as the refinements of thought and action that are a part of civilized life, and to lead them into the Christian fold.

Five centuries of effort had provided the Christians with a foundation on which to build efficient institutions through which these things might be accomplished. The sixth century found them with the Bible in the Vulgate form, translated by St. Jerome and his collaborators. Great xenodochia had been built which could serve as models for commercial teaching, charity, and nursing care. The Orders of Widows and Virgins had been absorbed into monasteries. As nuns these women would share in a new movement which would change the course of future history by making over the uncivilized. A time had come when the institution became a necessary protection. Life outside it was unsafe, and individual effort, or scattered organization of work in homes, could make little

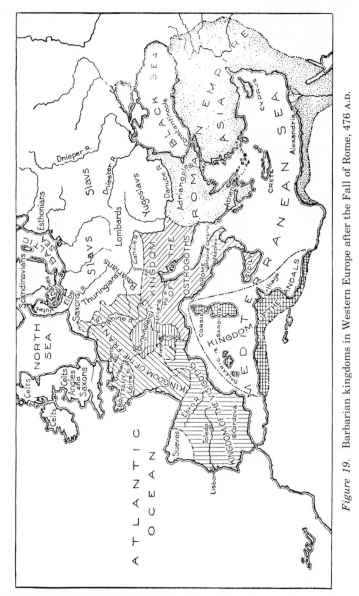

Figure 19. Barbarian kingdoms in Western Europe after the Fall of Rome, 476 A.D.

headway. Throughout Roman Europe, deaconesses sank into obscurity amid the general confusion. The church was beginning to assume guardianship over nursing, medicine, and charity, as well as of literature, science, and art.

Suggestions for Study

1. Who was Emperor of Rome at the time of the birth of Jesus, and what factors were contributing to the unhappiness of the people?

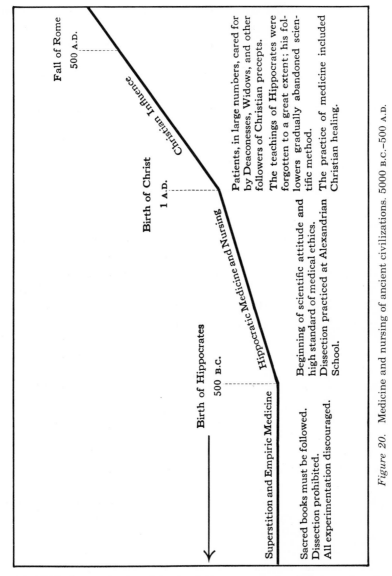

Figure 20. Medicine and nursing of ancient civilizations. 5000 B.C.–500 A.D.

2. (*a*) Show how the teachings of Jesus contained the seeds of social revolution. (*b*) What quotation from Matthew, Ch. 7, constitutes the Golden Rule of the Christians, and from Matthew, Ch. 25, shows their attitude toward prisoners?

3. What system of organization was adopted by early Christians in order to ensure a world-wide spread of Christian teachings?

4. Which apostle of Jesus became the first pope of Rome?

5. (*a*) What missionary preacher was largely responsible for carrying the teachings of Christianity to far-off places? (*b*) What was his influence on the position of women?

6. Who was entrusted with carrying the precious Epistle written by St. Paul to the Romans?

7. Who is known as the first deaconess and first visiting nurse, and why?

8. Describe the duties and responsibilities of early deacons and deaconesses.

9. (a) Make an outline of entrance requirements for each of the three Orders of women of the early Christian church. (b) Members of which group are considered the forerunners of nurses?

10. What is known of nursing methods of the time?

11. (a) Show how visiting nursing came to have its beginnings with the Christian movement. (b) Which order of women engaged in this work?

12. Discuss, from the following standpoints, the Roman matrons who were converted to Christianity: (a) Characteristics typical of Roman women. (b) Social life compared with that of the majority of early Christians. (c) Their noted friend and teacher. (d) Attitude toward asceticism. (e) Their individual accomplishments.

13. What well-known artist made a painting of Fabiola, a copy of which appears as the frontispiece of this book?

14. If you had been a citizen of the Roman Empire during this period, what opportunity for care during illness would have been available to you?

15. Show how institutional care of the sick gradually developed among Christians.

16. If you had been a visitor at the Xenodochium of St. Basil at Caesarea, what kinds of social work would you have seen going on about you?

17. What do you know of the plagues of the third century, and how do you account for them?

18. (a) Add a dotted line to the chart on page 71 to indicate the *general trend* in the practice of medicine from 1 to 500 A.D. (b) What two men made contributions of lasting value?

19. What factors contributed to the general stagnation in medical advance during this early Christian period?

20. Women of what class of society did the nursing during the first four centuries of the Christian era?

21. (a) What influences contributed to the breakup of the Roman Empire in 476 A.D. (b) What social institution was ready to assume guardianship of medicine, nursing, charity, and education, during the five hundred years of "Dark Ages" that were to follow?

References

Asch, Sholem: The Apostle. New York, G. P. Putnam's Sons, 1943.

Austin, Anne L.: History of Nursing Source Book. New York, G. P. Putnam's Sons, 1957, Chap. 2.

Brown, Lewis: The World's Great Scriptures. New York, The Macmillan Co., 1946.

Caldwell, Taylor: Dear and Glorious Physician. The Story of St. Luke. New York, Doubleday and Co., 1959.

Dana, Charles L.: The Peaks of Medical History. New York, Paul B. Hoeber, Inc., 1936.

Editorial Staff of *Life:* The World's Great Religions. (Special edition for young readers.) New York, Golden Press, 1958.

Fitch, Florence: One God; The Ways We Worship Him. New York, Lathrop, Lee, and Shepard Co., 1945. (Describes religious observances of Jews, Catholics, and Protestants. Many illustrations.)

Fosdick, Harry Emerson: The Man from Nazareth. New York, Harper and Brothers, 1949.

Friedlander, Ludwig: Roman Life and Manners. New York, E. P. Dutton & Co. and London, George Routledge & Sons.

Gibbon, Edward: The Decline and Fall of the Roman Empire. (Giant edition.) New York, The Modern Library, Vol. I (180–476 A.D.).

Goodspeed, Edgar J.: Paul. Philadelphia and Toronto, The John C. Winston Co., 1947.

Heaps, Isabel W.: Five Marys. New York, Abingdon-Cokesbury Press, 1942.

Kirkland, Winifred: Discovering the Boy of Nazareth. New York, The Macmillan Company, 1944.

Members of School for Graduate Nurses, McGill University, Montreal, Canada: Vignettes from the History of Nursing. The Canadian Nurse, March, April, May, June, July, 1928.

Miller, Madeline S.: Footprints in Palestine. New York, Fleming H. Revell Co., 1936.

Nutting and Dock: A History of Nursing. New York, G. P. Putnam's Sons, 1907, Vol. I, Part II, Chaps. 1 and 2.

Reinach, Salomon: Orpheus, A History of Religions. New York, Liveright, Inc., 1930.

Part Two

THE MIDDLE AGES

Circa 500 to 1500 A.D.

Chapter 5

EARLY MIDDLE AGES
Society in Small Cooperative Units

Broadly speaking, the history of civilization divides itself into three great periods or eras—ancient, medieval, and modern. Within these lie lesser periods, but dissolution of the greatest state that man had yet been able to bring under one rule destroyed a civilization representing many centuries of human development, and the process of building up a civilization to replace it covered other centuries. An interval of about one thousand years between social destruction and social restoration has been named the *Medieval Period* in European development, or the *Middle Ages*.

This is a good place to remind ourselves that dividing lines between what we call *periods* in history can never be looked upon as hard and fast boundaries. One of these so-called periods begins within another through the activity of changing influences that grow imperceptibly and operate at times with sudden force. Periods fade out. They do not end precipitately, but there are times when events occur to hasten a change in the trend of affairs.

The early centuries of the Middle Ages in European history are collectively known as "the Dark Ages." In order to understand this, we must try to imagine what it would be like to be surrounded ourselves by swarms of semisavage people who had descended upon our country, seized our property, and set about making crude homes for themselves right in our midst. No central government could interfere in our behalf, because there was none. The armies which we had become accustomed to looking upon as invincible in our support no longer functioned. The officials who had done our thinking for us had disappeared. Meanwhile, robbers made life unsafe, and roads, aqueducts, sewers, and bridges, in great numbers, had been ruined. Destruction of utilities, combined with crowding, put public health in the same evil plight as business, education, and government. Romans who could do so escaped to the eastern part of the Empire. Those whom circumstances forced to remain in the west settled down to a slow working out of a social compromise which would enable them to live together with the barbarians as citizens of a new world.

The fate of civilization rested upon health protection, a different form of government, and the education of thousands of barbarians to civilized standards. Time has shown that the Christian religion and its representative, the church, accepted the burden of these tasks and carried them to fulfillment. Its gospel of love for all human beings found new expression, and its leaders undertook to calm the excitement of people who had lost their sense of security and were beginning to herd together in search of safety. Many turned to the *monasteries,* which offered refuge and peace. These institutions began a period of great expansion and were able to hasten the return of order while they preserved the accomplishments of religion, education, medicine, and nursing.

At the same time secular units formed around strong men who helped individual members to establish a life routine by reviving, on great estates, an ancient governmental institution known as *feudalism.* This was a type of patriarchal rule which provided men with homes for their families and with food and bodily protection, in return for their service as farmers and, in case of war, as soldiers. Rome had encouraged the growth of a landowning class, and the number of great rural estates now increased. The immediate problem of all groups was to arrange for adequate protection from attack and to make themselves self-sustaining.

Social poise and trade were gradually restored to a noticeable degree by 800 A.D. and, following the revival of commerce, a third type of protective unit known as a *guild* began to appear as, for the first time in history, workers organized for mutual benefit. These forerunners of modern labor unions were to become, eventually, the core of a great guild system which would regulate craftsmen and traders, manufacturers, and commerce. *Monasticism, feudalism,* and *guilds* thus constitute pivots around which society learned to move during the Middle Ages, and the church emerged as chief authority, with feudal government and guilds under its control.

CHRISTIAN MONASTICISM

Monasticism is a system which we have found to be of very ancient origin and common to various religious beliefs. As a phase of Christianity it had developed to a considerable extent before the fourth century, when it received new stimulus from the enthusiasm of Marcella, Paula, Saint Jerome, and the altruistic group to which they belonged.

The primary purpose which the monastic establishment served was to house men who desired to live apart from the world and to promote their individual salvation, a purpose which did not change when Christianity brought into it the broader ideal of service to mankind. With the fall of Rome, Roman citizens of every class turned to the monastery for refuge, and barbarians, too, sought its help as they realized that an institution which resisted their destruction was also willing to show them kindness.

RISE OF BENEDICTINE MONASTERIES

To an Italian monk, history ascribes credit for fixing the trend of monastic development for several centuries to come. In 529 A.D. this monk, whom we now know as *St. Benedict of Nursia,* was busily making use of stones from ruins of an ancient pagan temple to build a monastery for a few followers. The site was a rugged mountain top between Rome and Naples, and his neighbors were many of them pagan, some barbarian as well. Gradually, Benedict induced all to become Christians and taught men who had been enemies to harmonize their customs and manners. An institution grew on Monte Cassino which was one of the most efficient of medieval protective monastic units, as well as a radiating center for monks whose numbers and success brought new hope and courage to other groups already hard at work trying to banish the barbarism which had deluged Europe.

Plan of Monastery Buildings and Grounds. Ultimately, many monasteries took on a characteristic arrangement. When a plot of ground of suitable size had been walled in with high stone walls, there slowly appeared a church, a storehouse, dining room or refectory, and a row

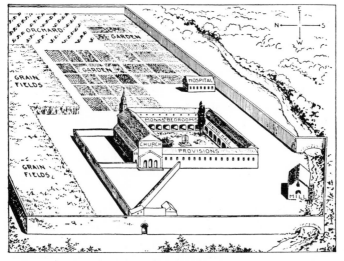

Figure 21. General plan of a monastery. (From Hayes, Moon, and Wayland, "World History," by permission of The Macmillan Co., publishers.)

of cells or bedrooms for monks, all arranged around a square court. Beyond this group of buildings were fields of grain, orchards, barns, workshops, a mill beside running water, and such other buildings as the activities of the institution might require. Here also were a hospital and quarters for strangers. None could be turned away, and charity extended to the poor grew to great proportions. By the ninth century the majority of monasteries maintained, in addition to such quarters, a school for children of the people who, as things settled down, began to live just outside its walls.

The Benedictine Rule. During the development of Christian monasticism numerous rules or codes regulated the daily life of monks. The Benedictine Rule was formulated to meet the needs of a new era. Manual labor, which Romans had relegated to slaves, had become a prime necessity for all men. It was a time when every man had to earn the right to live, and all Benedictines worked. The abbot (L. *abbas,* father) whom they elected to be the head of the institution worked side by side with the monks. Many monasteries were born of the motherhouse on Monte Cassino, and in the centuries following its inception, twenty emperors and forty-seven kings abdicated to become Benedictine monks. Ten empresses and fifty queens, with many princesses and ladies of the court, became nuns.

The path of the monastic novice was not easy. The Benedictine Rule made his novitiate a period in which he was tried out to determine his fitness for monastic life. Constantly under supervision, restrictions forbade him privileges accorded to those who had been accepted into the monastic organization. Accepted monks were divided into three groups according to the length of their experience. Seniors, or "wisefolk," had spent fifty years as monks, a middle class twenty-four to fifty years, and juniors less than twenty-four years. Privileges and duties were arranged in accordance with these divisions, the hardest work falling upon the youngest group, who were enjoined to love the seniors who, in turn, were to know them as brothers. Should monks fall ill, adequate care was assured them, for an *infirmarian* saw to their nursing and supervised a special hospital in which they were housed until recovery. The hospital provided for strangers occupied a separate building. In the words of St. Benedict:

"Before all things and above all things care is to be had of the sick, that they may be served in the very deed as Christ himself, for He hath said, 'I was sick and ye visited Me,' and 'What ye have done unto one of these little ones, ye have done unto Me.'"

Agriculture, Arts, and Crafts. Agriculture was necessarily a chief interest of monastic units of this time, and Benedictine institutions performed a great public service by improving farming methods and reclaiming vast areas of previously useless land. It became the custom for monasteries to rent pieces of their property to tenants at nominal rates. Further income was derived from gifts, and, gradually, poverty was left behind and great wealth took its place. As people settled down in orderly groups, highways became safer and trade slowly revived. Inside the wall, meanwhile, arts and skills were becoming highly developed and specialized. Among monks and nuns could be found artists in architecture, music and painting, expert silversmiths and goldsmiths, doctors and nurses skilled in the use of home remedies in sickness.

Preservation of Knowledge. From its earliest days the Christian monastery had known the influence of scholarly men and women. *Cassiodorus,* a patrician contemporary of St. Benedict, is credited with introducing the copying of religious and classic manuscripts to the monks of a monastery that he founded. St. Benedict took up the idea, and these two brought to their fellow monasteries of the Middle Ages the privilege of preserving knowledge likely to have been lost in that disturbed era. In times which anteceded printing or typewriting, all this tedious work was laboriously done by monks or nuns who worked in the chilly atmosphere of medieval buildings and, often, by the light of a candle.

As manuscripts were passed from one monastery to another, they exerted a civilizing influence. The thought of great minds among the ancients was spread abroad and eventually handed down to us. The books were used to found libraries in which they were preserved with studious care for scholars of the future. They provided monks and nuns with some scientific knowledge regarding care of the sick. They were the groundwork of universities.

The ninth and tenth centuries saw decline of this monastic prestige in some quarters. Within the church itself there was dissatisfaction with institutions which continually acquired wealth and, with wealth, a greater ease of life and greater freedom to mingle with a society which was finding it possible to move about once more. Monastic severity of life was becoming less attractive and more relaxed. However, a new Benedictine monastery at *Cluny* in France heralded a change of thought and a return to simple expression of Christian service. It also established a new tradition by making the various houses which branched out from this parent organization subject to its control. Its fruits appear in the late Middle Ages.

WOMEN OF MONASTICISM

The task of creating a civilization that would surpass that which had been destroyed drew women to share with men its difficulties and its satisfactions. Monastic houses for women grew in number and their founders were usually women of influence. Many were allied with royal courts, some were daughters of powerful, converted barbarians accustomed to such luxury and education as were known in their time. Great properties were brought to the church, and numerous women became heads of great institutions. Known as *abbesses* or mothers, they frequently assumed control of so-called "double monasteries" composed of men and women. In England, especially, this type was common, and a wall might be built through the middle of the church so that the sight of one another might not divert the worshipers from their devotions. Sometimes a cemetery separated their houses. Monks as well as nuns took the vow of obedience, and history honors the abbess for her skill as an executive in developing orderly institutions. She was recognized as an equal by rulers and church authorities, and she managed business with financial acumen. The church gave her equality with the abbot. Some abbesses traveled extensively, some had literary talent, some were teachers or preachers.

Of the many abbesses who with their nun associates availed themselves of this new opportunity which Christianity offered women for usefulness to society, we shall mention only one who belonged to this period of the early Middle Ages—*Radegunde of Poitiers*. Radegunde (? –587), a barbarian queen, fled from a husband who, after many other cruelties, had just murdered her brother. Pursued by the king's knights, she managed to make her way to Poitiers where she took refuge in the Christian Church. Here, in sanctuary, none could harm her. She persuaded the bishop to consecrate her to religion and, becoming a nun, devoted life and property to a convent which she established. Here two hundred nuns assisted her in care of the poor and the sick. The leper's misery already had caught her sympathy and, now that she was free to do so, she made him her especial charge.

Convent Dress.   Nuns of these early times, like the abbesses, were not wholly withdrawn from the world. Some of them lived at home; not all of them took vows. No distinctive dress was required until circumstances arose which seemed to make it necessary. The monastic ideal of humility pointed to the use of plain, coarse materials in clothing, an ideal further encouraged by the poverty of many of the earliest convents. Convent women spun the wool and wove the cloth for their garments. A criticism made about the seventh century has survived the ages and accuses nuns of paying too much attention to the making of fine clothes.

In itself, the costume probably reflected the fashion among aristocratic women of the time, and the wearers had but carried the ideas of their social set into convent life. Many of them, too, were not far removed from the barbaric stage. The significance of the dress lies in the fact that its incongruity with monasticism attracted notice, and criticism of it prepared the way for that ultimate reform which ended in uniformity.

The veil as an adjunct of woman's dress has a long history. As a means of keeping evil spirits away from brides, as a relic of ancient custom which made a woman don it to distinguish her in her married state, and as part of convent dress, its symbolism has been that of humility, obedience, and service. After being accepted by all nations of the ancient world, it gradually came to mean that the bride, forsaking all others, guarded her charms for her husband. By the time of the Roman Empire, custom demanded that, while in public, ladies conceal their hair with veils or caps, and prescribed such distinguishing features as a red veil or veil with red stripes for the newly married woman. Veils of Turkish, Hindu, and Arabian women were to be removed only in the presence of their immediate families.

Within the walls of the church Christian women veiled their heads. As the custom grew, added regulations in regard to the use of veils began to appear. According to social position, all women wore them, those of queens sweeping to the floor, those of plebeians reaching only to the waist. Among religious orders, where they came to be part of the prescribed habit, they are still worn, and veils of different types are accorded to nuns in the various stages of their service. In another form the veil is worn by nurses in many European countries, and by Red Cross workers everywhere. The cap of the modern nurse is a modification of it and is associated with the rendering of service to mankind.

FEUDALISM

Modified by Christian ideals, the ancient system known as *feudalism* began to take its place side by side with monasticism in western Europe. When dissolution of the state left the greater part of the populace adrift, it was natural that many Romans should seek protection from great landlords, many of whom had retired permanently to country life. It was natural, too, that powerful barbarians should set up similar estates and that, later, barbarian kings should parcel out land to favorite subjects. Such a land grant was known as a "fief" or "feud" on the continent, while in England it went by the name of "manor."

Before 1000 A.D., there were scattered all over the continent of Europe cooperative farming units, isolated from each other and governed by individuals known as lords, knights, earls, counts, or barons. Kings nominally owned the land and these warrior lords held it in fief or feud. The central government of each kingdom was still in its infancy and supported no standing army. The provision of a fighting force was left to the landlords, whose serfs abandoned the soil whenever called upon to do so. Abbots and abbesses, as heads of monastic organizations which often held lands in fief, had to meet the same obligation by maintaining similar forces of armed men, and monks at times were called upon to fight.

Wherever he chose to live, the landlord built his home. Its purpose was to provide shelter and protection for his family and a place of safe retreat for the families of his serfs who lived in a village outside its encircling wall. The location chosen for the castle was usually high up on the edge of a rocky precipice from which there was a full view of the land on all sides. Castles in the early days of feudalism were of wood or stone, built with thick walls, and surrounded by a water-filled ditch or moat, outside of which ran a second, strong, palisade-like wall. At intervals along this wall were towers for purposes of fortification. A drawbridge to connect the castle with the mainland could be lowered or withdrawn at will.

Life in these first feudal castles was hazardous and necessarily without luxury. The fine carvings, beautiful works of art, magnificent tapestries, and elaborate furniture that we associate with great stone castles of many stories belong to the latter part of the Middle Ages. Likewise, the lady of early days was far from being an idle, pleasure-loving beauty. Her days were full of hard work. She had to be capable of supervising the entire establishment. She had to understand cooking, sewing, weaving, spinning, general farming. She had to bear and care for chil-

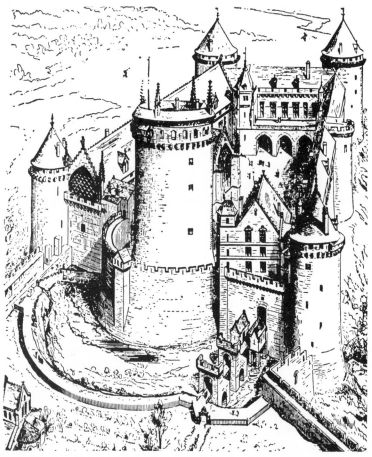

Figure 22. A castle of northern France built in the thirteenth century. A restoration by Viollet-le-Duc. (Gertrude Hartman, "Medieval Days and Ways," by permission of The Macmillan Company, publishers.)

dren, ride and hunt like a man, and command soldiers, or even fight, if that was necessary. Her knowledge of home remedies for all kinds of illness had to be extensive, and she was called upon to nurse family guests, or villagers, as need arose. First aid and surgical emergencies were all in her day's work. She was doctor and nurse combined. In the absence of organized charity, the duty of providing for the poor devolved upon her also. Her very name indicated this responsibility, for "lady" is derived from a word which means "she who looks after the loaf," while "lord" means "loaf-giver."

By the end of the tenth century some progress had been made toward social recovery, but two privileged groups had arisen, represented by the monk and the feudal lord. The former was being weakened by ease as wealth was acquired and discipline was relaxed to favor prominent persons who wished to enter monastic life. The feudal lord kept the continent in confusion through his determination to stick to the occupation he preferred, that of fighting. Agriculture suffered from the absence of his laborers; famine and disease accompanied the lack of adequate food. Farm animals became poor in quality and the bulk of meat was pork, fresh or salted. Few vegetables could be grown, for the women had all that they could do to keep other industries going.

GUILDS

The third form of protective unit which aided recrystallization of society was to be seen in the *guild*. In conformance with needs of the time, it became the first organization of workmen formed for the purpose of mutual benefit and it united individuals not attached to monastic or feudal groups. It reached its height about the twelfth century, and in it lay the seed of the modern labor union and of professional organizations as well.

When monasteries and feudal estates had set up their orderly units of society and made it possible to bring about some revival of trade, they emerged somewhat from isolation. Markets grew up outside the manor as well as outside the monastery. Goods were peddled about the country and exchange of wares gradually increased. Great fairs for the display and exchange of goods came to be events of importance to both institutions. Merchants then formed *merchant guilds* or societies which protected members as they traveled roads made dangerous by robber bands. Help was advanced to families if need arose. After a brief life merchant guilds split up into *craft guilds,* each of which represented one type of skilled workmanship. *Religious guilds* also came into existence.

Craft guilds gave encouragement to good work by a system of inspection, as well as by dismissal from membership of the inadequate or careless. Guild leaders held the title of *master*, which they won by producing a

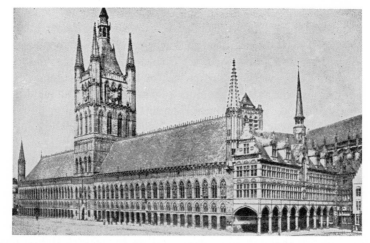

Figure 23. Hall of the Clothmakers' Guild at Ypres, Belgium. One of the most beautiful guildhalls in Europe. (Gertrude Hartman, "Medieval Days and Ways," by permission of The Macmillan Company, publishers.)

piece of work of outstanding excellence or by spending several years under the direction of a master workman. Under the *master* worked *apprentices* and *journeymen*. Apprentices were youths whose fathers paid a fee for their admission to the privilege of learning a trade. They lived in the home of the master, worked at a specific craft for a period gradually lengthened to seven years, and received in return for their labor board, lodging, clothing, and more or less character training.

On completion of training the apprentice became a journeyman. The name is derived from a French word meaning "day" (journée), and derives its use from the fact that the journeyman was free to earn regular wages in employment by the day outside the master's home. He frequently lived there, however, and paid his way by work done between times. When he had passed his examination and had enough money to set up his own establishment, he became a master. The degree of Master of Arts, still awarded by universities, is a survival of the system which gave him his title.

In the guild apprenticeship lies the origin of a system which has characterized the management of our schools of nursing. The director of nursing in the capacity of "Master" leads the instruction of her apprentices or student nurses who, in return, give care to patients. In some countries nurses graduated from a school have been permitted to remain in residence and give their services to the hospital when not employed in private duty outside it — true journeywomen.

ISLAM, A RIVAL OF CHRISTIANITY

While feudalism and monasticism built up little strongholds for the succor of distraught inhabitants of a disintegrating empire, a new barbarian invasion was preparing to advance upon Europe from the southeast. On the arid desert of Arabia, were thousands of nomadic people who, strangely enough, would be called upon by fate to play a part in the work of regeneration. They also lived in small protective units which we know as tribes. Patriarchal chiefs, or sheiks, took the part of rulers. Nature had made subsistence difficult for these tribes, and a settled manner of life impossible for most of them. Few and far between, in her sandy wastes were the fertile spots which offered the fruit of date palms as food, and water as drink, for themselves and their horses and camels and flocks of sheep.

Oases were the cause of frequent disputes over right of occupancy or use, and petty warfare over property, or blood feuds exacting a life for a life, were part of everyday existence. Distance, deep sand underfoot, and frequent sandstorms, forced the *Arabs,* as they were called, to resort to travel by camelback or horseback. Their horsemanship was unrivaled, and the animals that they bred had unusual hardiness, beauty, and speed.

Outside of raising flocks of sheep and herds of camels, the principal business of the Arabs, and their amusement as well, was the robbing of camel caravans plying between cities and villages developed by their more civilized brethren or by men of neighboring lands. The city of Mecca held a shrine to which they made pilgrimage for worship of a sacred stone in a temple known as the "Kaaba." In Mecca, too, and in Medina, great fairs were held which gave the desert dwellers opportunity to engage in trading. For four months each spring a truce was called to warfare so that all might make the most of these excursions.

About 570 A.D. there was born in the city of Mecca an Arabian child who was to be the prophet of a new world religion. The tribe to which Mohammed's family belonged was possessed of considerable influence and, like other Arab tribes, worshiped idols. When Mohammed was a young man, he was engaged by a rich widow of his tribe to manage a caravan for her, and so satisfactory was his work and so pleasing his personality that the widow became his wife. Her devotion to him led her to encourage an abstraction in religion which increased as time went on. It became his practice to withdraw frequently from life about him and give himself up to meditation.

Mohammed spent a great many years in the analysis of religions, especially Judaism and Christianity, but not until the age of forty did he begin to speak publicly on the subject dearest to him—a faith which would unite his countrymen and give them a better ordered life. When he did, he met indifference. Finally he left Mecca and took up his abode in Medina. Here his success was not marked until he enlisted the interest of the Arab tribe known as "Bedouins." Mohammed's ideas appealed to Bedouins, and it became their religious duty to force upon indifferent Mecca and commercial Medina a religion which their citizens had refused to accept. Desert Arabs were fighters, and Mohammed now sent them forth to fight a holy war, attacking all infidels who refused to come into submission to the will of Allah. "There is no God but Allah, and Mohammed is his prophet" ran his creed. Mecca was conquered and Medina, too. The followers of Mohammed went on into the Byzantine Empire, to Egypt, northwest Africa, and to Spain and France where at last their further progress was halted by the Christians a century after Mohammed's death.

By 637 A.D. the Moslem zealots had taken Jerusalem, thereby arousing a horrified and helpless resentment among Christians the world over. As Mecca was to the Arabs, so Jerusalem was to Christians — a place of pilgrimage, the lodestar of Christendom. Nevertheless, Moslem mosques arose for new worshipers, and a new religion held sway over this holy city for over four and a half centuries, although Arabs did not always rule.

What was this religion that could so speedily unite a disunited people, spread so far as to make itself a dangerous rival of medieval Christianity, and be embraced today by five hundred million followers? To the smouldering discontent with hardship which was felt by the average man, Mohammed had added the spark of religious enthusiasm. At his command men abandoned primitive gods and native animism, surging forth by thousands to spread the will of Allah, as it was interpreted for them by His prophet. Submission to this will was the core of the religion that Mohammed taught, and from this basic ideal it took

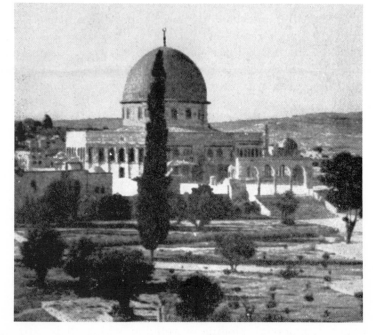

Figure 24. Omar Mosque at Jerusalem. (Photo by Burton Holmes, from Ewing Galloway.)

its name "Islam" (surrender—to the will of Allah). Its followers called themselves "Moslems" (submitters). From a balcony on the outside of each mosque, an official known as a *muezzin,* five times each day, called believers to prayer:

"Allah is Almighty . . . Allah is Almighty . . . I witness that there is no other God but Allah . . . I witness that Mohammed is his prophet . . . Come to prayer . . . come to prayer . . . come to the house of praise, Allah is Almighty . . . Allah is Almighty . . . There is no God but Allah."[1]

Through Mohammed the civil as well as the religious life of Moslems was directed. His teachings, incorporated in the "Koran," now the bible of Moslems, formulated rules for achievement of the good life. Gambling, lying, the charging of excessive rates of interest on borrowed money, wine-drinking, uncleanliness, and the eating of unclean food were sins to be shunned. Kindliness, honesty, hospitality, forgiveness of injury, almsgiving, cleanliness, and the eating of prescribed foods were virtues. No one could pray to Allah without first washing his hands. No confusing array of gods had to be pleased. For one month out of each year believers were required to fast, and at five stated times each day they must address themselves directly to Allah in prayer. At these times they were required to prostrate themselves upon the ground but always with face turned toward Mecca. This city, which had always been holy to Arabs, was still to be the shrine of pilgrimage. Indeed, under Allah's command, they were to make a pilgrimage to Mecca at least once in a lifetime.

Thus in a brief space of time, a great revolution was brought about in the land of desert dwellers. Religion brought isolated and individual tribes together in common ways of thinking and living and gave them a common aim. In a little over a century after the Bedouins undertook to spread Mohammed's teachings, not only had a Moslem empire sprung into being, but pilgrimage to Mecca of thousands of converts from many parts of the world was beginning to alter the face of society at large. Ideas were exchanged, people grew to know each other better.

All this serves to bring out a constructive quality not observed at first in militant Islam. Without it empire building would not have been possible. The fearless riders of swift horses, whose shining blades of Damascus steel had stricken terror into the hearts of people of many lands, began to realize the foolishness of destroying those things which made civilization different from the barren life of the desert. They became interested in what other people did and their uncluttered minds absorbed readily all kinds of knowledge.

Medicine and Science under Islam. Eventually many of the sciences, and particularly that of medicine, became indebted to Islam. As people in the west tended to discard the teachings of Hippocrates and Galen and

---

[1]Lamb, Harold: The Flame of Islam. Reprinted by permission of Doubleday, Doran & Co., Garden City, New York, p. 11.

to revert to superstition, Moslems, Moors, Saracens, or Mohammedans, as they variously have been called, assumed responsibility for the advancement of science with eagerness. Their caliphs, who succeeded to leadership of Islam on the death of Mohammed in 632 A.D., began to find time and opportunity to encourage learning, including that associated with the practice of medicine. The works of Hippocrates and Galen were translated into Arabic.

To this Islamic interest in learning medicine owes a great deal. Physiology and hygiene were studied and an extensive materia medica developed. Although Moslem belief in the uncleanliness of the dead forbade dissection, surgeons practiced and learned to use hyoscyamus, cannabis indica, and opium as anesthetics. Great physicians were produced, the following Persians among them: *Rhazes* (860–932), who contributed material of lasting value on measles and smallpox, as well as an encyclopedia of medicine; *Hunayn,* an oculist who translated parts of Hippocrates and Galen; and *Avicenna* (980–1037), who wrote a "Canon of Medicine," in use for centuries after his death. In this medical treatise love has a place among the mental or cerebral diseases, where it finds company with insomnia, amnesia, mania, hydrophobia, and melancholia.

With advancing knowledge of medicine, great hospitals were built and those of Bagdad and Cordova became famous. We hear of women working in them, but instruction seems not to have gone beyond bed-making. In the following description is conveyed a sense of beauty and of psychological and spiritual values as well as of a wide scope of institutional development:

"It possessed four courts, each having a fountain in the center; lecture halls, wards for isolating certain diseases, and dispensaries for out-patients were also found. Among the most novel attractions was a hall where musicians played day and night and another where story-tellers were employed for the benefit of those who suffered from insomnia. Those religiously inclined could listen to the reading of the Koran, which went on day and night uninterruptedly in certain rooms. Each patient, upon being discharged from the hospital as cured, received some gold pieces that he might not be obliged to attempt hard labor at once."[2]

Status of Women under Islam.   Certainly, desert life could not offer much to woman outside her all too uncertain home. Commonly, education was denied her and her husband chosen for her. Marriage was her duty and fruitfulness her glory. If she proved faithless, she could be beaten. Polygamy to the limit of four wives was permissible, but no woman might have more than one husband at a time. Divorce was denied a wife, while her husband could procure it on slight grounds and with the privilege of taking her back as often as twice after such separation.

On the other hand, Mohammed improved woman's position in some

---

[2]Quoted in "Four Thousand Years of Pharmacy" by Charles H. LaWall, Philadelphia, J. B. Lippincott Co., 1927, p. 115.

respects. He forbade infanticide, and made parents include daughters in the privilege of inheritance. It is even said that a few rich women were permitted to learn to read the Koran. Nevertheless, woman's care during childbirth, and in case of gynecological disease, remained as it had been, traditionally, in the hands of untaught midwives.

MEDICINE AND NURSING, 500–1000 A.D.

The inundation of western Europe by barbarism in the latter part of the fifth century brought to a standstill any scientific advance in medicine. Primitive people brought primitive beliefs and habits with them. They destroyed books, they upset public hygiene, and they made wretched the life of the man who wished to devote himself to learning. If they could do so, studious men of all professions fled to Constantinople where scholarship still throve and conditions of life were little disturbed. If they could not, they sought the peace to be found in monasteries.

In the west, monasteries and feudal estates could not immediately expand to their ultimate organization as social units. Meantime, even the provision made by Romans for public hygiene through sewers, water systems, and public baths was ignored, and these utilities were destroyed or allowed to fall into disrepair. The teachings of Hippocrates and Galen were lost sight of, and talismans, incantations, amulets, charms, astrology, and primitive media from as many sources as there were races were restored to favor in treatment of disease.

In monasteries monks and nuns, confronted with the task of giving medical care to large numbers of sick people outside their cloisters, had to find some way to do it. Manuscripts which they secured were copied, used in teaching, and preserved. Books were compiled of recipes, plants useful as drugs, and commonly used home remedies. The foundations laid by Hippocrates and Galen were retrieved in part, but no further progress was made along scientific lines.

In the eastern division of the old Roman Empire, interest in science was little disturbed by happenings in the west. Jewish students continued to carry medicine to various parts of the known world. Translation of medical writings into Arabic enabled Moslems to return medical lore to Europe by way of Spain. Medicine's further advancement under either Moslem or Christian influence was hindered by restrictions placed on human dissection.

Little distinction was made between medicine and nursing. The novitiate served by both monk and nun anticipated the probationary or preclinical course of modern schools of nursing. Nuns studied the same works as monks, and in the monastic institutions treated or nursed women, while monks treated and nursed men. Both spurred themselves on by an ideal of hard work as Christian work and, like St. Jerome,

Paula, Fabiola, Marcella, and other famous ascetics who shunned no task however disagreeable, they expiated sin and experienced personal uplift in service to God through service to man.

Isolation of feudal manors and monastic groups, together with a general cessation of travel, kept these free for a time from recurrent outbreaks of pestilence. Skin diseases due to faulty diet became prevalent and were often confused with leprosy. As far back as the time of Jesus, the leper had aroused the sympathy of Christians. St. Basil had arranged for his segregation from other patients in the xenodochium. Lazarettos are mentioned in western church history during the sixth century and, as time went on, they increased with spread of the disease. Nevertheless, the pathetic figure of a human outcast, forced to warn men of his approach by means of horn or bell, was a familiar sight which touched the hearts of queens and knights who went out of their way to give him alms.

As a major portion of the population retreated into isolated protective units, the nurse deaconess of an earlier day was able to continue her work only here and there. Dangers of life when Roman protection was gone inevitably idealized the security of a nunnery. The medieval girl, who might have served as a deaconess, became a nun. The monastery brought into the nursing field the young man also. Nun and monk became, preeminently, the nurses of western society during the early Middle Ages. With the advent of feudalism, the lady of the castle, aided by nursing lore handed down by her mother, rendered corresponding service to the sick on her lord's estate. She nursed or supervised the nursing of the sick in her family and among tenants and serfs.

In the guilds general funds raised among members, provided nursing care for those who needed it and, in time, built and supported hospitals. The isolation of these and of the feudal groups necessarily threw upon each, responsibility for care of its sick. The burden of public charity and the nursing of the poor were gradually turned over to monasteries, although three famous hospitals are known to have been built outside of monastic walls. These were the Hôtel Dieu of Lyons in 542, the Hôtel Dieu of Paris in 650, and the Santo Spirito of Rome in 717 A.D. One bright spot in the general darkness surrounding medical practice was the birth of the first school of medicine at *Salerno* in Italy where men, and women too, were helping to inaugurate a return to truth.

Suggestions for Study

1. (a) Describe conditions at the beginning of the Dark Ages which made it necessary to seek the protection of an established institution. (b) To what cooperative units could appeal for help be made?

2. If you had entered a Benedictine monastery as a novice, to what types of activities would your attention have been drawn, and what would have been some of the ethical principles that you would have had to learn?

3. Compare the novice and the novitiate of medieval monasteries with the preclinical student and preclinical period of a school of nursing.

4. Compare the three stages of service following the novitiate with those following the preclinical period.

5. What was the attitude of St. Benedict toward care of the sick?

6. Discuss the women of monasticism from the following standpoints: (a) Social status; (b) Ability and position of abbesses, and (c) Manner of dress.

7. Explain the statement that the arts, education, religion, medicine and nursing were preserved in the monasteries through the disturbed conditions of the Middle Ages.

8. Show a possible relationship of the nurse's cap to the veil as a part of woman's dress.

9. If you had belonged to a peasant family on a medieval manor, to whom could you have looked for care during illness?

10. Show how continuous warfare carried on by feudal lords led to malnutrition and disease.

11. Compare the guilds of the Middle Ages with labor unions and with professional organizations of today.

12. How did the name of the degree of "Master of Arts" originate?

13. What circumstances led to the establishment of Islam as a rival religion to Christianity?

14. How did the conquest of great territory by Moslem invaders affect the prevailing practice of medicine and nursing?

15. Discuss medicine and nursing of the early Middle Ages.

16. Why is our system of nursing education considered to be related to the apprenticeship system?

17. Make your own adaptation of the first part of the chart on page 123 and add a dotted line for the general trend in medicine.

References

Davis, William Stearns: Life on a Mediaeval Barony. New York, Harper & Brothers, 1923.

Hartman, Gertrude: Mediaeval Days and Ways. New York, The Macmillan Co., 1937.

Hayes, Moon, and Wayland: World History. New York, The Macmillan Co., 1955.

Scott, Sir Walter: The Monastery. New York, Funk & Wagnalls Co., 1900.

Thompson and Johnson: Medieval Europe. New York, W. W. Norton & Co., Inc., 1937.

Wells, H. G.: Outline of History. Garden City, New York, Garden City Publishing Co., 1931.

Zahm, J. A.: From Berlin to Bagdad and Babylon. New York and London, D. Appleton & Co., 1922.

Chapter 6

LATE MIDDLE AGES
Society Becoming Mobile;
Detachment of Individuals

The opening of the eleventh century shows western Europe still holding the foreground of the world picture by virtue of difficulties besetting it after monasticism and feudalism had helped it to take its first steps toward a new and better social order. Less obvious than organized grouping had been the social process of race fusion by intermarriage which had been going on for five centuries. Barbarian women had proved to be an unexpected influence in furthering the cause of Christianity, for this religion appealed to them. As women adopted Christian ideals and a change came over their manners, many of them were able to induce men to become Christians also. Whole kingdoms often followed in the footsteps of a queen who had led her king away from pagan gods, but it was still too early to expect more than a partial change in barbarian outlook.

Meanwhile some of the enthusiasm of early pioneer days had vanished from the monasteries. Feudal lords had checked barbarian invasions, and now kept up a petty warfare among themselves as a matter of entertainment as well as a satisfaction for ambition. The whole land had been cut up into a picture puzzle of little kingdoms. Many people made laws, but there was no central power which could enforce them. The church remained the chief guiding influence.

PILGRIMAGES TO PALESTINE

Pilgrimages to places associated with persons or things assuming a sacred character from their association with beliefs had been a means of expressing zeal among adherents of all religions. Pilgrimages to Palestine, with its treasury of associations with the life of Jesus, began in the first century. St. Jerome, Paula, and others of the fourth century made this pilgrimage and prolonged their stay in order to improve conditions for other travelers in this foreign land, providing hospices as temporary dwelling places and giving care in hospitals to those overtaken by illness.

The beginning of the Late Middle Ages saw pilgrims in great numbers on their way to Palestine once more. Merchants of Italy already were reaping the economic advantages of a midposition on travel routes, and we find that country providing comforts at her ports and establishing an inspection of ships to prevent overcrowding. The pilgrim who had reached an Italian port, however, had probably met and overcome dangers to which other fellow travelers had succumbed. Highways throughout Europe were not only few in number, but they were in poor repair and infested with robbers. A journey on foot was a hazardous adventure. The few scattered hospitals in existence were insufficient to take care of the many overtaken by sickness or failing strength.

Education for Knighthood. An increasing stress on education for knighthood now becomes apparent, and ethical ideals modify more and more the military objectives of feudalism. Patiently a new conception of knighthood is developed, one in which ethical qualities combine with physical prowess in an ideal of glorious achievement which places the worth of general welfare beyond that of selfish ambition. Eventually the noble youth goes from stage to stage of growth. Ceremonies, ever increasing in brilliance, mark his progress until, at twenty-one, he attains the goal of knighthood.

The stimulus toward service to others which this new form of education brought to the knight turned his energies more and more to the adventure of making a pilgrimage to Palestine. More and more, too, did the everyday pilgrim have need of his protection for, with the advent of more settled conditions, the general public was beginning to follow man's roving instinct again. Reviving trade as well as religious enthusiasm encouraged it. Monasteries experienced a dwindling of population, for those least fitted to stand the dullness of their seclusion began to leave. The incidence of sickness and accident and the profits of robber bands both increased with the traffic on forest-bordered highways, for there were long, lonely stretches between settlements.

THE CRUSADES (1096–1271)

At the beginning of the eleventh century Arabia enjoyed the prestige of world power. South and east of the Mediterranean all lands belonged to Moslems, and Spain also had fallen into their possession. Since 637 A.D.

they had held the city of Jerusalem. The original Moslem empire, however, had weakened itself by splitting up into three sections, each under the rule of a different caliph. In turn it now found itself attacked by invaders from Turkestan – wild and savage people who seized the eastern division and, with it, the Holy City of Christendom, Jerusalem. Although they adopted Islam, the Seljuk Turks, as the new rulers were called, did not show the same tolerance to Christians as had other Moslems. The world was stirred to hatred and fear of the Turks, and when they appeared in the neighborhood of Constantinople, threatening it with destruction, the emperor of the old eastern division of the Roman Empire sent out to the west a call for help.

In the papal seat at Rome was a forceful, charming man whose education combined the ideals of chivalry with the stern solemnity of the monastery of Cluny where he had formerly been a monk. Urban II answered the appeal of the east by calling an assembly of several thousand people at Clermont, in France. This, in part, is what he said to them:

"From the borders of Jerusalem and the city of Constantinople ominous tidings have gone forth. Often, before now, have they come to my ears. An accursed race, emerging from the kingdom of the Persians, a barbarous people, estranged from God, has invaded the lands of the Christians in the east and has depopulated them by fire and steel and ravage. These invaders are Turks and Arabs.

"Come forward to the defense of Christ. O ye who have carried on feuds, come to the war against the infidels. O ye who have been thieves, become soldiers. Fight a just war. Labor for everlasting reward, ye who were hirelings, serving for a few solidi.

". . . and more – whosoever shall offer himself to go upon this journey and shall make his vow to go, shall wear the sign of the cross on his head or breast."[1]

Urban's remarkable oratory moved the audience so that even before he had finished, they arose shouting. "Dieu lo vult!" – "God wills it." The pope asked for volunteers and to every man of these he issued a red cross which, as a soldier of Christ, he was to wear on his head or breast. "Dieu lo vult" became a battle cry and, in 1096, the first of a long series of Crusades, or expeditions of cross-bearers, set out for the Holy Land, to rescue Jerusalem for Christians. Romance gave lustre to each venture, and a common aim united classes. Chivalry further enhanced the colorful march of medieval humanity. Troubadours sang songs. Lords and their knights rode the highways on splendid mounts, coats of mail jingled, and gay plumes floated from helmets glittering in company with shining shields and swords. More drab in attire, and often wearily, a motley throng of men, women, and children trudged on foot along the highway. Over all hovered sickness and death, but these were ignored for two

[1]Lamb, Harold: The Crusades: Iron Men and Saints. Garden City, New York, Doubleday, Doran & Co., 1930, pp. 39–41.

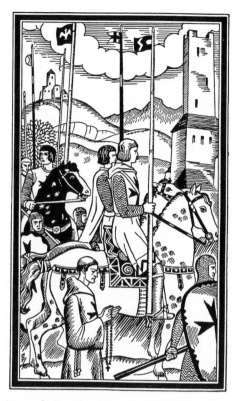

Figure 25. Crusaders. (From Reinach, Salomon: Orpheus—A History of Religions. New York, Liveright, Inc.)

reasons. Enthusiasm for the Christian religion had reached a peak, and men moved under the spell of a common spiritual impulse, their childlike hearts filled with childlike faith. At the same time, this unruly family of the church had endured for five hundred years the repression of its native instinct for motion, and it quickly discovered satisfaction in a general uncontrollable sweep toward the east.

ORDERS OF MILITARY NURSES

In an age when brigands infested forest-lined roads, and sanitary precautions were unknown or overlooked, wounds and sickness soon demanded attention. Crops failed as men abandoned the fields, or hungry Crusaders ruined them. The general nutrition was low, and multitudes were exposed to contact with diseases for which they had no acquired immunity. Hundreds of thousands died on their way to Jerusalem. More hospitals and nurses must be forthcoming. Existent xenodochia and monasteries were far apart and unable to fill the emergency in spite of heroic efforts to do so. Monasteries, too, declined in male population, for many monks sought the activity of crusading experience.

Christianity and feudalism together worked out a solution of the problem. The church promoted hospital construction, and cities and towns in time raised common funds to support city hospitals. Feudal knights assumed a large share of responsibility for relief of sickness and poverty in Europe as well as in Palestine, and nursing saw the introduction into its ranks of great numbers of men, for enormous institutions were founded and run by *military-monk* groups. Unavoidably, these brought into hospitals their military ideals. A change in hospital and nursing personnel first took place in two hospitals in Jerusalem, one for men, the other for women, that, as early as 1050, had been financed by private charity to meet the needs of pilgrims. They were named, respectively, the Hospital of St. John of Jerusalem and the Hospital of St. Mary Magdalene.

Secular in the beginning, these hospitals became part of a monastery in which monks and nuns subscribing to the rule of St. Augustine did social work and nursing. So kindly was the spirit of these workers, who made no distinction between friends and enemies when help was needed, that sympathizers all over the world enriched their institutions with many gifts. Early in the twelfth century, necessity urged the monks of St. John of Jerusalem to serve the interests of Crusaders in an unusual way. Mounted on horseback, they began to ride out from the monastery to assist in battle with the Moslems. When the emergency passed they returned to continue with their work of nursing. Because of this dual role of warrior and nurse, they became known as *Knights Hospitallers* or Military Nursing Orders.

During the two centuries of warfare that comprise the Crusades, numerous orders of knights hospitallers met varying needs of the times, as rescuers of sick and wounded along the highways, in first-aid stations, or in hospitals. The Order of *Knights Hospitallers of St. John of Jerusalem* remained the best known. A second famous order of hospitallers also had headquarters in Jerusalem, where a new hospital had risen about 1131 and had been named the "Hospital of St. Mary of the Teuton." The monks who were nurses in this hospital formed the Order of the *Teutonic Knights Hospitallers.* A third and equally famous order of nursing monks confined its activities to the care of lepers and derived its name, the Order of *Knights of St. Lazarus,* from the Lazarus mentioned in the New Testament as the object of Christ's sympathy.[2] Institutions known as "lazarettos" became fairly common. Many of their officers were lepers.

The soldier monk was for two centuries one of the outstanding figures in human society. His activities were by no means confined to Palestine, but orders originating there speedily spread east and west. Orders of Hospitaller Sisters also developed in connection with some groups. Money, land, even principalities, often came under their control through bequests of grateful pilgrims or other sympathizers and great fortress-

---

[2]Luke 16:19–31.

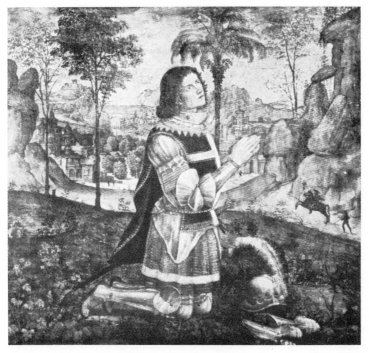

Figure 26. A Knight Hospitaller of St. John of Jerusalem. In armor with the tunic of the Order over his breastplate. Portrait in Chapel of St. John in Cathedral of Siena. (Painting by Alberto Aringhieri from Hume, Edgar Erskine: Medical Work of the Knights Hospitallers of Saint John of Jerusalem. The Johns Hopkins Press, Baltimore.)

like hospitals began to arise wherever one of their branches was organized.

The youth of all Christian countries yearned for opportunity to join in work that appealed to youth's admiration of a uniform, to its love of the adventurous, of the chivalrous, and of that ascetic sacrificing of self for the good of others which expressed the soul of religion in a time when religious spirit dominated men. Perhaps the earliest outward sign of military influence on hospitals and nursing was apparent in an ideal of uniformity in dress that had been gradually forming in monastic groups. Like all who joined the Crusaders, the various orders bore the cross of Christianity. However, to differentiate themselves, they began to present variations in the form and color of the cross. Their choice of robes and cloaks further helped this necessary differentiation. The variety of these, and of their accessories, exerted the same spirited charm as does the variety in military or nursing uniforms today.

MEDIEVAL SOCIAL PROBLEMS

The thirteenth century began with stirrings of change. The Crusades, which had been under way for a century, had brought a progres-

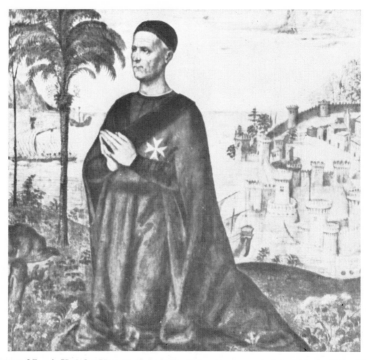

Figure 27. A Knight Hospitaller of St. John in convent dress. Portrait in Chapel of St. John in Cathedral of Siena. (Painting by Alberto Aringhieri from Hume, Edgar Erskine: Medical Work of the Knights Hospitallers of Saint John of Jerusalem. The Johns Hopkins Press, Baltimore.)

sive disintegration of those small protective units formed for protection against barbarism. With scattering of population and freeing of slaves, and often of serfs too, great numbers of bewildered men found themselves without protection. New conceptions of religious leadership and civil government were necessary as monastery and feudal fief declined, and greater power was centered about kings. A sudden acceleration in growth of towns with strongly commercial ideals, a youthful independence, and the moral recklessness of "boom" were significant of a change in needs.

For several centuries before the Crusades the inner life of many monasteries had been approaching a state of decay. Earlier days of hard work had been replaced by wealth gained through increasing land values and gifts. A great missionary task had been accomplished, and pioneering days were far behind. Monks abandoned manual toil for other pursuits, and abbots became politicians who enjoyed the privileges of great lords and vied with royalty in the pomp and luxury of their mode of life. Though scholarship managed to retain its place in some monasteries, an insufficient discrimination in selection of monks and nuns often replaced industry and austerity with idleness and levity. As among our modern hospitals and schools of nursing, there were groups who maintained high standards, and there were others who brought criticism on the whole social institution to which they owed their origin.

Public opinion turned gradually against an institution which seemed to be lending itself to private rather than public ends, and people began to criticize the church which it represented. Efforts to reform abuses tended toward stricter discipline and attempts at reversion to the ascetic life. Some headway was made, but the times called for other means than revival of austerities within the monastery. There was lacking still an influence in the everyday life of the masses that would help to straighten out a world that had changed since the sixth century — a society even more confused in its needs than that which was left to find itself after the Fall of Rome.

Another medieval problem of great magnitude was the control of leprosy. During centuries in which people of the west had been gathered into immobile, compact groups separated by considerable distances, disease had been under a natural control. When they were set into motion by the Crusades and subsequent trade activity, both acute and chronic infections increased. Over and over society was visited by epidemics which gained in severity and, among chronic diseases, leprosy or diseases mistaken for leprosy, became more and more widely diffused. The Knights of St. Lazarus were now taking it upon themselves to provide many more of their leper hospitals, but the failure to cope with what had become an immense social problem was still apparent.

A cruel policy of segregation of the leper had come to be popular. He was a social outcast, with none of the rights of other men. Officially, he was dead, and the church read a burial service for him. He had no home, no belongings, no family, no way to earn a living. Denied the simplest comforts of life, he must beg his way without intruding the sorry spectacle of himself even on those who might help. Whenever he approached a human being he must ring a bell, sound a horn, or cry the warning word of "Unclean." His plight met sympathy here and there, and individuals of the noble or royal groups had done much for his relief. As a problem of public health he continued to be a menace.

Two other social problems of acuteness hinging more or less on the problem of medical care were *infanticide* and the *orphaned or abandoned child.* The tragic number of adult deaths by war or disease left multitudes of children homeless. Moral laxity prevailed and was encouraged by long-continued war with its unfailing trail of illegitimate babies. Babies were often left on doorways or abandoned in alleys. Little children wandered about, homeless beggars. Parents lived in no fear of the law. Harsh times made orphans of thousands. The abandoned child of early and medieval times suffered cruelly. He could be picked up and sold for money and so was at the mercy of slave-traders.

RISE OF MENDICANT ORDERS

During the Late Middle Ages, a unique development of the monastic idea found expression in traveling religious missionary bodies pledged to literal poverty. As exponents of Christian ideals they did not live apart from the world of men, but trooped barefoot through it. They depended upon the uncertainties of begging for their food, and this custom earned for them the name of *Mendicant Orders*. The asceticism of the Mendicants was a sacrifice of personal desires and devotion of self to the good of others without retirement from the world. Church authorities sanctioned this innovation which strengthened the peoples' faith in Christianity by keeping before them the ideal of a Christlike life.

Changing conditions brought forth almost simultaneously, in Spain and in Italy, two young social leaders who opened the way to better things. Both brought religion directly to the people by living among them as mendicant monks, and one also stimulated a movement in the interests of public health as far as leprosy was concerned. They founded the Dominican and Franciscan Orders of the Church.

St. Dominic (1170–1221), of the noble family of Guzman whose castle stood in a village of Castile, gave up his plan of becoming a monk in a monastery. Famine in Spain and its resultant misery brought him the opportunity to serve the mass of poor men through closer contact. He set forth hoping to restore to the fold of the church those who had succumbed to anti-religious influences at work among them, and to convert others. Like-minded men, and women too, gathered around him and became known as *Dominicans*. These he sent abroad as traveling preachers, seeking to make Christianity the one religion through Christian teaching and example.

St. Francis of Assisi (1182–1226), on the other hand, belonged to that middle class just emerging from a society which had known only two classes, nobility and slaves or serfs. His father was one of the merchants who profited by the trade revival accompanying the Crusades. The family accumulated some fortune in the business of selling cloth, velvet, and embroideries, and the son, when old enough, helped to manage the shop in the market place of Assisi in central Italy. Legend tells us that while he was waiting on a customer, a beggar appeared, asking for alms. Etiquette required a salesman to stay with the firstcomer, and the poor man left impatiently. As soon as he could, the kind-hearted boy rushed off through the winding streets to find the beggar and make up lavishly for his sense of failure in being kind.

Like many another son of a father who works industriously to gather riches, St. Francis' sense of money value was not well developed and neither did he settle down to the humdrum of business. Youthful irresponsibility finally brought open trouble with his father who forbade him to use the family name ever again. Then it was that St. Francis left home to live in the woods as a solitary, vowed to the service of God.

The friendly boy, who loved flowers and trees as well as people, found it easy to be happy, singing with the birds, making friends of all the wild folk. St. Francis busied himself in repairing the local church, earning his meager necessities by doing any task that offered, and still found time to give devoted service to a small colony of lepers who lived nearby. Three years passed and the life of Jesus, literally followed, became for him the life ideal. He was fired with a determination to help all men share with him the good life and to bring peace to this unpeaceful age.

A merchant friend joined him, and then a church official. They decided to go forth among the people, and Francis unwittingly established an historic costume when he robed himself humbly in a rough, woolen peasant's tunic and tied a piece of rope around his waist. The others with equal humility bound themselves to utter poverty and the service of the poor. Because there were so many lepers, miserable and neglected, and because, too, the task of caring for them was so completely disagreeable, these men chose to identify themselves with the care of this group. Many lazarettos owed their establishment to the efforts of the *Brothers Minor* or Little Brothers, as Francis called members of the group which continued to gather about him. When they numbered twelve, all set out for Rome, where receipt of papal sanction gave the *Franciscan Order* a place in the church. Each of these men accepted his task of traveling from place to place, preaching along the way, and doing the work of a religious revivalist, nurse, or social worker as he went.

Uniform Dress. The Dominican robe was of white wool surmounted by a black cape made with a hood which could be pulled over the head when necessary for warmth. This cape caused the brothers to be known, popularly, as *Black Friars*. The habit of the Franciscan was the same loose, rough, wool peasant robe with rope girdle which St. Francis himself had once donned on impulse. Its shade might be brownish or grayish, and the wearers were called *Gray Friars*. Gray Friars began to spread ever farther through the land. Lepers were gathered up, surrounded by an encouraging sympathy and sometimes cured. Whereas segregation without care had failed to curb the progress of leprosy, the Franciscans were able to contribute greatly to a public health movement which has ended in almost universal control.

The Second Order of St. Francis. While young Spaniards, young Italians and other youths of medieval Europe were leaving home to join the Crusades, military orders, or brotherhoods, were they leaving behind all the equally ardent and attractive young women? Many types of women followed the trail toward Jerusalem, women everywhere became nurses in the ranks of the hospitallers, and women soon joined Dominicans as teachers and Franciscans as nurses, although they were not permitted to be beggars. One young friend of St. Francis came also from Assisi. Beautiful, a lady of the noble class, and only seventeen, *Clarissa* waited with girlish eagerness for news of the work with lepers. Watchful parents had arranged a marriage for her and did not encourage any interest that might develop into the wish to be a nurse, but their daughter saw St. Francis now and then and had already made up her mind to leave the world to work for God.

In the awesome darkness of night in medieval Assisi, Clarissa ran away from home and found her way to the little church that owed its restoration to her good friend's enthusiasm. Francis and his followers, by torchlight, were there lifting up their hearts in prayer. It must have been with some fear of the consequences that they welcomed Clarissa into their group, but St. Francis himself consecrated her at the altar and himself cut off her long, beautiful hair to encourage her in humility. She threw aside her jewels and the expensive dress worn by girls of her rank and wrapped herself, like the others, in a rope-bound robe of wool.

Then Clarissa was taken to the safety of a Benedictine convent in the neighborhood, where she remained under protection of the nuns until the Franciscans were able to establish her in an abbey of her own. It eventually stood by the small church where she had dedicated her life to a service of the poor that was to continue for forty difficult years. Huts adjoining this church were filled with lepers by the Brothers. Nursing care was provided by Clarissa and a group of Sisters who gathered about her. They received the name of *Poor Clares* or the second order of St. Francis. The begging of the Brothers Minor or Little Brothers supplied all with food. Youth had discovered what the times had need of and set about the business of providing it.

RISE OF SECULAR ORDERS

Third Order of St. Francis. While Mendicant Orders were being welcomed, other groups of men and women interested in a religious life without seclusion began to appear. From the end of the eleventh century they had been coming forward in different parts of Europe, and the term "secular orders" now describes religious organizations of laymen or laywomen who took no perpetual vows, and might work under the church or outside of its authority. Membership was composed of citizens who, frequently, did not leave either home or business to join any separate community. To a great extent they identified themselves with nursing in hospitals or in private homes and, in the latter aspect, their work reverted to that of the once loved but now almost forgotten deaconess.

In Italy the wave of religious interest among the laity became, on one occasion, a matter of embarrassment to St. Francis. In one of the towns through which he passed everybody insisted on becoming a Little Brother or Sister. Anxious as he was to win workers, he could not accept them at the cost of home life and with the consequence of childhood suffering. He therefore begged impulsive fathers and mothers to practice the principles of Christlike living as they went about their customary tasks, thereby improving home and community relations. Then he formed among them a secular order and named it the *Order of Tertiaries* because it represented the third group in his following.

St. Elizabeth of Hungary. Famous names are found among the Tertiaries of St. Francis. One of the first to ally herself with the order, as it spread beyond the confines of its native Italy, was *St. Elizabeth* (1207–1231), a daughter of the royal house of Hungary. Beautiful and high-minded, this young woman had been reared in the tradition of good deeds, and among her family were some who shared the current interest in lepers. Fortunately, marriage at the age of fifteen made her the wife of a true knight who did not fail her in sympathy when she wished to ease the burdens of poor people about them. He helped her to build hospitals in his native Germany, and she went into peasant homes to assist when babies came or to take food to the hungry.

The kindness of St. Elizabeth has inspired many legends. Time lends variation to these, and the following is only one of several versions of a popular tale. The unearthly beauty of soul radiating from Elizabeth was miraculously revealed to her husband. Pulling aside her cloak one day to see what she carried beneath it as she started out to visit his tenants, he beheld a basket of roses. Roses were out of season, and Elizabeth herself had filled the basket with food, and yet, there it was, overflowing with the

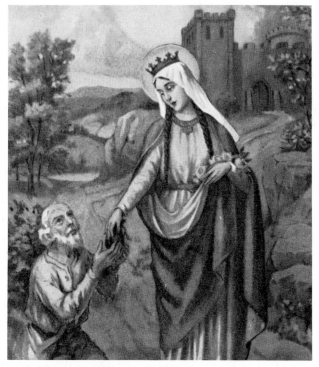

Figure 28. St. Elizabeth of Hungary and a beggar. ("Miniature Stories of the Saints," Book Two, by Rev. Daniel A. Lord, S. J. [Catholic publications].)

lóvely flowers which had blossomed to protect her from the possible pain of his displeasure. The chivalrous knight is said to have chosen one with reverence, that he might carry it through life as reminder of his wife's goodness.

Difficulties with relatives-in-law who criticized her charities as extravagance, an enforced separation from her children, the death of her beloved husband in a Crusade—all were personal trials which served to throw the interest of St. Elizabeth of Hungary more and more into nursing and social work. Twice every day it was her custom to visit, in hospitals or in their homes, patients suffering from any malady, for she feared none. She gave baths, did surgical dressings, fed the helpless and delighted, above all, in the care of children. The saddened young noblewoman earned for herself a place beside her friend, St. Francis of Assisi, and the early church deaconess as a forerunner of the visiting and public health nurses of modern times.

The work of St. Elizabeth of Hungary and many of her friends or contemporaries serves to illustrate a growing interest in charitable work on the part of laywomen. Indirectly, it speaks of the introduction of welcome occupation into the lives of many women of the thirteenth century. During more than a hundred years of wars that continued to destroy many millions of men by disease as well as by the sword, the possibility of woman staying with her traditional business of homekeeping grew more and more dim. The most eligible of their marital prospects were in monasteries if not in battle. Just as they have done in later days, women set out to find new work.

Beguines.   Coincident with the development of secular orders in central Europe was an even more marked development in Flanders (now Belgium and parts of France and the Netherlands) with establishment of a model community of independently organized laywomen of religious purpose. Within an enclosure just outside the city wall of Liége arose a church, and around it rows of little cottages began to pop up. Women called *Beguines* (bĕg′ēns), members of an order dating back to the seventh century, came to live in them and called the new establishment a "Beguinage." They kept house together, three or four to a cottage, and took simple vows of chastity and obedience. However, some Beguines preferred to remain with relatives in town, and residence in the Beguinage was not insisted upon. No one vowed poverty or gave up property, and all were free to marry, but no married member lived in community.

Busily Beguines of Liége, with the help of the bishop, set about finding jobs that would earn a common fund for upkeep of property, support of members, and charity. Sewing, lacemaking, the tending of children, teaching, and other tasks associated with woman's industry were undertaken. *Visiting nursing* in neighborhood homes was started, and families able to pay for this service did so. When a hospital was added to their responsibilities, the Beguines nursed the patients who quickly filled it and here, too, collected fees from those who could pay. Whole hearted devotion to public service by thousands of women in such centers brought its reward, and many gifts found their way into the treasury to provide for an ever widening scope of work.

The fame of the Beguines spread about and their cottage communities appeared elsewhere in Flanders as well as in other lands. By the end of the thirteenth century there were two hundred thousand of these lay workers whose settlements were spread throughout great and little towns so that the townspeople might be reached in days when transportation and communication, too, were so difficult that the nurse had to rely on being within easy walking distance. This made some Beguinages very small, and in large cities the number of them might run up to forty or fifty. *The scattering of, and not the concentration of, medical and nursing activities was the aim of the secular order of Beguines* which reached its height of usefulness in the fourteenth century.

Long ago the Belgian people learned to depend upon this secular order during national emergency, for Beguines on many occasions assumed obligations connected with distribution of food, clothing, and supplies, now included in the functions of Red Cross Societies. They have been ever ready to provide special nursing service when epidemic or disaster occasioned a need, and the two World Wars found them once more actively at work among soldiers. Their houses stand as memorials to a little group of high-minded, resourceful women who, in the later Middle Ages, opened an avenue to useful service for thousands of women.

GAINS AND LOSSES OF THE CRUSADERS

Three years after they left home, the first Crusaders were in possession of Jerusalem. The Cross, emblem of Christianity, supplanted the Crescent, emblem of Islam. Christians held their prize for nearly a century but in 1187 it was taken from them by *Saladin,* a cultured Moslem of Armenian birth who showed sufficient lenience to permit those who could afford to pay ransom and finance their journey to return to Europe. Several thousand of his prisoners were freed. Pilgrims were no longer excluded from the Holy City, and something was done toward improving conditions for those who continued to make the journey.

SOCIAL CHANGES ASSOCIATED WITH THE CRUSADES

Many changes were to be observed in western society after two hundred years of religious warfare. Some came through natural growth but others came directly as a result of the mingling of peoples and the contact of a young civilization with a mature one. Half barbaric Europeans of varied races learned a great deal as they drew together in a common cause. Inevitably, all were touched by refining influences that emanated from eastern empire culture, which had known no set back such as the western empire had suffered.

The magnificence of a great city like Constantinople amazed these sightseers when they passed through it, as did the commercial efficiency of cities like Venice, Genoa, and Pisa. Naturally, they assimilated ideas of art, government, and business. In far eastern countries they met people who knew many things that they did not know, and numbers of them lingered in Palestine to set up homes beside the Moslem and the Jew. Such crusaders learned a tolerance for religious and racial differences that was at variance with the ideas that brought them to Palestine. There was some intermarriage between east and west.

Buying and selling were inseparable from movement of peoples and gave stimulation to commerce. Travelers learned to use and like new articles. The demand for luxuries spread, and luxuries soon became necessities. Western Europe wanted salt and spices, silks, fine muslins, luxurious rugs, and rare fruits, just as men want automobiles and all kinds of electrical conveniences today.

Shopkeepers, like the father of St. Francis, became rich men conscious of the independence that riches gave them. As a group they were forming what soon became known as the "middle class." In towns and cities which grew rapidly as these men pushed the development of industries, the middle class gradually learned to use its voice in government as well as in business. The guilds, protecting former peasants or serfs whom the new industrialists employed as workmen, reached a high level of organization. The abbot of the monastery and the feudal lord both were being shorn of considerable power by an urban group which was learning to look to a king as its guide in civil affairs.

As early as 1215 the doctrine of individualism, or the determination of standards for any social group by the individuals who comprise it, was strong enough to set the will of the people against the will of *John, King of England,* and force his signing of the Magna Charta. In this document he acknowledged certain rights as belonging to all his subjects and, in so doing, abandoned any dream that he might have had of ruling as an absolute monarch.

National governments soon supplanted church and feudal government, and kings became responsible to the people. Individualism, nationalism, and democracy became a part of western social development as a result of changes during the Crusades. They affected all institutions. The east taught western merchants improved methods of finance, and great banking systems grew. Successful business stimulated the dreams of adventurous men who wished to follow to their source the things which Europe had learned to crave.

The western world, by the thirteenth century, had reached the beginning of a great era of discovery. In 1271 two brothers of a Venetian family named Polo who had already been to China set out again. One of them took along his son, Marco Polo, a boy of seventeen who entered with spirit into all the adventures of a long and dangerous trip which culminated in residence among the Chinese for seventeen years. It was while a prisoner of war, shortly after returning to his native Venice, that Marco told to a fellow prisoner the well-known tales of his travels. The story was put into book form and its firsthand information of exotic lands gave stimulus to the adventurous men of Europe. Two centuries later the book fell into the hands of Christopher Columbus.

CHIVALRY INFLUENCES THE POSITION OF WOMEN

In spite of the independence and position attained by a relatively small number of abbesses, and the executive position often forced upon the feudal lady, women in general throughout the Middle Ages were becoming more and more servile in their attitude toward men. The freedom of action that had come to the fore in ancient Rome slipped away. However, from the time that knights became busied with Crusades, a spiritual influence representing a blending of ethics, etiquette, and romance began to soften the crudity of the times. France called it *chivalry,* and *troubadours* helped it along by singing about it. To castle halls or gardens and the village greens, they brought music and lyrics of war and brave men, of spring and flowers, of beautiful, good, and gracious women who had the undying love of noble knights.

The woman of the Middle Ages, still a half-savage like her husband, began to realize as she listened to these songs that she might develop qualities to match those of the ideal in knighthood. Loveliness, the charm of courtesy, grace of motion, and beauty of dress became more important, and although for centuries after this she would still have to accept her lot in marriage without choice, the period of Crusades marks the beginning of something different for her. She learned the possibility of giving herself instead of being taken as a wife. She was led to a sense of romantic love with spiritual values which could give color and enchantment to marriage even if it remained for her an economic necessity.

Taken all in all, the woman of the Middle Ages had little chance for happiness. If she avoided marriage and was religious, she sought a convent. To whatever class of society she belonged, she found hard work her lot. Always, one baby followed another in a procession cut short, usually, by her own early death. For her care when they were born, she must accept the midwife in lieu of the physician. A husband's appreciation of his wife was based on the number of her sons. If she survived to bring them up, she was so ignorant of child hygiene and household sanitation that a brood of fifteen or more might diminish to two or three as she watched them die one after another.

GREAT PLAGUES OF THE FOURTEENTH CENTURY

After the Fall of Rome the isolation of those units into which men banded for mutual protection had given almost complete defense against infections from outside the group. As these slowly passed through a stage of disintegration, contagious diseases increased. Travel and war brought people into contact with diseases for which they had acquired no immunity. When, with industrial changes, families crowded together into towns, malnutrition increased the seriousness of a problem attendant upon urban growth as well as upon neglect of land and failure of crops. Epidemics became frequent, and on several occasions reached the pandemic stage.

If we stop to consider the elaborate machinery in use today for the control of communicable disease, it will not be difficult to understand how helpless the people of the Middle Ages were when it came upon them. The laboratory has now become the scientific core of a great system of diagnosis, prevention, and treatment. An army of public health workers guards the public of today, and departments of public health see that protective laws are enforced. Travel between countries is subject to restrictions of quarantine. Tremendous effort is made to spread information regarding prevention and cure. In spite of all this protection scientists know, even today, that their best efforts may be rendered ineffective by the fallibility of the human element.

The people of the Middle Ages had none of these protective forces, and few escaped communicable disease whenever it appeared in the community. It is little wonder, then, that terror seized any group among whom appeared a communicable malady of deadly virulence. Smallpox, bubonic plague, typhus, pulmonary tuberculosis, influenza, erysipelas, anthrax, trachoma, and leprosy were well known. The latter was often confused with scabies or psoriasis. Repeated outbreaks of mass hysteria and epidemic chorea led to the inclusion of epilepsy with communicable disease.

In 1348 appeared a terrible epidemic of bubonic plague which was popularly known as *Black Death* because of the dark hemorrhagic spots which appeared under the skin of its victims. The disease had already passed through Asia and Africa before reaching Europe and its fatalities are estimated to have totaled, in the end, one-fourth of the population of the earth. When the epidemic began in medieval Europe people either shut themselves up or fled before it. The malady was in such acute form that victims seldom survived three days. Most of them died without medical attention or nursing. They were buried in great pits or thrown into the river or the ocean which returned diseased bodies with each tide.

It is not surprising that in the fifteenth century the populace of Europe, descendants of those who had undergone for centuries hardships such as war, famine, and disease, should develop emotional disorders in

many forms, including a *dancing mania* which spread throughout town
and country. Everywhere, over the length and breadth of Europe, groups
of people began to dance. Faster and faster they danced until they
twitched and frothed at the mouth and, in the end, dropped from exhaustion. St. Vitus was chosen as the patron saint of these wandering
dancers, who left homes and kindred to follow one another. Their afflic-
tion has since been diagnosed as chorea, or St. Vitus' dance.

About the same time a virulent disease, now thought to have been influenza and known to its time as *sweating sickness,* began in England and
spread over the continent. Again great numbers died, and the care received by many hastened the end. Belief was current that the patient
must sweat continuously for twenty four hours in order to have any
chance of recovery. Windows and doors were carefully closed, the stove
was kept going, feather beds and furs were piled upon the patient and,
to ensure their remaining in place, sheets were sewed to the bed. Beside
him sat attendants ordered to keep him awake that he might retain his
senses, and these did their best, even to whipping him with a branch,
or dropping vinegar into his eyes. "Once for all, the patient must not have
his own way; what he would have you do for him, that must not be done."[3]

There were occasional physicians who disapproved of such treatment,
and some who sensed irregular living and overeating as incidents
affecting resistance. Some even advocated fresh air and fewer bedclothes.
The undue weight of most people of medieval times stood in the way of
their recovery from any of the acute diseases mentioned. Lacking dietetic
science, and consuming excessive amounts of many foods, they suffered
much from constipation, headaches, sourness of the stomach, and, undoubtedly in many cases, from an overworked heart.

SAINT CATHERINE OF SIENA; HOSPITAL NURSE AND VISITING NURSE

Two benefits may be traced to the miseries which tortured human
beings in the late Middle Ages. The modern practice of quarantine grew
out of experiments in restriction of travel which were made during the
progress of the Black Death. There was a material increase, too, in the
number of institutions for care of the sick and in the number of volunteers
who did nursing. One of the outstanding examples of the efficient volunteer nurse at this period was a young Italian girl who has come to be
known as *St. Catherine of Siena* (1347–1380). Siena is a town near
Florence, and Catherine was one year old when the Black Death first
appeared in Europe. Unlike many other volunteer nurses who so far had

---

[2]Quoted in "Epidemics of the Middle Ages" by J. F. C. Hecker. Trubner & Co., London,
1859, p. 249.

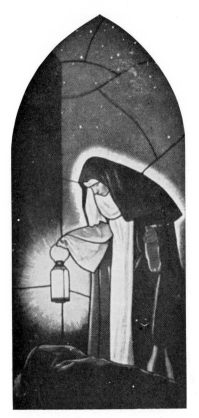

Figure 29. St. Catherine of Siena. A present day conception. (Courtesy of Will Ross, Inc.

gained fame in history, she was not of noble birth. Her parents were of the middle class and only moderately well-to-do.

Apparently little Catherine grew to be a capable, willing girl with a decided bent toward asceticism. She formed the custom of flogging herself thrice daily, in expiation of her own sins and of those committed by all persons living or dead. Tired out with the labor of the day, she laid her head at night on a pillow of stone. Her spare time she spent in making visits to the sick in the town's hospital. Here one of her first undertakings was bathing and dressing a leper. Like many another young nurse who has since begun a career with a task equally distasteful, Catherine discovered that even the most difficult of patients yielded to her patience and her earnest desire to be helpful.

Nursing brought great happiness to Catherine, but it was natural that parents should find it hard to understand a daughter who did not choose to be just like the other young girls about her. They tried to dissuade her, but with tact and sweetness she won her way with parents, too. Back and forth, morning and evening for several years, she walked between her home and the quite distant hospital, until her lamp at night came to have for the sick poor of Siena very much the same significance as would attach itself to a lamp in the hands of another nurse when

Florence Nightingale visited her soldier patients of the Crimea. Catherine of Siena made the hospital of La Scala a blessed place because of her presence there.

By the time she was twenty four this unusual girl had succeeded in obtaining sufficient education to be able to read. She had to wait four more years to learn to write, and then she was possessed of accomplishments confined almost wholly to the upper classes. She became, too, a tertiary of the Order of St. Dominic, and member of an organization of women within that Order whose objections to her youth had to be overcome before they would allow her to go around the streets on errands of mercy, nursing cases of minor ailment, and seeing that acute cases were taken to the hospital. The young woman whom they thus grudgingly admitted to their circle soon increased its efficiency by organizing a corresponding body of men to provide a needed ambulance service. As volunteer stretcher bearers, this group carried sick and wounded to the hospital whether they found them at home or by the wayside.

In 1372 the plague reached Siena and while it lasted St. Catherine no longer took time to go home but worked day and night in La Scala Hospital. Her few hours of rest were spent in a friend's house nearby. Even though many townspeople fled the city she was able to gather about her zealous helpers in response to her courageous example. With them she nursed the sick and, by selflessness, skill, and organizing ability, won a great name throughout Italy. In later years, as they looked about for a way in which to honor her, citizens of Siena rebuilt the hospital of La Scala which still stands as her memorial. The home in which she once lived is still tended carefully and her room, her lamp, and the stone pillow are there to remind the traveler of one of earth's gifted children whose talents were well used.

In divers ways young Catherine, the mystic, rendered service to her community as a citizen and she came to deplore the exhausting and unchristian prevalence of long continued feuds between families, which made street quarrels and wounded men a feature of everyday life in the Italian town. So many of these did she contrive to settle that reputation drew her into political affairs of national and international moment, and her ability won for her such influence with the Pope that she succeeded in ending a prolonged strife within the church itself.

MEDICINE DURING THE LATE MIDDLE AGES

As the Middle Ages progressed, a returning fluidity of population from the seclusion of monasteries and feudal estates increased the danger from infectious diseases, and epidemics raged. Towns grew, but sanitation remained in woeful state. The people were fear ridden and, even as they submitted to disgusting forms of dosage and the most heroic of wrong treatment, they died by millions. The western world seemed in danger of losing forever all that heritage of medical science which had been derived from Greece. That it did not do so was due to the guardianship of three groups who preserved Hellenic medicine until the strangely mixed peoples of Europe were culturally ready to use it. These groups were monks and nuns of Christian monasteries, progressive physicians of Constantinople, among whom were many Hebrews, and physicians who entered Spain with the Moslem invaders.

Monastic Medicine.   The western church, by copying and re-copying pieces of classical learning had taken the works of Galen and Hippocrates into its keeping. The manuscripts were in monastic libraries even if they could not always be interpreted as the physician would interpret them. There were always in the monasteries some men and women who became experts in healing. Monks found their way to the University of Paris, and even before this they were among students in Spain.

St. Hildegarde.   In the twelfth century there appeared among the Benedictines in Germany an abbess, *St. Hildegarde* (1098–1179), who has been accorded an honorable place in both medical and nursing history. Born into the nobility, Hildegarde was educated from the age of eight in a double monastery ruled by an abbot and situated near Bingen, a town on

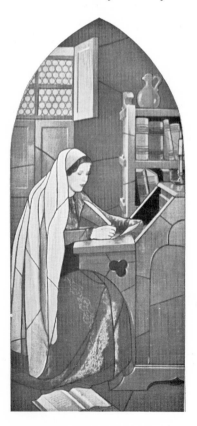

Figure 30. St. Hildegarde. A present day conception. (Courtesy of Will Ross, Inc.)

the Rhine. As a young woman, circumstances placed her in charge of the convent under the abbot's direction. She met the situation ably, and her superior intelligence was acknowledged by all about her during the eleven years in which she occupied the position.

By the end of that time Hildegarde wished to be free to arrange her own life and devote more time to study. Gathering about her a group of noblewomen, she established a new convent where she ruled as abbess for many years. Like other abbesses, Hildegarde was influential in Germany and was able to foretell certain of its political developments. A student of many forms of learning, Hildegarde devoted herself especially to medicine, nursing, and natural science.

So skillful did she become in the practice of medicine that she went far beyond the men of her time and produced works which anticipated later scientific discoveries. People from far and wide sought her advice, and her cures were famous. They were attributed by some to miraculous power, by others they have been explained as the result of keen observation of the sick under her supervision in the convent, and lifelong study. She was a strong believer in fresh air and the free use of water, wrote a number of books on medical subjects which described, among other things, jaundice, some worm diseases, lung diseases, and dysentery.

Byzantine Medicine. The eastern school of medical learning at Constantinople, which served as a second custodian of scientific medicine, preserved that carried to it in early days by Greek scholars, and later by scholars from Alexandria or Rome. Some of these Byzantine physicians remained permanently in Constantinople as teachers or copyists. Others carried what they learned to far-off lands. Some traveled to Arabia, some to Europe. Their services were sought by rulers and men of wealth and, wherever they came together with other scholars, they aroused interest in Greek medicine.

Moslem Medicine. The third custodian of medicine was Arabia. In Arabic form the works of Galen and Hippocrates were carried back to the west by Moslem invaders. Great cultural centers developed in the Spanish cities of Cordova and Toledo, where medical manuscripts were among the treasures of Arab libraries. Through students of the physician Avicenna, Galen became the medical authority of Spain, and Spain a Mecca for students of medicine from other parts of Europe. Spanish Jews proved efficient translators of Arabic manuscripts into Latin, and Europe steadily approached conditions of social development favorable for the revival of science in medieval medicine.

By the time the medieval period was half over, there had passed several hundred years of assimilation of barbarian neighbors by the Roman population. There was evidence, too, of the spread of new ideas as people gradually ceased to be shut off from one another in small social units. The influence of travel was toward new ways of thinking. Gradually, success came to the medical school in Salerno, Italy, and sick

Crusaders who were treated there as they passed through Italy advertised its methods. Those who had experienced the care of eastern physicians joined with these in demanding better medical care when they returned home.

Rise of Universities.   A revival of interest in all learning was already becoming apparent, and learned men, many of them friars of St. Dominic or St. Francis, were being surrounded by groups of eager students. The consolidation in units of numbers of such groups was an innovation to which medieval scholars gave the name "university" (all turned together). In 1110 the University of Paris was started; in 1158 Bologna, in Italy, had another; in 1167 England organized the University of Oxford, from which a group migrated to start Cambridge; and in 1181 came Montpelier in France. By the fifteenth century Italy had sixteen universities, one of which grew around the medical school at Salerno, and similar institutions were scattered all over Europe and beyond it in England, Ireland and Scotland. Medicine had become a branch of study widely pursued, and some of the great hospitals of the present day had been founded.

Barber Surgeons.   One serious drawback to scientific progress during the late Middle Ages existed in the objections to dissection held by both Moslem and Christian. Another was the inferior position accorded to surgery by Avicenna who advocated use of the cautery wherever possible, and supervison of lay helpers by the physician when cutting was unavoidable. About the same time the church forbade the wearing of beards by monks and, unwittingly, introduced a popular mode for men and a new vocation. By the thirteenth century barbers (FR. *barbitonsores,* or shavers of beards) are found organized as a Guild of Barber-Surgeons some of whom, in addition to barbering, did bleeding, cupping, leeching, tooth extractions, and treatment of surgical wounds. The physician held himself aloof from this group to which he relegated surgery, and although he gained for himself the protection of a license as well as the backing of universities, the surgeon remained unskilled and unrecognized for centuries.

In 1453 A.D. Constantinople fell before the Turks, and this time fleeing citizens of a falling Roman Empire turned back to the west. They took Greek learning with them and added their quota of medical knowledge to that of the monk and the nun, the Hebrew and the Arab. Christians, Jews, Moslems — to these followers of the world's great religions, modern scientific medicine owes contributions toward restoration of that Greek foundation on which its superstructure rests. Although the first signs of returning consciousness after what has been called the "Age of Coma in Medicine" were apparent as early as the twelfth century, its full recovery was not seen until the nineteenth. It took all of that time to unearth scientific methods of thought and to do away with slavish adherence to tradition.

GROWTH OF HOSPITALS

Uncontrolled communicable disease, fluid population, and a hasty development of urban life have been noted as outstanding factors in medical problems of the late Middle Ages. Solution seemed to focus on provision of increased facilities for segregation of lepers and an adequate supply of beds in institutions maintained, primarily, for care of the sick. Secular orders and private citizens made great public contributions as they supplied more and more lazarettos or hospitals and volunteered a nursing service to cover them. When people flocked townward in the wake of industry, the church, too, recognized the limitations of a system that left responsibility for medical care to isolated monasteries or crowded xenodochia.

In 1198 A.D. Pope Innocent III established in Rome what was intended to be a model institution designed for the sick and named the "Hospital of the Santo Spirito" (Holy Spirit). The secular Order of Santo Spirito was asked to take charge of administration and nursing. Church executives or influential citizens who visited the Papacy on official business were invited to study the building and the plan of operation and encouraged to organize similar institutions in towns from which they came.

The idea of city hospitals met with hearty cooperation, Germany adopting "Heilige Geist" as the equivalent in name, and France using

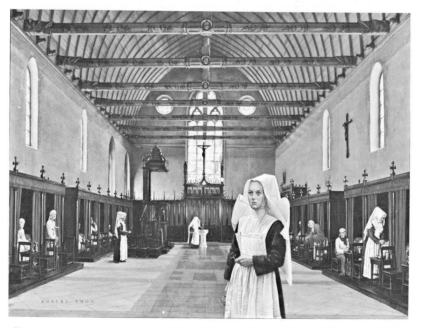

Figure 31. A Ward of the Hôtel-Dieu of Beaune, France, founded in 1443 and believed to be the World's oldest Hospital. A Chapel is at the end of the Room. (From "Great Moments in Medicine," produced by Parke-Davis and Co., Detroit, 1961.)

the designation"Hôtel Dieu" (House of God), which had been applied earlier to two great institutions, one in Paris, the other in Lyons. In England, among others, there appeared the beginnings of three famous hospitals, St. Bartholomew's, Bethlehem (for the mentally ill and better known as "Bedlam"), and St. Thomas, in which Florence Nightingale was to revolutionize nursing. English, and also continental, hospitals early tended to pass over to city control.

Meantime, some of those military orders which had originated in the emergency of pilgrimage and war made use of their accumulated wealth by furthering the development of hospitals. When seven hospitallers of the Order of St. John of Jerusalem escaped death in the final struggle to repossess the Holy City, they and their successors lived for a time on the island of Cyprus. Later they were transferred to the island of Rhodes and ruled there for two centuries. About the end of the late Middle Ages, they came into possession of the island of Malta. Here, in the seaport town of Valetta, in 1575, they built a famous hospital.

This hospital of the Order of St. John at Valetta accommodated somewhat less than a thousand patients. One ward was a hall, five hundred feet long, thirty four feet wide, and thirty feet high. Tapestry or wool hangings helped to take the chill from bare, cold walls in wintertime.

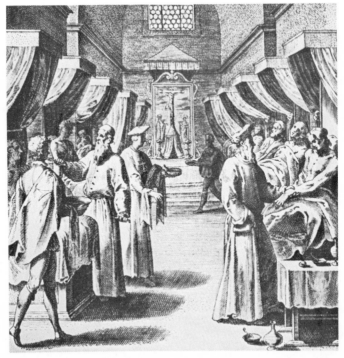

Figure 32. "Knights Hospitallers ministering to patients in the great ward of the Sacred Infirmary at Valetta, Malta, in the sixteenth century." Woodcut from Statutes of the Order, 1584.

Paintings enlivened them. To prevent drafts and ensure privacy, each bed was enclosed in a tentlike curtain. Wealth permitted luxuries, and the food service included bowls, plates, and covers of solid silver, as well as a few forks — implements just coming into use.

A well perfected organization provided for department heads in charge of silver, linen, wine, diet, phlebotomy, buying and accounts. Nursing, almsgiving, distribution of food to the poor, care of foundlings and of the insane were among institutional functions. Patients were segregated according to their status as pilgrims, as members of religious groups, or as belonging to the laity. Cases of slight indisposition were not placed with acute cases. A tailor's shop saw to the mending of clothing worn by indigents. A medical staff was assisted by a barber-surgeon who took charge of bleedings, the application of leeches, and blistering. Paid physicians instructed knights in anatomy and the care of the sick. Ten chaplains attended spiritual wants.

The architecture of this remarkable hospital repeated a tradition of the hospitallers in its fortress like characteristics. Windows, small and narrow, were sunk deep and high in thick stone walls. The patient, even when not imprisoned within a tent of curtains, saw nothing of the world outside. He was also deprived of fresh air. This forbidding type of structure long influenced institutional building in Europe. Fortunately, however, other forms of architectural development made themselves apparent, for men traveled abroad and saw the products of Moslem or Byzantine culture. Hospitals of the medieval period took on some of their architectural features.

New Gothic forms, such as were produced in magnificent cathedrals of the time, also appear in hospitals. Especially in the south, gardens or colonnades gave patients access to the outdoors. In Spain, Moslem influence showed in lavish external ornamentation, while interiors here and elsewhere introduced much beauty in tiling. Often the hospital was a great ward built like a church, with lofty supporting arches, perhaps a gallery, and with an altar at the end which made it possible for the sick to be present at celebration of mass. Beds were commonly placed end to end along the side walls so that nothing might interfere with their seeing the holy place at all times.

The social problem of the abandoned child was also met by these medieval hospitals. His welfare was among the considerations of those men and women who were eager to better social conditions. Additional separate foundling hospitals were the result, but the reception and care of foundlings was usually part of the program of all medieval hospitals. From the twelfth century the crèche (cradle) became a feature of charitable work in the medieval city, and a cradle was kept inside the portal of hospital or church in readiness for the mother who wished to consign her baby to the care of others. Sometimes the children remained until grown, the boys learning trades, the girls being taught household duties including spinning and weaving and, often, provided with a dower by the hospital when they married.

NURSING OF THE LATE MIDDLE AGES

Looking back over the late medieval period as a phase in the development of nursing we find interesting changes, each due to an accompanying change in society; for nursing care, like any other service to the public, must continually adapt itself to ever-changing social needs.

From the great need for nurses to care for the sick and wounded during the Crusades came those units of Knights Hospitallers who nursed the sick only during intervals when they were not busy fighting. Great numbers of men became nurses, and the military ideal of order and discipline became apparent. There were women, too, who organized as auxiliary units of these orders, like the Sisters of the Hospital of St. Mary Magdalene and the Sisters of St. Lazarus. When the Crusades ended, the monasteries of military orders extended over the land from Palestine to England, their men and women nurses carrying on under the influence of the leper movement and a novel war against disease. With the military order a harsher element entered nursing. The vow of unquestioning obedience had long been incident to monastic organization, but monastic organization was on the family basis with abbot or abbess as father or mother. Emphasis was now placed on rank and on deference to superior officers.

The many unsolved social problems of changing times, and especially the plight of those cast out as lepers, were causing criticism of conditions as they were and an awareness of need for developing among the people the simple faith and kindly service of the early followers of Jesus. This need was met by the Franciscan Mendicant Order founded by St. Francis of Assisi.

Gradual disintegration of the protective units of the monastery and the feudal estate brought further changes. The new social need arising from redistribution of population and urban growth now brought nursing out of the institution and back into the home, where the deaconess first found need of it. This situation was met by the Beguines of Belgium, the Tertiaries of St. Francis, and other secular orders which included private duty nursing and visiting nursing with hospital activities.

In the late twelfth and early thirteenth centuries, as the city hospital under civilian direction came on the scene, a tendency to develop civilian nursing groups in hospitals accompanied the innovation. At the same time medicine was becoming differentiated from surgery and nursing. The newly organized medical schools were turning out men who had devoted much time to study. Learning brought distinction to this group, while it gave them a new viewpoint on their work and new methods. Procedures which had once occupied them were now given over to assistants, and became special functions of barber-surgeon or nurse.

All medieval monastic nursing was necessarily simple. It featured shelter, regular hours, simple food, pure drinking water, herbal medicine (mysterious often, but harmless), the washing of sores, the dressing of wounds and a few simple nursing procedures. To these were added the mental solace of kindliness, music, and religion. Equipment, like procedures, had been accepted by tradition. Beds were large ones of wood, pillows or rings were covered with leather in lieu of rubber, and feathers, moss, or horsehair provided their filling. Long-handled warming-pans heated with hot coals or hot water anticipated the hot water bottle. Catheters and enema bulbs had been in use even among ancient people. There were no thermometers, and nurses trusted mainly to their hands in determining temperature, although the bare foot was used as an extra precaution in testing water for the newborn baby's bath.

Sweet-smelling herbs, perfumes, odors arising from burning of fragrant woods, and such things as orange peel were favorite deodorizers which availed little in face of bad ventilation and a prevailing aversion to fresh air. The omnipresent fireplace made the hot shovel and hot coals readily available for carrying these about. Little oil lamps, still seen among relics of antiquity, were in use at night. Even the simplest procedures in bedside nursing were difficult and time consuming for lack of conveniences which we take for granted. Among institutions for care of the sick then, as now, there were always some that were very good and some that were very bad.

There were not always enough nurses, and there was a change in their caliber as the later medieval monastery opened its doors to men and women who were the unfortunate product of a phase of low social morality and low standards of home life and education. With passing centuries the sickbed came to hold more than one patient and, at last, even as many as six. Medieval sensitiveness to bed crowding was not keen, for this was a home custom. The difficulties that it added to changing of linen for the sick are obvious. Patients were sometimes not only dirty but ill-fed. Indifference met those who dared to point out dangers in this crowding and poor nursing. The civilian hospital sometimes introduced women of low character to augment inadequate nursing staffs, thereby completing the range of medieval nurses from high-bred, intellectual men and women to the most inferior.

Nursing had begun a decline which was to persist for a long, long time. Contemporary medicine, however, was in the ascendancy as capable physicians from medical schools were added to that scattered group of doctors, usually Jews or Saracens and sometimes learned men from the school at Alexandria, who had been handing medicine down from one to the other throughout the Middle Ages. A revival of Greek science was beginning, and as universities arose everywhere to quicken medical interest in it, medicine and nursing separated.

Nevertheless, the tradition of early Christianity, which made nursing the vocation of the finest type of individual, persisted through the Middle Ages and did not die with them. Early monastic leaders in nursing had been men and women of intellect, their lives significant of culture, refinement, and democracy. Individual queens like St. Rade-gunde and princesses like St. Elizabeth, ladies or knights, idealists of the middle class like St. Francis and St. Catherine of Siena, all con-tributed to establish a conception of the care of the sick as one of the finest expressions of interest in the common good. Henry II, king of England, established a lazaretto for women in Rouen, France, on condi-tion that noblewomen only should nurse the patients. As late as 1492 Queen Isabella of Spain whose jewels went to finance the discovery of America appeared in person on the field as she directed her own ambu-lance and nursing service. These names have been remembered, but there were many, many others who worked with those who bore them to make strong and resistant the roots of a vocation that would not be publicly recognized for nearly four centuries.

Uniformity in Dress.   There is observable during the progress of the Middle Ages a decided tendency toward uniformity in the dress of nurses. No uniform had been worn by the deaconess and none distinguished the early nuns. The lady of the court or the castle who became a nurse con-tinued to wear her fashionable clothes. Wool or linen was her common choice of material, but silk and velvet were not considered out of place, and the abbess dressed in accord with her feudal rank. The uniforms adopted by the military nursing orders encouraged uniformity in other nursing groups.

As early as the ninth century, a distinctive dress had been recom-mended for monastics and during the Crusades it became quite common. As they were then developed, monastic uniforms or habits savored, natu-rally, of period fashions. These were both gay and luxurious. Were the foundation of the habit black or brown, it followed that color would be used to offset dullness. Scarlet, bright blue, white, or purple was worn by men as well as by women. Robes took on the long, flowing lines favored in the east, and cloaks were freely bordered with ermine. In fact, the availability of all types of fur, combined with the chill of thick-walled stone buildings heated only in spots, encouraged its use not only as trim-ming but as full lining.

Headdresses varied from the plain pointed hood or cowl of cloth, or the Roman veil assumed by the married woman on her bridal day to much more elaborate designs. The wimple, or folded piece of linen drawn up under the chin and tied on the head under a cap, veil, or hat, was common to civil society and monastery. As groups grew in number, details of uniform increased and changed with the effort to distinguish them from one another. The cross of Christianity, worn in common by all religious orders, took many forms.

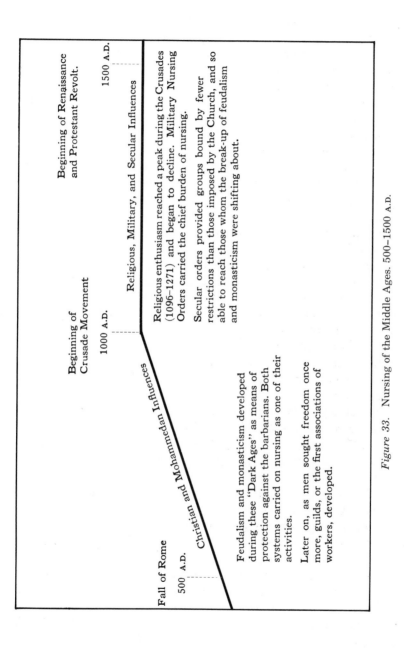

Figure 33. Nursing of the Middle Ages. 500–1500 A.D.

Suggestions for Study

1. While a large part of the population of western Europe was shut up in monasteries and feudal estates, what changes were going on outside which became evident after several centuries?
2. (a) What is the purpose of a pilgrimage, and why were so many undertaken during the late Middle Ages? (b) Do you know of any other type of pilgrimage than that of Christians to Jerusalem?
3. What were the objectives of the series of wars known as the "Crusades"?
4. What organization, corresponding to our army nurse corps, provided nursing care to sick and wounded soldiers of the Crusades?
5. (a) How did the military nursing orders differ from the usual orders of knights and monks? (b) What new influences did they bring into nursing?
6. Name a number of social problems confronting people of the Middle Ages?
7. What criticisms led people to welcome development of mendicant orders?
8. (a) How did the mendicant orders founded by St. Dominic and St. Francis differ from other established orders of the church? (b) What three orders were ultimately founded by St. Francis? (c) Are any of these active today?
9. What influence did the military nursing orders and mendicant orders have on the dress worn by nurses?
10. What third type of nursing order, representing a wide departure from the usual restrictions of the Church, was founded during the latter part of the Middle Ages?
11. What famous nurse of this period became a member of the secular order of Tertiaries of St. Francis, and why might she be considered one of the first visiting nurses?
12. (a) What other secular order became famous, and what type of nursing service was rendered by it? (b) In what way did it provide for reaching as many people as possible?
13. (a) Were the Crusades a success or a failure in regard to regaining Jerusalem from the Moslems? (b) What social changes resulted from the vast movement of population in an easterly direction?
14. Give reasons for the fact that the late Middle Ages are considered to be the period of beginning of romantic love.
15. Quote the lines about a knight and a drawbridge from "The Vision of Sir Launfal," by James Russell Lowell.
16. Account for the great epidemics that swept over Europe during the fourteenth century.
17. (a) Tell what you know of St. Catherine as hospital nurse and

visiting nurse in her home town of Siena. (*b*) To what mendicant order did she belong?

18. By what three groups was Greek medicine preserved during the difficulties of the Middle Ages?

19. What contributions to the practice of medicine and nursing were made by St. Hildegarde?

20. Discuss the advantages and disadvantages of being a patient in the Hospital of St. John at Valetta.

21. (*a*) What circumstances led to the development of city hospitals? (*b*) What provision was made for nursing care in them?

22. (*a*) Tell what you know of nursing of the late Middle Ages. (*b*) Give reasons for the fact that nursing entered a long period of decline.

23. Why was contemporary medicine in the ascendancy?

24. Give an account of the origin of uniform costumes for those engaged in nursing.

25. (*a*) Through reference reading in the encyclopedia and elsewhere show under what circumstances the word, "Saint," is authorized to be used before the name of an historical character. (*b*) How many nursing saints can you name, and with what special type of work is each associated?

26. (*a*) What illustrations can you find that show the general tendency of architecture of the time, including that of hospitals? (*b*) Compare the emphasis on beauty with that on provision for carrying out principles of hygiene.

27. (*a*) Can any form of society be expected to remain stationary? (*b*) Discuss the necessity for ability to make good adjustment to changing conditions.

28. Complete your own adaptation of the chart on page 123, adding a dotted line for the general trend in medicine.

References

Austin, Anne L.: History of Nursing Source Book. New York, G. P. Putnam's Sons, 1957, Chap. 3.

Briffault, Robert: The Days of Ignorance. New York, Chas. Scribner's Sons, 1935.

Chesterton, G. K.: St. Francis of Assisi. New York, Geo. H. Doran Co., 1924.

Farrow, John: Damien the Leper. New York, Sheed & Ward, 1927.

Frank, Sister Charles Marie: The Historical Development of Nursing. Philadelphia, W. B. Saunders Co., 1959.

Haggard, Howard W.: The Doctor in History. New Haven, Yale University Press, 1934.

Hume, Edgar Erskine: Medical Work of the Knights Hospitallers of Saint John of Jerusalem. Baltimore, The Johns Hopkins Press, 1940.

Hutton, Edward: St. Francis of Assisi. New York, Longmans, Green and Co., 1950.

Lamb, Harold: The Crusades: Iron Men and Saints. Garden City, New York, Doubleday, Doran & Co., 1930.

Lamb, Harold: The Flame of Islam. Garden City, New York, Doubleday, Doran & Co., 1931.

Major, Charles: When Knighthood Was in Flower. New York, Grosset & Dunlap, 1907.

Nutting and Dock: A History of Nursing. New York and London, G. P. Putnam's Sons, 1907, Vol. I, Part II, Chaps. 3–9.

Peattie, Donald: A Cup of Sky (St. Francis of Assisi). Boston, Houghton Mifflin Co., 1950.

Rayner, Edwin: Famous Cathedrals and Their Stories. New York, Grosset & Dunlap, 1935.

Riesman, David: The Story of Medicine in the Middle Ages. New York, Paul B. Hoeber, Inc., 1935.

Schimberg, Albert P.: The Larks of Umbria (St. Francis). Milwaukee, Wisconsin, Bruce Publishing Co., 1942.

Stewart and Austin: A History of Nursing. New York, G. P. Putnam's Sons, 1962.

Part Three

THE MODERN ERA OF
SCIENTIFIC AND SOCIAL
EVOLUTION

Beginning Circa 1500 A.D.

Chapter 7

RENAISSANCE, REFORMATION, AND A DECLINE IN NURSING

When the year 1500 dawned on the western world, men were thinking of many new things. The spirit of revolutionary change filled the air as it had five and also ten hundred years before, and as it does today. The world had suddenly become very much enlarged by land and sea trade with the Orient and the discovery of America. Old ways of doing things would not work under new conditions. The individual was just making it known that he had had enough of cooperative living. A secular spirit, arising in commercial towns, had invaded the church. People were ready to discard old ideas and were seeking some new form of the old religion that had been a mainstay in darker times. Kings by this time ruled supreme, each little nation speaking a different language and developing different customs from the neighbors round about.

THE RENAISSANCE

By 1577 *Sir Francis Drake* had found his way around the world, his ship only one among many that had been bringing home to Europe and Britain tales of wealth beyond the seas in India, China, the East Indies and, above all, in America. Ambitious businessmen and nations saw profit in permanent trade with this new land and power in its colonization. The compass and ships of better build had already improved transportation, and expedition after expedition was equipped and sent on its way. Gunpowder changed fighting methods and increased kingly power by weakening feudal lords. Castles could now be blown up, and the use of guns required new skills. Gunpowder affected surgery and nursing also, for it brought new types of wounds and new difficulties from infection.

129

The recent invention of the printing art was putting books into the hands of many people and spreading ideas with strange rapidity. An astounding machine made it possible to turn out quickly great numbers of books, each one of which would have occupied a skilled copyist for at least half a year. The Bible, which even in its Latin form had been read up to now chiefly by monks or other scholars, became before long the object of intensive study by the general public. The art of printing also gave to students of literature access to the works of their predecessors.

THE CLASSIC REVIVAL

A classical revival began in Italy where wealth derived from an advantageous trading position during the Crusades had brought a leisure that came more slowly to other countries. Caesar, Cicero, Virgil, Aristotle, and Homer became part of European and British curricula. People copied the ancients, becoming more and more worldly under their pagan influence. The emphasis placed by medieval forbears on the virtues of self-sacrifice and self-denial was cast aside. Men questioned everything, "debunked" existing ideals, exacted accuracy, and even doubted the church. The new state of mind reflected itself in the general attitude toward charitable works and, in particular, on medicine and nursing.

In the realm of literature the Renaissance stimulated men, and women too, to classical scholarship. Leading trends of thought during these times were expressed by famous writers. *Erasmus* (1469–1536), the wandering scholar of Holland, encouraged education while he derided medieval ideals and superstitions. The Englishman, *Sir Thomas More* (1478–1553), dared to frame a "Utopia" just as men of our day dream and write of the abundant life for all; *Martin Luther* (1483–1546), in Germany, translated the Bible into his own language and led a revolt against contemporary Christianity which ended in a division of the church into Protestant and Catholic sections; *Cervantes* (1547–1616), a Spaniard, made fun of feudalism and chivalry in "Don Quixote"; *William Shakespeare* (1564–1616) drew upon life rather than upon the classics for his philosophy; and *John Milton* (1608–1674) gave to the world his "Paradise Lost," and in other works argued for political and religious freedom and a free press for utterance of public opinion. These are a very few of the names which stand out in a period of brilliant intellectual activity and reorganization of human values.

In the field of art a corresponding awakening was taking place among painters, architects, and sculptors. Its wealth and natural beauty made an artistic center of the city of Florence, one day to be the birthplace of Florence Nightingale, whose fame as a restorer of the nursing art would equal that of the painters, sculptors, and architects gathered there. A school for artists developed, and two students in the school of Florentine art stand out as geniuses. *Michelangelo* (1475–1564) and

Leonardo da Vinci (1453-1519) were architects, sculptors, engineers, and painters. Both took part in supervising the building of the greatest of churches, St. Peter's at Rome. For four years Michelangelo painted frescoes in the Sistine Chapel of the adjoining Vatican, palace of the Popes. As these were on the ceiling, he was forced to work hours at a time, lying on his back on a high scaffold.

Leonardo da Vinci painted "The Last Supper" on a wall of the refectory in a monastery at Milan and he, with like intensity, worked from dawn to dark forgetting to eat. In this masterpiece Jesus is shown seated with his twelve disciples at a long table. Marvelous variations in expression on the faces reflect the individual reaction to the words that have just been heard: "One of you will betray me." Da Vinci's "Mona Lisa," a portrait of a lady of lifelike beauty and an enigmatical smile, hangs in the Louvre at Paris.

Botticelli (1447-1515) made delightful representations of Greek gods and goddesses. One of the best known among these is "Spring" in which appear Venus, Cupid, and the Three Graces. *Raphael* (1483-1520), another student of Florence and among the "moderns" of the sixteenth century, is best known for his Madonnas, most famous of which is the "Sistine Madonna." The great *Titian* (1477-1576) led a group of students in Venice. The Venetian school was noted for its mastery of color, as the school at Florence was noted for form and grace of line.

A school arising somewhat later in Flanders produced *Rubens* (1577-1640) and *Van Dyck* (1599-1641). Spaniards were led by *Velásquez* (1599-1660), and the Dutch by *Rembrandt* (1606-1669). The English did not evolve their own school of painting until the time of *Sir Joshua Reynolds* (1723-1792) who painted the well-known "St. Cecilia," and *Sir Thomas Gainsborough* (1727-1788) who painted the "Blue Boy" and the "Duchess of Devonshire."

"Blue Boy" and "Duchess of Devonshire," however, were significant of other changes going on in society. The former pictured the son of an ironmonger, the latter a member of the aristocracy. The times permitted a class of newly rich to dress its children in blue satin, with rich lace and plumed hats. These children lived in homes where fine portraits were no longer out of place. Their fathers and mothers had leisure to acquire appreciation of the arts and to enjoy the privileges which wealth once had given only to the class which the duchess represents.

POLITICAL REVOLUTION

During the medieval period the great family of the mother church had grown up to a considerable extent. Strong men now ruled kingdoms which they felt they should be allowed to manage without parental interference and by right of divine power in themselves. Under kings a system of private ownership and private enterprise was taking shape. An era was beginning in which desire for wealth and the grasping of opportunity would hold chief place in men's minds. Kings of nations were now testing out autocracy, the popularity of which England (already nearer to democracy than other countries) was able to disprove through Parliament and the ancient Magna Charta.

In France the once all-powerful feudal lords soon found that they could get nowhere without royal favor. It became the fashion among them to take up residence near the royal person so that no opportunity for gaining this favor might be lost. As courtiers they were flattering accessories, but often financially dependent. *Louis XIV* (1643–1715) used them and their ladies to build up around him such a royal court as overshadowed the colorful one of Queen Elizabeth of England. He made himself the center of a great machine representing power. Around him were thousands of richly dressed, often very attractive and clever, men and women, all basking in a glory created from the labor of the French common people.

The marvel of Versailles, with its glittering gold, its crystal and mirrors, its paintings and tapestries, was conjured into being. Its gorgeous drawing rooms were used for many gay and frivolous pastimes. A precedent of regal magnificence had been established that all the royal courts of Europe tried to emulate. Idleness reigned. By the time *Louis XVI* became king of France the country was nearly bankrupt. His vain queen, *Marie Antoinette,* loved Versailles, and gaiety, and luxury, and indulged herself to the limit. All her extravagances, great or small, every bit of foolishness or display only made more bitter the hatred of those men and women who were getting ready to do away with it all.

The ambitions of kings led to war, and a spirit of national competition was fostered in the people. Germany, Spain, England, and France kept Europe in uproar. One great struggle followed another until the Seven Years' War (also known as the French and Indian War), beginning in 1754, made England the leading power. In that struggle France lost Canada, which thereafter was an English colony. The poverty which followed the wars brought a discontent that flamed up in a series of great revolutions: the American Revolution (1775–1783), the French Revolution (1789–1795), the Latin-American Revolution (1800–1825). While the disturbance was not yet over, there arose from the angry masses a dictator who undertook to unify Europeans and manage their affairs for them. The Napoleonic wars began in 1797 and ended in 1815 when the Duke of Wellington, at the battle of Waterloo, buried dictatorship for a time. At the beginning of the nineteenth century, England and democracy were in the lead.

INDUSTRIAL REVOLUTION

War and revolution affected the political aspect of two continents. Individuals of the time, as well as generations following them, were called upon to make many and difficult adjustments. These adjustments, however, were minor in comparison with those which accompanied a revolution of a different kind which began in England about 1750 and upset long accustomed modes of life by changing modes of work. For this reason, it has been named the "Industrial Revolution," and with ever-increasing momentum it still goes on. A revolution in transportation and communication has followed in its wake.

All countries of the world now experienced the stress of constant change, but England was first to be affected. The raising of sheep and the manufacture of cloth from their wool had long been a chief industry of her people. Spinning and weaving were done in farmhouses by slow hand processes. Machines were now invented that speeded up production and reduced the number of people needed to make cloth. Factories were built where the machines could be placed. If the farmhouse family wished to earn a living it must move to the town where the factory stood. Its members would have to adjust to new ways of working as well as to the confinement of life within the narrow limits of tenement flats and city streets. Guild principles of fairness would no longer control the price asked for cloth, and wages would be kept at a minimum so that the owner of the factory might have a maximum profit.

The skill that it might have taken a lifetime to acquire in order to turn out an especially fine article no longer had the same value. The machine could standardize quality. Before long the independent master of apprentices bound to him to learn his craft in his little shop, and the farmer who held a strip of cultivable land, were forced to give up craft and land and become laborers for rich men. These changes heralded corresponding ones in other industries. The efficiency idea took hold of agriculture and business. An era of inventions began, the number of manufacturing cities grew.

THE REFORMATION

The Reformation or Protestant Revolt, beginning in 1517, helped to precipitate the disaster toward which the vocation of nursing was headed. The church had tried to overcome a waning enthusiasm for religion but there were those who insisted on finding their own way to a truthful expression of a simple Christian belief, and they had been gathering energy to assert themselves. Two outstanding groups of reformers, by this time, were at work — those who stayed with the church and those who were throwing in their lot with revolutionist *Martin Luther,* once a German mendicant monk, now leader of a separatist group called "Protestants" (those who protested). Whole countries began to emerge as distinctively conservative or protestant in their bent. Where there had been only one church, there were henceforth two, differentiated by the names, Protestant and Catholic.

In areas where the popular majority held to old beliefs, there were reformers who continued their efforts to cure abuses by slower methods than those of upheaval. Representative of this group was one *Ignatius Loyola,* a Spanish soldier who, in 1534, inspired the organization of an order of teaching clergy who would help to solve the problem through the channel of education. The missionaries of his Society of Jesus, commonly known as *Jesuits,* were militant preachers upholding orthodoxy, but they were also among the earliest of trained teachers and equipped with an unusual thoroughness of method. Wherever they went they won respect for scholarship and took a leading place as educators, especially in institutions of the higher grades. In this time of stress the Catholic Church welcomed their support which was augmented, shortly after, by the foundation of the *Order of St. Ursula* (patron saint of maidens), a woman's order dedicated to the education of girls. Many convent schools were founded by the Ursulines in Europe.

In 1545 a general council of church authorities was called at Trentino, in Italy, for the purpose of discussing ways and means of removing causes for criticism and clarifying the church position. This meeting lasted eighteen years, and so much was accomplished during that time that this *Council of Trent* has since been looked upon as one of the most famous and decisive of ecclesiastical gatherings. Doctrinal issues were re-stated, financial relationships discussed and the position of the Catholic group thoroughly identified.

The two religious bodies, however, failed utterly to reach a middle ground of tolerance. Also, each country's ruler tried to make all of his people think and worship as he did. The result was an era of cruel hatreds, with a tremendous development of sects as an outlet for budding individuality. Civil conflicts were induced and the climax was reached in an international conflict known as the "Thirty Years' War" (1618–1648). Political, economic, and religious issues were fought out, and a state of comparative religious tolerance was reached. To ensure themselves true freedom in religion, people had begun to leave the Old World for the New.

TRANSFER OF EUROPEAN CULTURE TO AMERICA

Not long before America was discovered, the spirit of adventure pervaded Europe and led men to India, China, and Japan. The most far-reaching result of these foreign contacts was the awakening of Europe to the advantages of commerce and increased power through wealth coming from the outside. Real expansion began when a new continent was discovered unexpectedly. By that time Spain, Portugal, and England stood ready and eager to grasp the hand of opportunity. France finished one of her wars and followed them.

A New Spain, a New France, and a New England grew up on the other side of the Atlantic, and Portugal appropriated what is now Brazil. The northern continent, before three centuries had passed, was divided among European nations in almost transverse sections. The southern section belonged to Spain, the middle one to France, and lands in the far north, Newfoundland and a strip of Atlantic coast were English. What is now California was far across great deserts, rivers, and high mountains and one of the most remote spots on earth.

If Spanish or French, the pioneer in America was of the Catholic faith and, usually, a man who loved adventure. If he was a friar or priest, he was zealous for Christianization of the Indian. The English colonist was a Protestant and determined to set up a permanent home for himself and family in a land where he had come to seek religious freedom. Each national group brought national customs with it and hoped to transfer European culture to America. Old ideas and new ones, superstition and wisdom, monasticism and Puritanism — all established themselves in new soil. The spirit of the sixteenth century Renaissance, however, came too.

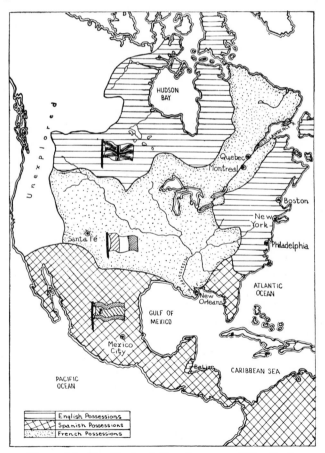

Figure 34. New England, New France, and New Spain.

Of all the nations speculating in colonization Spain appears to have been, easily, the luckiest in her beginnings. In Mexico and Panama she found a land already possessing a high degree of civilization as well as mines of fabulous wealth and stores of mined gold. She could begin shipping fortunes to the homeland at once, and she did. Many of her noble adventurers found personal fortunes and set up homes in a land which offered freedom for initiative. They established a university, a medical school and a magnificent hospital in Mexico City. They introduced Spanish art, dressed with the richness of famed grandees, and made life gay for everyone with music and dancing, ribbons, gilt, and bright colors. Gay-plumed cavaliers made love to beautiful señoritas.

French neighbors of triumphant New Spain brought gaiety with them, too, but did not find so ready an opportunity for wealth, power, or ease. Both climate and North American Indians were less friendly, and the extraction of wealth was more difficult. Some of the new settlers ruled tracts of land as lords of miniature feudal manors, or "seignories" as they were called. Only a few French women dared to leave their beloved France and build up a social life in such austere surroundings. Like the Spaniards, however, Frenchmen were not at all averse to assimilation with the people about them. French-Indian populations soon matched the Spanish-Indian combination that was the first of many mixtures to enter the American melting pot.

The influence of the Englishman was different and lasted longer in the life of America. His religion was simple and often harsh in its expression. Sabbath observance was strict, and he advocated the virtue of work with all his might. He brought his wife with him from England, and his ideal was a good home—a better one, if possible, than he had left in the "old country." His was a substantial type of character that wore well and fitted him to meet the heavy odds against him. Northern Indians were fiercer; northern climate was harsher; and the rocky New England soil produced food grudgingly and held no gold.

The Protestant Church led the intellectual life of New England as the Catholic Church led that of New Spain and New France, and any citizen on occasion took on additional functions of farmer, lawyer, physician, or political adviser. The life of the American pioneer, to whatever nation he owed allegiance, remained under the influence of Europe. Separation did not free him from the burden of her political troubles or cut the currents of her thought. The ships which made their way so slowly and with so much danger across a great ocean did what the radio does today—they supplied a means of transmitting both good and evil. Wars fought at home by colonizing nations had to be fought in America, too. At the same time a great era of manufacturing development, beginning in England and manifesting itself on the continent, was causing a rapid evolution in modes of living. America, whose trade was partially responsible for this, felt, inevitably, the influence of changing trends in her own industrial organization as well as in the lives of her people.

MEDICINE OF THE RENAISSANCE

As in the fields of art and literature, so in the field of medicine came a rebirth of the science of a classical past, with new viewpoints, new methods, and outstanding men to exploit them. Throughout the Middle Ages, scientific thinking had given way before the unscientific, and Galen had eventually shared the earlier fate of Hippocrates. Superstition and quackery superseded both, and both had been almost forgotten. Knowledge of the anatomy of the human body was very meager, and surgery had come to be looked down upon. For several centuries, however, there had been evidence of returning scientific interest in the study of Aristotle, master of all learning. In some monasteries, as in the universities, many a patient plodder made ready for a new day. *The sixteenth century Renaissance included medicine.*

Numerous names now became prominent where no name had equaled that of Hippocrates for two thousand years. Old theories were disproved. The new era announced itself though *Paracelsus* (1493–1541), a Swiss educated in Italy, who threw to the winds all time-worn medical tradition, did his own thinking, and urged others to do the same. His progressive spirit reinvigorated the practice of internal medicine. He introduced new drugs, among which was mercury as a cure for syphilis; he improved treatment and shared with those of his time the deductions which he was able to draw from a wide experience.

The work of bringing the fundamental science of anatomy into medicine fell to *Andreas Vesalius* (1514–1564), a German who studied in Paris, and whose belief in the need for dissection led him to do it in secret and in defiance of the law. Vesalius' part in progress was that of proving that Galen's theory was based on animal, rather than on human anatomy. His own book, "De Fabrica Humanis Corporis" is the foundation of present-day anatomy. One of Vesalius' favorite pupils was *Gabriele Fallopio* (1523–1562) who went further than his master, describing among other of the minute organs the ovaries and the Fallopian tubes.

The life of *Ambroise Paré* (1510–1590), a French radical, was bound up with the advancement of surgery to a position of greater dignity. In youth he was apprenticed to a barber, and later was accepted into the Guild of Barber-Surgeons. It was he who brought back to use the ligature for bleeding vessels due to gunshot wounds, which his contemporaries treated with boiling oil. He stood also for less interference with nature than was customary, and the inscription on a monument which France erected to his memory explains this attitude in his own words: "Je le pansay, Dieu le guarit" (I dressed him, God cured him).

About this time the raising of social and professional distinctions between barbers and surgeons manifested itself in England and on the continent. Requirements were being set for preparation to practice. The physician was a man with university accomplishments, while the surgeon was a skilled craftsman. More and more restrictions were placed on the work of the barber, although complete separation of his function from that of the surgeon did not take place for some time.

In the seventeenth century *William Harvey* (1578–1657), an Englishman, gave impetus to the study of physiology when he discovered the system of blood circulation with the heart acting as a central pump. His only reward from many of his time was ridicule and receipt of the appellation, the "Circulator." *Athanasius Kircher* (1602–1680), a Jesuit monk, used a microscope and connected microorganisms with contagion. *Anton van Leeuwenhoek* (1632–1723) made improvement of the microscope his contribution and wrote many scientific treatises of value to medicine on microscopic life and plant histology.

While science was securing its foothold in a field where quacks flourished, her adherents tended to become argumentative and scholastic and to lose sight of the welfare of the patient in speculation about the source of life and health. In reaction to this tendency an Englishman, *Thomas Sydenham* (1624–1689), stressed the ancient Hippocratic practice of observing symptoms with great minuteness and recording them accurately and was able to revive the clinical point of view. He also influenced the trend of medicine by his detailed description of prevalent disease, by advocating fresh air in place of the stuffiness of sick rooms, and by simplifying prescriptions and abandoning disgusting ingredients generally relied upon.

Treatment of the insane up to the latter part of the eighteenth century was notable chiefly for its inhumanity. In England, at that time, a Quaker by the name of *William Tuke* introduced more understanding methods in a retreat or sanitarium which he himself established. In France *Philippe Pinel* followed a Belgian example by abandoning the use of restraining chains and also instituted other humane reforms.

In 1798 *Edward Jenner,* an Englishman, discovered a satisfactory method of vaccination against smallpox, thus making it possible to avoid one of the many epidemics which had long harassed mankind. Innovations like these serve to illustrate a trend in medical thought indicating eagerness on the part of enlightened men to discard old ideas for new ones. Scientific machinery remained incomplete, however, and superstition still ruled the practice of the average physician as it did also the beliefs of the public. While here and there men hit on cures which withstood the tests of later science, others were giving out theories which did not withstand them. Meanwhile, both doctor and layman retained faith in the power of individuals to work on one another for good or evil, and in two instances, at least, the seventeenth century saw this faith gain emphasis.

Great importance was now given to the ceremony of the King's Touch, which offered the victim of scrofula a promise of cure if a royal ruler laid his hand upon him. For this reason scrofula was known as the "King's Evil." The modern dictionary defines it as "tuberculosis of the lymphatic glands, and sometimes of bones and joint surfaces, with slowly suppurating abscesses and fistulous passages, the inflamed structures being subject to a cheesy degeneration." The superstition growing up around it degenerated into the use of touchpieces of medals touched by the king's hand and worn around the neck of the scrofulous person.

In opposition to the beneficence of the King's Touch stood out the harmful influence of the evil spirit, and imagination endowed it with the form of an old woman and name of "witch." People of the seventeenth century placed ever more responsibility upon this worker of evil when disease appeared. Their helplessness expressed itself, at last, in a form of mania which discovered such evil spirits in neighbors, especially any who showed peculiarities in personality, and their destruction was demanded. Thousands of innocent victims of public apprehension, often mildly insane, were put to death in one way or another. The favorite method was that of hanging and the mania spread to America where it ended in the scandal which gave fame to Salem, Massachusetts.

MEDICINE IN AMERICA

Far off in America, dangerous and isolated country that it then was, the health of explorers or immigrants had had no guidance. Dominican or Franciscan friars or Jesuit priests accompanied Spanish expeditions and, usually, were possessed of some medical skill. Nuns as well as clergy went with the French and supplied the luxury of nursing care. Most ships carried one of the inferior type of surgeons who might be fortunate in possessing the medical equipment gained by an apprenticeship. The English colonist companies appointed company physicians, but the professional medical practitioner seldom stayed in the colonies more than a year, for it was unusual if he possessed the pioneering enthusiasm required to endure their hardships.

The result was that colonial medicine, especially in New England, found itself in the hands of any man who possessed education, once the capable mother of a household felt a case beyond her skill. Clergy, schoolteachers, and political leaders alike shared responsibility as sources of advice. Some of them had studied a little medicine, others depended on the few books of home medicine then available, and all mixed their intelligence with prevailing European or Indian superstition and much prayer.

"Of medicine the Puritans knew little and practiced less. They swallowed doses of weird and repelling concoctions, wore charms and amulets, found comfort and relief in internal and external remedies that could have had no possible influence upon the cause of the trouble, and when all else failed they fell back upon the mercy and will of God. Surgery was a matter of tooth-pulling and bone-setting, and though postmortems were performed, we have no knowledge of the skill of the practitioner. The healing art, as well as nursing and midwifery, was frequently in the hands of women. . . . There were a number of regularly trained doctors—though not a physician had more than a smattering of medicine."[1]

Disease lurked always in the white man's neighborhood. His earliest houses were ramshackle shelters lacking in sanitary protection and with poor water supply. Yellow fever proved a deadly enemy. Measles, scarlet fever, smallpox, and diphtheria were often epidemic, and typhoid was especially prone to appear whenever the snow melted. Indians in contact with white communities succumbed readily to their diseases. The Pilgrim and the Puritan continually mourned the dead, in whose memory they erected the thousands of headstones that still seem to be lined up inescapably before all New England. The names and ages inscribed thereon offer a perpetual reminder of the inadequacy of care received by mothers and their children in the early days of a country that was to attain international prestige in the practice of medicine.

As time passed, living conditions improved. Fine homes often came to replace poorly ventilated, badly drained shelters, as men grew prosperous. It is these homes of the second growth that we are accustomed to associate with the colonial period. Still the colonies had few doctors, and profiteering quacks sometimes had to be punished.

Medical Apprentices. Opportunities for medical education were limited to personal instruction by individual physicians. Sometimes a doctor handed down what he knew to a son; sometimes he accepted an apprentice. This apprentice might or might not be equipped with the bachelor's degree. The doctor permitted him to read his medical books, discussed points in medical practice with him, had him visit patients, and between times kept him busy with chores such as cleaning the office or grooming and feeding the horse. Just as in industry, the medical apprentice worked up slowly through a period of almost wholly practical training, usually lasting five or six years. Then, if he could afford it, the new doctor undertook a long, expensive trip to Britain or Europe where he studied in medical schools and observed procedures in hospitals. If this was beyond his means, he went immediately into practice and shared it often with men who had no training at all.

The apprenticeship method had advantages, for the aspirant to medical practice came into close contact with patients who represented the master's private clientele and usually dwelt far apart. The apprentice had to take much personal responsibility for their care and improvement of their condition. Social distractions were few, and the intimacy of private conference with the master illuminated texts and cases. As an educational system apprenticeship depended too much on the proper combination of instructor and apprentice and offered no standard of

---

[1]Andrews, Charles M.: The Fathers of New England. The Chronicles of America. Copyright, Yale University Press, New Haven, Vol. VI, p. 82.

practice or theory to the latter. It did not protect the public from inefficiency. In Europe, where the physician could study at a university, and
the surgeon learned a manual craft by apprenticeship, it was this very
difference that privileged one to belong to a group which did not acknowledge the other. In America this distinction automatically disappeared under conditions requiring both functions to be filled by the same
man.

Development of Medical Schools. The Revolutionary War and its
aftermath exposed the inadequacy of medical protection and stimulated
provision for it. Departments in medicine, however, did not find a place in
colleges and universities until after Harvard, the first American university, was over a hundred years old. Then they were organized in rapid
succession at the College of Philadelphia in 1765 (later a part of the
University of Pennsylvania), at Harvard in 1783, at Dartmouth in 1798,
and at Yale in 1810. The Middle West followed with its own schools,
and there were commercial medical schools that sprang up as if by magic.
Four hundred schools of medicine were founded before 1860, and many
of them were responsible for inflicting very poorly educated doctors on
the public. Little was done to regulate them, and there were short courses
and easy ways of attaining the status of physician. Instruction was very
frequently of poor quality, libraries were inadequate, there were no
laboratories and little or no opportunity for dissection. Often the school
had no connection with a university or even with a hospital.

Doctors in the early colonies must have been lonely men, deprived
almost wholly of contact with those who were interested in medical work
and progress. To remedy this condition nineteenth century America saw
a great development of medical societies organized on college, city,
county, or state basis. The earliest were formed for discussion of common
problems and some reports of meetings were developed. A group consciousness was being built up and a group pride sustained that made
possible elimination of abuses in the medical practice and improvement
of educational opportunities in America.

American Medical Association. By 1846 the time was ripe for concerted action, and a congress of physicians was held in New York City.
Certain improvements in medical schools were advocated, and in 1847
the *American Medical Association came into being for the avowed purpose
of advancing medicine and rendering service to humanity.* Among its
committees was one called the "Committee on Medical Education," which
worked toward the elevation of medical standards. Medicine in the
United States now had the strength of organization to back needed
reforms and to push plans for educational advancement along medical
lines.

Advances in Medicine. Individual effort toward improvement of
medical procedure was not lacking. *Oliver Wendell Holmes,* Professor
of Anatomy at Harvard University, was also a general practitioner of

medicine who, from observation of maternity cases, arrived at an opinion that anticipated modern obstetrical asepsis. In 1843 he published it for his associates under the self-explanatory title, "On the Contagiousness of Puerperal Fever." Applause was not immediate; in fact, professional approval was withheld and the idea ridiculed. Over in Europe *Ignaz Semmelweis,* physician of Vienna, had managed in 1867, through practice of cleanliness, to reduce the death rate in a maternity ward from 10 per cent to a little over 1 per cent. He, too, published a paper under the title, "The Etiology, Nature, and Prophylaxis of Puerperal Fever," which European contemporaries likewise refused to accept. Not only did they make fun of their progressive colleague, but so persecuted him that he suffered a mental breakdown. In 1846 *Dr. Crawford Long* and *Dr. W. T. G. Morton* introduced the use of ether as a general anesthetic. A year later *Sir James Simpson* made chloroform serve a like purpose in England.

American affairs, meanwhile, in spite of wars had moved swiftly on. Great projects of engineering and agricultural development were put through. Frontiers moved continuously in a westerly direction until, in 1849, the discovery of gold in California placed them on the shores of the Pacific. Vacancies in the field of labor, which pioneers of the west left behind them, were filled by immigrants. Millions of people changed their abode in a comparatively brief space of time. Always medicine went with them, and always it passed through pioneer stages of development as they did. Always it was a little further ahead when the pioneering began until, eventually, it caught up with Europe. Men who acquired wealth in America found pleasure in endowing universities after the manner of European princes.

ERA OF SANITATION

Up to 1837, when Queen Victoria ascended the throne of England, government had not made health one of its responsibilities. Disease prevention was a rare dream. No one had grasped the principles of hygiene and sanitation. Epidemics continued as of old, and a few quarantine regulations which had grown out of the Crusades were the accepted and wholly inadequate medium of control. Boards of health were unknown in spite of the fact that population now centered in cities. Garbage was thrown into the streets where pigs did their best to remove it. There were no city sewers, and city water supplies were drawn from dirty rivers or exposed wells.

Individually, the rich, the learned, the poor, and the ignorant were alike in their dirty habits. Personal cleanliness was a difficult thing to attain, and people got along happily without it. Private bathing facilities were far from adequate. The open fireplace furnished limited supplies of hot water. Cold water often had to be carried from a considerable distance. The public bath was not accessible as in old Roman days. Clothing was heavy, hard to wash, and worn for long periods. No dry cleaning was used on feminine apparel which was often handed down from one generation to another. Straw provided beds for all who could not afford the monstrous wooden structures in use among the well-to-do. Fleas, rats, mice, and lice traveled with all classes of society.

The time was very ripe for men interested in public welfare to begin to apply some of the laboratory achievement of the scientists who had been at work for what seems now to have been a long period. To *Sir Edwin Chadwick* (1800–1890), an English *lawyer,* is credited the initiation of a great sanitary era about 1830. A commission began to study the health of towns and cities, and the government assumed the role of promoter of national health. Emphasis was placed on disposal of sewage and garbage and water purification. Many germs were disposed of with proper disposal of decaying matter, and health conditions began to improve. Men and some women in various parts of the world came forward then to help make legislation possible, to demonstrate statistical methods, to improve the quality of medical service, to study epidemics, and to hunt out the sources of disease.

Among the new sanitarians was *Sir Sidney Herbert* who, as Secretary for War when war broke out in the Crimea in 1854, was able to rely on his friend *Miss Florence Nightingale* for an understanding interest in military hygiene, and intelligent cooperation in developing it as far as the scientific resources of her time, and military conservativeness, would permit. In America *Lemuel Shattuck* (1793–1859), a socially minded *layman* with an interest in statistics, was laying the foundation for a corresponding movement which led eventually to founding of the United States Public Health Service.

WOMEN OF THE RENAISSANCE

The Renaissance was a period when Europeans had time to think. Great wars and little wars were over for a time. Roman imperialism and feudalism had been lived through, and a young and energetic society had grown up sufficiently to take its place as a group of nations. Men now wanted to be free, to live their own lives, to be individuals and to be happy. An enlarging world increased their opportunities and satisfied those adventurous longings which had subconsciously actuated much of their fighting.

The passive role which women had had forced upon them began to change as the privilege of learning was extended to them. They began to expect from men the gentle manners and devotion which decadent chivalry had introduced and shown desirable. There were prominent figures, like Elizabeth of England and Mary of Scotland, whose position or beauty made it possible to exact these from courtiers and set standards for all men to follow in their approach to women. Chivalry was not allowed to die. There was much writing of poetry, romantic drama, and songs dedicated to the charms of women who were both beautiful and good.

There were now three social groups, upper class or aristocrats, middle class or bourgeois, and lower or industrial class. By the time of Florence Nightingale (1820–1910), women of the upper classes had become part of an aristocracy which disapproved of manual labor. They played with languages, knew some music, and often dabbled in painting. A wave of romanticism, finding its expression in sentimental literature, surrounded their girlhood with an intriguing rosy glow which was subdued by the formality that set women apart for worship. There were some women who longed to use their intelligence more actively, and these unconventional ones found ways to do so.

The new educational opportunities of the period beginning with the Renaissance were confined to women of the nobility and well-to-do families of the middle class. Teaching was done at home, at first by tutors and later by governesses. Sometimes learned fathers, like Mr. Nightingale, undertook to give additional instruction to their daughters. Among the Italians an occasional woman won public recognition as orator, preacher, doctor, or the lawyer typified by Shakespeare's *Portia* in the "Merchant of Venice." In other parts of Europe women remained in greater seclusion.

Formal education for women did not advance to any great extent for a long time. Always, a few ventured into intellectual fields because they had the independent urge to do so. Among them were some who dared to pioneer the rights of their sisters. On the whole, however, although the feminine status showed a tendency upward, and woman had received some recognition as a being of intellectual capacity, she as yet had no legal equality with men. Women were minors in the eyes of the law. They could not own property, and all business of a legal nature must be done through their husbands. Man's ideal woman had the loveliness and dependence of Juliet rather than the wisdom and fearlessness of Portia.

In America, by the time the pioneering movement turned westward, the children of early settlers had grown up to a greater hardihood and self-reliance. The pioneer wife worked side by side with her husband, doing whatever came to her capable hands to be done. Less hampered by the traditions of older societies, she found it easier to adapt herself to the wilds and, as far as her individual conservatism permitted, she slipped away from conventionality and class distinction.

RISE OF FEMINISM

As early as the beginning of the seventeenth century there began to be heard from women, and from men here and there, brave statements in regard to the equality of women with men, and even broaching their right to an education. Little by little the voices became louder and the chorus of greater volume—great enough to drown out the voices of those who opposed it. While men took their places on either side, a group of courageous, persistent women, now famous for championship of their sex, earned for themselves the name of "feminists."

Feminists eventually stood for things which it took time and struggle to procure, including legal and academic privileges for women, a reform of marriage that would put it on a basis of preference rather than arrangement, and the right to vote and to hold office. As time went on, the Revolutionary War in America and the French Revolution made people conscious of the rights by which men could share more equably the good things of life; it was natural to begin to think and talk more forcibly about the rights of women.

The era following the close of the Napoleonic wars in 1815 was one of comparative peace in which social unrest, economic and intellectual feverishness, sudden release of inventive genius, and the great improvements made in communication and transportation were all reflected in the lives of women. In a steady stream they emerged from the seclusion forced upon them by dangers of the Middle Ages and subsequent religious conflicts. Many among the infants, born about this time, were to spend their lives in unusual activities. Some became world figures who will always be remembered because they made the world a better place in which to live.

The extension of suffrage was one of the moot questions of the time. Women rallied to advance their right to this privilege when they found that social reforms which they desired required voting power to achieve them. Some sponsored with equal vim a temperance movement. Prominent in the two groups were *Elizabeth Cady Stanton* (1815–1902), *Susan B. Anthony* (1820–1906) and *Frances E. Willard* (1839–1898).

Some women set about the improvement of educational opportunity. Numerous schools were founded and books written. *Emma C. Willard* (1787–1870) started a seminary for girls, while she found time also to write poems which include the popular "Rocked in the Cradle of the Deep." *Catherine Beecher* (1800–1878), sister of the famous preacher, Henry Ward Beecher, also established a seminary and wrote under constructive titles such as "True Remedy for the Wrongs of Women" and "Letters to the People on Health and Happiness."

Philanthropy touched even more closely the lives of still another group of women. *Elizabeth Fry* (1780–1845) undertook the reform of prisons, a loathsome task. *Harriet Beecher Stowe,* sister of Catherine Beecher, wrote "Uncle Tom's Cabin" in the interests of Negro emancipation. *Julia Ward Howe* (1819–1910), whose husband shared her friendship with Florence Nightingale, became a preacher and lecturer interested in prison reform and world peace and was author of "The Battle Hymn of the Republic."

Three girls in the brilliant circle found their sphere among the sick and wounded. *Dorothea Lynde Dix* (1802–1887) devoted her life to the welfare of those afflicted with mental illness. *Florence Nightingale* (1820–1910) uncovered the disgrace of poor care of the sick in hospitals and developed a means of assuring good nursing through systematic education of selected young women as nurses. *Clara Barton* (1821–1912), who saw hospital service during the Civil War in America, directed her work and influence afterward toward organization of the American Red Cross Society. Into the midst of these ardent reformers, chiefly middle class women, came another woman, *Victoria,* queen of an Empire, friend of international good will and human betterment, exponent of temperate living. By the social standards which she set for them, she sustained their efforts in the "Victorian Age."

WOMEN OF THE INDUSTRIAL REVOLUTION

The women outside of these two groups — aristocracy and wealthy middle class — belonged to that great group whose husbands were craftsmen in the towns, small farmers, or laborers. These women suffered much from the social evolution of their time. The Industrial Revolution brought strange, new problems into the life of the countrywoman. She who had managed her household and directed the industries of spinning and weaving saw these industries moving away from her. Independence and social prestige were lost to her if she remained in the country. If she was young enough to be acceptable as a factory worker, she joined the wife of the craftsman in the new town, working side by side with her in the big factory. If she was too old to do this, she stayed in the country to watch a wretched poverty close in about her as her handwork grew costly and people learned to prefer the machine-made goods.

Women who became factory hands fared as badly as the countrywoman, even if they were a little more independent as wage earners. They, their husbands, and even their children, were swallowed up by the mechanistic processes that invention had set going. Fourteen hours a day of work that was always being speeded up left little energy or time for the demands of life. Homes must be made in rickety, unsanitary houses with no privacy for a family, no village green in the neighborhood where friends might gather, no opportunities for children's play and only the barest subsistence for all.

As time passed, the hastily thrown together towns lost their newness, and the degradation of human beings began to show. No nuns in nearby convents taught the children, no schools took their places for a long time. The townswoman, without education, toiling in never-ending drudgery, knew that her tired children were sometimes whipped to make them work too. No laws prevented child labor; in fact, for many years no legislation gave protection to any worker in industry. Terrible accidents befell the laborers while they learned to manage power machinery, for safety devices were lacking in the early days of industry, and weary, undernourished children and adults were ready victims. Medical and nursing care were unorganized, and no compensation plan existed.

The lower class woman lost morale in this atmosphere, and it is not surprising that the public house attracted her as well as her man. She coarsened and grew hard. When the French Revolution broke out in protest against the insane extravagances of her sister, *Marie Antoinette,* and the court which surrounded her, women of this class betrayed an almost inhuman desire to get even with her and her kind. In fact, the vindictiveness of spirit with which they entered into this disturbance is not only an expression of the harm which industry unwittingly had wrought, but promise of a demand for rights for women as well as for men.

A DECLINE IN NURSING

Disturbed political conditions, the Renaissance, the Protestant Revolt, the general low status of medicine, and the position of women all affected nursing of the period between 1500 and 1860 A.D. The essential spirit of the Renaissance, intellectual enlightenment, could touch it only indirectly, since nursing was an art still outside the intellectual or the esthetic realms, although sensitive to influences from both. Continued withdrawal from the church of vast numbers of tributary supporters who allied themselves with Protestants reduced the number of nurses in monastic institutions. A general lack of interest in monastic life lowered it further, and monastic suppression ushered in the climax of its decay. To Luther and other Protestant leaders, the existence of many thousands of offending monasteries seemed an obstacle which could be met only by forcible removal.

A widespread movement toward suppression of monasteries brought about conditions similar to those produced in England by Henry VIII (1491–1547). He did not even trouble to change his religion, but took advantage of Protestant disaffection to free himself from papal authority. With covetous eyes fixed on monastic properties that represented one-fifth of his kingdom, he based his revolt on the petty excuse of church refusal to sanction his divorce. On the strength of reports made by a royal commission appointed to inspect them, he wantonly destroyed over six hundred monasteries. Beautiful old buildings were wrecked, their gaping wounds left for the gentle ivy to cover reverently. Precious vessels, art treasures, splendid windows — everything of value even to the ornamental utilities of hand-wrought iron and the lead on the roofs — was either ruined or taken away.

The immediate result of monastic dissolution was that hospitals and inns were suddenly snatched away from a public dependent upon them for many centuries. The poor were left without the principal organized system of relief. Substitute provision for the burden of charity was overlooked, and while wars were waged for religious opinion, the care of the sick and the poor, a supreme trust of Christianity, was neglected. A general lack of interest in monastic life hindered successful introduction of reforms in those institutions which remained.

Another effect of the Reformation was to complete the withdrawal of medicine from monastery to university. Medicine thus found a refuge denied nursing. Medical advance was assured while the techniques of nursing remained unchanged in the guardianship of the Beguines and other secular orders and those relatively few nuns who found it possible to continue their practice. Prominent among the latter were the Augustinians of the Hôtel Dieu and Heilige Geist hospitals. University learning in medicine, however, affected but faintly the activities of the general practitioner. While a few physicians realized the need of something better, apparently the average among them was satisfied with a low type of nursing service.

Except when compelled by dire necessity to become a teacher of children, no woman worked outside her home unless she was a member of the industrial class. Women who found places in hospitals as nurses were not acceptable even to industry. They were usually immoral, drunken, illiterate — the very lowest grade of human society. A decline in quality of public service for the sick, noticeable toward the end of the Middle Ages, became deeper and deeper.

A change was apparent now in the organization of hospital service. What had been for so many centuries gratuitous was changing over slowly and grudgingly to a paid service. The public would take painful centuries to adjust to the idea of paying money for care during illness, and to restore vocational desirability to nursing, inevitably a pivotal hospital function. The public had to learn, too, to separate nursing from domestic service, for with this it had become entangled. Meanwhile, the situation was being made worse by mismanagement, inadequate staffing, and even by deliberate exploitation. Women lost control of nursing as men, who were civil appointees, undertook leadership and withheld authority from women called *matrons* whom they put in charge of a secular riffraff taken on as nurses. The fact that among the latter were some whose responsibility for ward management dignified them by the title "Sister" was a concession to policy. "Sister" was a word retained to please the public, for among rich and poor it had come to be associated with a sympathy and encouragement radiating from the nun in the monastery.

The latter half of the period between 1500 and 1860 A.D., saw nursing conditions at their worst, and has been called "the dark period of nursing." New hospitals had been built, but unsanitary conditions made them a source of outbreak for many of those epidemics which served to keep life expectancy down to an average of about eighteen years. The poor, or the paupers as men called those for whom they provided the great, sinister, dirty buildings, associated them with extremity of wretchedness. Within those dreary, almost windowless walls were great wards holding as many as a hundred patients each. Women and men were not always segregated; diseases seldom. It was not uncommon for the sick to be thrown into beds already occupied by several bedfellows—the dead or the delirious, side by side perhaps, with those who still lived and retained their reason. In a room leading off such a ward, a nurse who had been on duty all day slept at night so that she might be within hearing and call of her patients.

In wards like these beds were so close together that, even had there been people to do it, cleaning was almost impossible. All kinds of rubbish collected and remained under them. Only a few iron beds were in use, and the wooden bedstead, the straw or feather mattress, and the bedbug were well known. Nursing procedures, simple as they had been up to this time, became simpler. Feet and faces that had once been washed before a stricken beggar entered a hospital bed from the dirty street, now went unwashed. Bed baths were not attempted. The usual treatments ordered for all conditions were bleeding and purging, a fact which at least spared harassed nurses the present-day rapid-fire adjustment necessitated by more individual consideration.

While respectable women were not expected to undertake nursing under such conditions, there was still criticism of drunkenness, heartlessness, and immorality in those who did. Such women received very small pay and very poor food. Much was expected of them in return. Housework, scrubbing, and laundry took up a great part of the time, and the hours of service fluctuated from twelve to sometimes forty-eight at a stretch. For night duty, old women were commonly engaged. For day duty, they were somewhat younger. No previous training was looked for, nor was character a consideration.

No change was to come until the middle of the nineteenth century. This was the influence that went with the Pilgrim emigrants to New England, and this was the background for their development of hospitals and nursing. Indeed, few discernible differences are to be met in descriptions of hospitals of this period, whether their location lay in Britain, in continental Europe, or in New England.

The person who suffered from mental illness was even worse off than he stricken by bodily disease. In spite of attempts to free him from restraining chains, he was far from being treated as a human being. His cell was apt to be small and damp, his food poor, the accepted remedies harsh. Fly blisters or mustard plasters might be applied to the head, strong purgatives or emetics given, or he might be ducked in cold water or beaten. The family to which he belonged was made to feel itself disgraced.

Prisons. Among all unfortunates to be institutionalized, however, the worst off were those who became prisoners. Society felt it had a justifiable grudge against them and dealt with them accordingly. The following descriptions of prisons, one continental, the other English, present what are conceded to be faithful pictures of their methods:

"A prison taint was on everything there. The imprisoned air, the imprisoned light, the imprisoned damps, the imprisoned men, were all deteriorated by confinement. As the captive men were faded and haggard, so the iron was rusty, the stone was slimy, the wood was rotten, the air was faint, the light was dim. Like a well, like a vault, like a tomb, the prison had no knowledge of the brightness outside."[2]

"Brandon was taken to Newgate, the most loathsome prison in London at that time, it being used for felons, while Ludgate was for debtors. Here he was thrown into an underground dungeon foul with water that seeped through the old masonry from the moat, and alive with every noisome thing that creeps. There was no bed, no stool, no floor, not even a wisp of straw; simply the reeking stone walls covered with fungus, and the windowless arch overhead. . . . I protested and begged and tried to bribe, but it was all of no avail; the keeper had been bribed before I arrived. Although it could do no possible good, I was glad to stand outside the prison walls in the drenching rain, all the rest of that wretched night, that I might be as near as possible to my friend and suffer a little with him."[3]

Augustinian Nuns. In the twilight and the darkness that enfolds nursing in these centuries between 1500 and 1860 gleams a tiny light. It is borne by an order of nuns following the rule of St. Augustine. This first purely nursing order of the church, established in 1155, bore a heavy share of difficulties arising in hospitals in times when religious and political strife kept disease-ridden countries in seemingly endless turmoil. Their nursing was carried on chiefly in the great city hospitals and they were under close direction of the clergy, sometimes working also under a lay hospital board. It is not surprising that they incurred criticism for disobeying orders given by doctors and that it was found necessary to teach them that good nursing of patients involves loyal cooperation with physicians. It must be acknowledged, at the same time, that the asceticism which motivated stern devotion to their chosen work has placed us in their debt for preserving nursing procedures as monasteries disappeared and secular nursing was yet imperfectly developed.

The life of the Augustinian nun was strictly monastic. She renounced the world and home ties following a novitiate which lasted twelve years or longer. Her life, henceforth, was passed in a hospital, its monotony broken occasionally by service as a private nurse in a home. She wore a white robe and, when a full sister, donned a hood. In the notorious "Hôtel Dieu," as Paris strangely named the great hospital they ran, these nuns became heroic figures, although the precedent for unremitting toil that they established proved, in some ways, unfortunate for nurses of a

---

[2]Charles Dickens, in Martin Chuzzlewit, 1911.
[3]Charles Major, in When Knighthood Was in Flower, 1907.

later day. From one to another the Augustinians passed on a routine of nursing, from year to year their duties of housekeeping and management increased. There were no lectures, no classes, little or no recreation. They nursed and scrubbed, cooked, sewed, and washed clothes without benefit of any of our modern facilities. It is difficult, perhaps, to picture their method of performing the function of laundresses, and it is also difficult to imagine the choice of white uniforms under prevailing conditions. Every day there was a "little wash" for their household of over six hundred patients; every six weeks there was what must have been named very correctly, a "great wash." The work was done in the river Seine, regardless of season or water temperature. Knee deep in the stream the nuns dipped, soaped, slapped, and rinsed until all was done. Then they went back to confusion and the care of sick people lying, often, six in a bed. When they asked for assistants for the sake of these patients, the now classic reply came that they were "always trying to do nothing."

Suggestions for Study

1. Give a description of general social conditions as the year 1500 dawned on the western world.

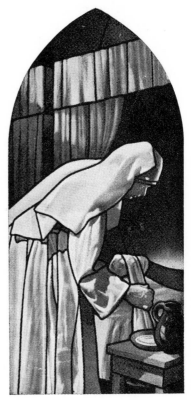

Figure 35. An Augustinian Nun. ("They Caught the Torch." Courtesy of Will Ross, Inc.)

2. (a) Make an outline of famous authors, sculptors, and painters of the Renaissance, adding several names to those mentioned in the text, giving the principal accomplishments of each. (b) Add the names of several scientists of the period, including Copernicus, Kepler, and Galileo.

3. Procure from an art store or from the Perry Pictures Company, Malden, Massachusetts, copies of famous paintings such as the following:

Spring—by Alessandro Botticelli
Pinkie—by Sir Thomas Lawrence
The Blue Boy—by Sir Thomas Gainsborough
The Duchess of Devonshire—by Sir Thomas Gainsborough
The Last Supper—by Leonardo da Vinci
Mona Lisa—by Leonardo da Vinci
The Sistine Madonna—by Raphael

4. (a) Compare the activities of Martin Luther of Germany and Ignatius Loyola of Spain during the Protestant Revolt. (b) What was the relationship of the Ursulines to the Jesuits?

5. Give an account of the colonization of America by Spanish, French, and English governments.

6. Tell what you know of the Industrial Revolution and its effect on the average citizen.

7. (a) Make a list of famous physicians and their contributions during this period. (b) Show how superstition lingered in spite of progress in some directions.

8. (a) What do you know of the practice of medicine in colonial America? (b) Name several of the early medical schools of this country.

9. What general conditions in regard to sanitation prevailed?

10. Discuss the status of women of the Renaissance from the following standpoints: (a) Type of life expected of a good woman; (b) Attitude toward work outside the home; (c) Circumstances under which she married, and (d) Attitude toward the feminist groups.

11. Discuss the Dark Period of Nursing from the following standpoints: (a) General causes; (b) Type of women employed, and their preparation for the work; (c) Title by which the nurse was known and its significance; (d) Type of person by whom nursing work was supervised; (e) A purely nursing order of the Catholic Church that carried on courageously amid many difficulties.

12. What was the contribution of the Augustinian nuns during this period?

References

Austin, Anne L.: History of Nursing Source Book. New York, G. P. Putnam's Sons, 1957, Chap. 4.

Dark, Sydney: The Story of the Renascence. Modern Readers' Bookshelf. New York, George H. Doran.

Dexter, Elizabeth Anthony: Colonial Women of Affairs. Boston and New York, Houghton Mifflin Co., 1924, Chap. 4.

Dickens, Charles: Martin Chuzzlewit. New York, Charles Scribner's Sons, 1911.

Fox, Ruth: Great Men of Medicine. New York, Random House, 1947.

Hayes, Moon, and Wayland: World History. New York, The Macmillan Co., 1955.

Kent, Rockwell (editor): World-Famous Paintings. New York, Wm. H. Wise and Co., 1939.

Nutting and Dock: A History of Nursing. New York and London, G. P. Putnam's Sons, 1907, Vol. I, Chap. 14.

Raynor, Edwin: Famous Cathedrals and Their Stories. New York, Grosset and Dunlap, 1935.

Raynor, Edwin: Famous Statues and Their Stories. New York, Grosset and Dunlap, 1936.

Schoolman and Slatkin: The Story of Art: The Lives and Times of the Great Masters. New York, Halcyon House, 1940.

Schubert, Marie: Famous Paintings and Their Stories. New York, Grosset and Dunlap, 1934.

Chapter 8

EARLY HOSPITALS OF
THE AMERICAS

NEW SPAIN

When Italian *Columbus* enlisted the aid of Spain's Queen Isabella in his scheme to open up western trade routes to the Orient and ended the adventure by setting foot on an island near the edge of a strange new land, he brought opportunity within reach of many a dashing cavalier. Stories of fabulous wealth inflamed adventurous hearts. Stories of benighted Indians fired anew the Crusading spirit. Spain's bravest took ship for a new world as soon as they could.

Hernando Cortez, efficient soldier of the King of Spain and organizer as well, conquered what we call Mexico. He met with cruelty the approach of the well-meaning Aztec ruler, *Montezuma,* whom legend had taught to believe in a white god, presumably now appearing in the form of Cortez. Spaniards soon profited from the wealth, not of the Aztecs alone, but also of those Toltecs, Mayas, and Incas whom we have found in territory stretching from Mexico into Peru. In Indian cities a civilization existed that included systematic provision for care of the sick, physicians, nurses, and hospitals. Indian culture had made some advance also into adjacent regions, north and west, inhabited by Pueblo Indians. These had reached the agricultural stage; but elsewhere, on mountain and plain, were roaming tribes whose friendliness to the stranger varied, apparently, with the harshness or gentleness of the climate in which they lived.

Among these hunter tribes were men still in the Stone Age of development. The medicine man of primitive peoples was their doctor; the

154

squaw or herbwoman his assistant and their nurse. Some lived in wigwams or in teepees, others in caves side by side with animals. Northern natives were energetic, fierce, and warlike. Those whose surroundings were semitropical were slothful and indolent, but frequently docile. The majority seem to have been dirty in habit, the Indian of northerly regions where cleanliness was most difficult, especially so. To women, Indians usually accorded the position of burden-bearer, cook, manager of the home, and helper in the fields. Among certain Indians, however, women were accorded the dignity of seats in the tribal councils, and often the tracing of descent through the mother gave her prestige.

Need for additional provision for care of the sick was created when the first boatload of adventurers started out from Europe. Crude conditions of travel led to deadly outbreaks of scurvy, as well as of disease contracted before leaving the homeland. On his second trip Columbus was careful to bring a physician. Explorers, conquerors, and conquered— all were exposed to infections for which they had no immunity. Unfortunately, almost simultaneous with this urgent need a period of depression in European nursing was being induced by the Renaissance and the Reformation and prolonged by revolutions to establish religious freedom and the civil rights of man. A great era of discovery facilitated the spread of disease at a time when opportunities for its control were less adequate than ever.

Spanish, French, and English colonizers met the problem of medical care and nursing in different ways. Spain, whose immediate financial rewards were greatest, was also best prepared for pioneering abroad. Protestantism had not weakened her church as it had in other countries. The three new missionary groups which Europe had brought into being— Dominicans, Franciscans, and Jesuits—stood ready, organized, and eager to help. Spain made use of them, and so did France. Protestant England had no corresponding support, and medicine and nursing were left in the hands of individuals. Orders of the Catholic Church accompanied the Spaniards to America, pushing back frontiers by exploration, supplanting paganism by Christianity, protecting, as far as they could, the public health. As they penetrated wildernesses and lived among tribal peoples, they devoted themselves with a will to any necessary task, encouraging the weary pioneer, teaching his children and often, as nurses or doctors, caring for the sick and injured without distinction between friend and foe. The Jesuits kept especially systematic records. In diaries called "Relations" they transmitted minute details of everyday happenings to their home office. These Relations have become a valued source of early American history.

Rise of Missions and Hospitals.   The problem which faced all Orders was very similar to that met by monks who long before had dealt with the barbarians who brought about the Fall of Rome in 476 A.D. The key to solution was the same, for the native American had to be brought to a state where he and the white man could live side by side. In the absence of established monasteries, a monastic type of institution known as the "mission" sprang up in the path of the missionary from Spain or France. Friendly advances were made to the Indians, a place of worship set up, and natives gathered about it in self-supporting communities that might reach the number of several thousand. Agriculture and trades were taught as well as religion. Well-organized care of the sick in these earliest missions could hardly be expected. There were overwhelming epidemics of measles or smallpox, times of stress during which the well had to help the few friars with the nursing.

The first real hospital in America, the Hospital of Immaculate Conception, was built and endowed by Hernando Cortez in 1524, on the spot where he had met Montezuma and the men whose land and gold he had come to take. As the Hospital of Jesus of Nazareth, it stands today in Mexico City, reflecting all the beauty and spaciousness of Spanish hospital architecture under Moslem influence. To Cortez it represented thanksgiving for victory and the expiation of sins that he might have overlooked as he made his peace with God. He intended it to shed its mercy on white and Indian alike, and put their care into the keeping of a nursing Brotherhood.

Seven years after the founding of the Hospital of Immaculate Conception in Mexico City, the hospital of Santa Fé (Holy Faith) was built in what is now New Mexico. This was the undertaking of padres (fathers) whose ambition led them to expand their mission to the scope of an ancient monastery.

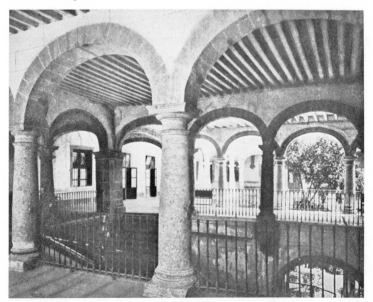

Figure 36. Hospital of Jesus of Nazareth, Mexico City. The first real hospital known to have been built on the American continent. Founded by Cortez, about 1524, as the Hospital of Immaculate Conception. (Guillermo Kahlo.)

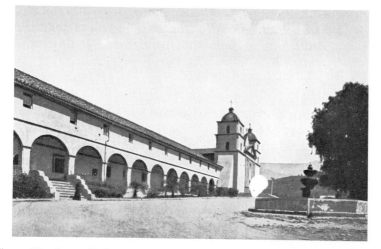

Figure 37. Santa Barbara Mission, Santa Barbara, California. Founded in 1786 and still occupied by Franciscan Fathers. (Published by Cardinell-Vincent Co., San Francisco.)

Missions gradually became part of the Spanish scheme of colonization, with control centered in the homeland. Military protection was afforded them by a line of presidios or forts. In little more than two hundred years the line of missions and forts was extended about six hundred miles along the coast of what is now the state of California. *Junípero Serra*, a Franciscan friar, was made responsible for this great project and, by 1776, when England's colonists were declaring their independence, his arduous zeal had placed his paternally governed missions with their schools and manual training centers as far north as the Mission San Francisco, so named in honor of St. Francis of Assisi.

With a determined little group of brown-robed followers of St. Francis, Father Serra brought Christianity to the California Indian. Through the brush and over the hills of California he had made his way on foot, laying out the route that would be the El Camino Real, or King's Highway, and make communication between his twenty-one missions a possibility.

The California missions ultimately gathered thousands of Indian children into the Christian faith, making them followers of the cross that Father Serra planted on the hills. He had opened a new land to the white man. His work was hampered continually by outbreaks of white men's diseases, of which mission cemeteries tell the story. Only occasionally was a doctor's help available, and the burden of medicine and nursing fell, in the main, on him and his friars.

NEW FRANCE

Not long after Cortez began the colonization of Spanish America,

France hastened to claim the lands adjacent to two great waterways – the St. Lawrence River with its source in the Great Lakes, and the Mississippi flowing south almost from that point into the Gulf of Mexico.

CANADA

In 1535 *Jacques Cartier* erected a cross and set up the flag of France at Cape Gaspé near the mouth of the St. Lawrence. Explorers, Franciscan friars, Jesuits, and settlers followed him to what is now Canada (Huron Indian for "settlement"). By 1607 there were settlements in Nova Scotia and Quebec, and Frenchmen had reconciled themselves to the work of getting their share of gold out of the fur trade instead of from mines or ready hoards of native treasure. Theirs was a difficult task, made worse by Indian hostility.

The same complications of disease arose as in New Spain. Measles, smallpox, and tuberculosis played havoc among the natives to whom Europeans transferred these diseases. The native rightly blamed the white man for the blight that fell upon his race. Dirt and cold, both of a degree beyond their experience, made it almost impossible for the friars to combat disease that swept like forest fire, let alone to advance religion among the roving groups that lived during long winters in smoke-filled wigwams crowded with men, women, and children, all infested with lice, and surrounded by flea-ridden dogs. In his zeal for saving souls the poor priest even tried living in these surroundings, but found that he must content himself with less close contact. His days were more than filled as he moved about baptizing the dying, doing what he could for the sick.

Hôtel Dieu and Ursuline Convent of Quebec. The idea of establishing in Canada a permanent hospital came from one of the Jesuits, and it caught the attention of a socially minded woman, the wealthy *Duchesse d'Aiguillon*. Niece of *Cardinal Richelieu,* one of the most influential political figures in France as well as in the Catholic Church, she made it her business to obtain a grant of land with permission to start this hospital in the city of Quebec, then a community of about two hundred and fifty people, principally Indians. Three nuns of the Augustinian Order, then supplying so many of the great city hospitals of Europe, were selected as nurses.

Meantime, the value of an orphanage and a school for the education of the little Indian and French children was suggested, and another member of the nobility pledged herself to this scheme. *Mme de la Peltrie's* enthusiasm carried her farther than that of the Duchesse d'Aiguillon. She determined to go in person to Canada to start the work. The order of St. Ursula answered her appeal by supplying nuns who were trained teachers. In May, 1639, Mme de la Peltrie and the little company of Augustinian and Ursuline nuns sailed from Dieppe. It took them two and a half months to reach the trading post of Tadoussac at the mouth of the St. Lawrence River. The tiny ship which buffeted them about on the great and little known Atlantic, left them there. The seasickness, shortage of drinking water, threatening sea, and floating icebergs faded from memory as they traveled wearily up the great river in a little boat, subsisting for two other long weeks on a diet of uncooked salt cod.

It was August first when they reached Quebec where the guns of the fort saluted, the village went on holiday. As they landed, Mme de la Peltrie and the nuns kneeled down to kiss the soil of that dreamed-of land they had dedicated themselves to save and keep for God and France. After mass they were taken to Sillery, four miles beyond, to view the pride of the Jesuit priests, the nucleus of a mission. Within a palisade built for protection against attack by hostile Iroquois bands stood a church, a mission-house, an infirmary, and the log-cabin dwellings of converted Indians. As no buildings had been provided for the new missionaries, the infirmary at Sillery was given to the Augustinian nuns for their temporary use as a hospital.

Before the Augustinian sisters unpacked their few belongings, the sick gathered about, besieging them for help. The bed linen brought from France was insufficient even when they attempted to eke it out by cutting it into pieces. The beds overflowed so that log-cabins had to be built and the church used for extra patients. August heat can be almost

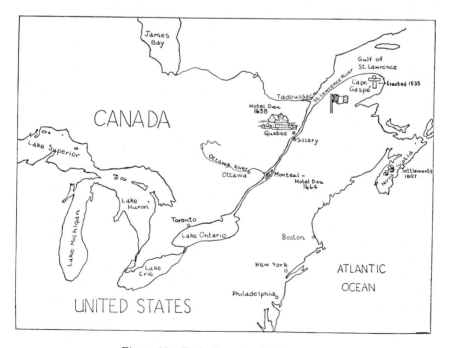

Figure 38. Early Canadian Settlements.

unbearable around Quebec, and the nurses had no time to recover from a long, hard trip. They felt it keenly, and as their work became even more emergent in character following an outbreak of smallpox, they were sorely tried. The effort to carry out accustomed nursing procedures for relief of dirty Indians crowded into inadequate quarters, unfamiliar customs, difficulties of providing suitable and sufficient food, lack of sleep, all told on them.

Their companions, the Ursulines, were no better off. They had been housed in an empty wooden warehouse on the bank of the St. Lawrence River just below the heights on which stood the fortifications of Quebec. Indian children overran the school-to-be just as their relatives had overrun the hospital. Smallpox broke out here also, and the Ursulines had to be nurses before they could be teachers. Fear of the epidemic drove the Indians from the surrounding country into Quebec. The Ursuline shack, as it really was, had to have berths put up along its interior walls for rows of patients, and mattresses laid close together on the floor for others. The nuns did their best and, fortunately, were not infected. "In those days of peril and catastrophe nobody had time to catch a disease. So it was with the Ursulines. Like Hotspur, they lacked the leisure to be sick."[1] In both of these emergency hospitals many Indians died — so many, in fact, that others stopped coming. Some months later the disease ran itself out, and enough peace descended upon all the harassed first nurses of Canada to allow them to make progress at last.

The Augustinians applied themselves enthusiastically to development of the work at Sillery. They called their hospital the "Hôtel Dieu," and here they were free, as they had not always been in Europe, to make the spirit emanating from it that of a true House of God. Its goodness penetrated the palisade and touched the entire community. The Indian, sick or well, could rely upon friendship; and kindness to him helped to protect the colony. Old Indian women and children, to whom fortune and the winter weather alike showed no mercy, found a home. An out-patient service in which the nuns dispensed quantities of medicine drew many others to their door and sent them away cheered by the helpful words dispensed with it.

Never did there seem to be enough room or enough time for all good works that the generous nuns found to do, and every arriving ship brought more patients, and more complicating infections. The year 1658 saw them moved into a new Hôtel Dieu of Quebec built near the fort where they would have protection in case of attack by their savage and uncertain neighbors. Here they built up an institution that endured many hazards and remains, to the present time, a mainstay for the city that grew up about it, and a suitable monument to three capable nurses

---

[1]Repplier, Agnes: Mère Marie of the Ursulines. Copyright, 1931, reprinted by permission of Doubleday, Doran & Company, Inc., New York.

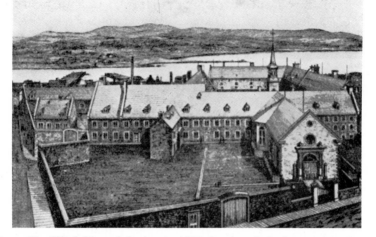

Figure 39. Hôtel Dieu of Quebec in 1825 showing stockades as protection against Indian attack. (From Hospital Management, September, 1939.)

who a long time ago were called upon to make a great adjustment and accomplished it.

Meanwhile, in the hospital which they had been called upon to organize so suddenly, the Ursulines were especially successful in utilizing the help of Indian women. Their teacher training, doubtless, set its own stamp of quality on this *earliest instruction and supervision of nurses in America.* As soon as it was possible, they returned to the work that they had set out to do. Little Indian girls sorely needed teachers if they were to grow up in the ways of civilization and Christianity and make good wives for French and Indian men. They had to learn how to keep their small bodies clean, how to wear and take care of the queer French clothing, how to behave in a mannerly fashion while eating at table, at the same time that they learned how to cook, sing, and read, and how to pray and give the right attention to chapel service. They must be led to practice kindness instead of cruelty.

The staunch little group of Ursuline nuns had a long struggle with poverty before a beautiful stone convent replaced inadequate quarters. In 1660, set high on the cliff of Quebec in seven acres of ground, the finest building in New France was erected. Quebec had given them the land, and friends had sent workmen from the homeland to fashion the buildings out of native rock. The great convent of the Ursulines stands on the same site today. Here the young women who braved the Atlantic storms to become wives for French colonists found protection. This was the locus of the marriage mart where they chose their husbands.

Settlement of Montreal. The next phase in development of Canada, after Quebec had been established, was foundation of a second settlement about two hundred miles farther up the St. Lawrence on what already had been named the "Island of Montreal" (Mount Royal rises behind it). Promoters of the new colony profited by Quebec's experiences. They included in their original plans a hospital and a school, and decided that the hospital was the immediate necessity if choice had to be made. In 1641 the first ship sailed from France carrying a governor, forty colonists, and four women. One of these, *Jeanne Mance,* since childhood had shown herself to be of unusual religious bent. She had not become a nun, however, and the inspiration that drew her now to far-off Canada she owed to reading the popular *Relations* and the example of Mme de la Peltrie. Her own fortune had not been sufficient to supply funds necessary for her venture, but the generous donations of *Madame de Bullion,* who became interested in her, had made it financially secure for the present.

The colonization party was forced to land at Quebec because August was too late in the year for clearing land, for sowing, and for building cabins of logs from great trees that must be felled. The winter would close down upon them and, perhaps, destroy them before their task was finished. A settler made room for them at his farm near Sillery and the Augustinian nuns. Mlle Mance saw at close range the life of a pioneer, in health and in sickness. She learned intimately the problem of dealing with the savage Indian. Mme de la Peltrie at the Ursuline school became her friend and extended her kindness to the little group of enthusiasts who were busied with boat-making in preparation for their trip up river in the spring. When that happy time arrived, Mme de la Peltrie went with them. In May, 1642, they reached the island on which they were to develop the tiny settlement that would grow into the great city of Montreal.

Hôtel Dieu of Montreal. By October, 1644, Mlle Mance was established in a building measuring sixty by twenty-four feet, divided into a hospital of two wards, servants' quarters and kitchen, and a room for herself. A palisade surrounded all, for the fierce tribes of the Iroquois were ever-threatening neighbors who prowled about and shot arrows from forest hiding-places and shared with other savages the delights of torturing captives. From France came hospital supplies, household and chapel furnishings, and animals to stock a small farm. Provision for medical aid was overlooked, and the colony depended on the common sense of Mlle Mance and the knowledge of medicine possessed by missionary priests. Fortunately, pioneer life made men rugged, and they seldom needed care unless they were beset by epidemic disease or were victims of accident or war.

For the next fifteen years, in the little mission hospital, Mlle Mance nursed the sick and stretched resources to interpret Christian hospitality to all who came her way. In 1659 the difficulties surrounding colonial organization and its support impelled her to visit France to see what could be done to improve them through a closer contact. While there she procured the services of three hospital nuns from the Society of St. Joseph de la Flêche, one of whom was made the first superior of the hospital. Mlle Mance did not withdraw completely from management of the institution and was the actual administrator of its affairs until her death in 1673. Within the next century all French developments at Montreal, and at Quebec also, passed into English control as a result of the Seven Years' War, and French support of its Canadian missions was suspended.

The change in political administration naturally created economic disturbances that shook the lives of all who had tried to make a place for themselves in this section of the New World. The nuns of Quebec were close to the hazards of war, for its decisive battle was fought at their very door. In the Ursuline convent and the Hôtel Dieu wounded French and English soldiers found nurses to care for them, and it was to the Ursuline chapel that France's hero, *Montcalm,* was carried for burial.

The nuns at the Hôtel Dieu of Montreal were at a loss to know how to keep their hospital going at all until one of them, resourcefully, devised the idea of selling bread. Their ovens immediately became a source of income and, before long, produced hundreds of loaves daily. In time also the great kettles began to turn out quantities of soap, and two household industries had been developed on a major scale. With sewing, candle-making, and other lesser activities, they went far toward maintaining an institution which the general poverty made more and more essential to community health.

The story of pioneer life of women in America, in the church and out

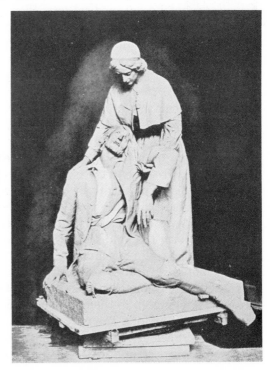

Figure 40. Statue of Jeanne Mance tending a wounded soldier. (From "History of Medicine in the Province of Quebec" by Maude E. Abbott, McGill University, Montreal, Canada, 1931.)

of it, appears unutterably hard until we remember that in pioneer living at any time and place will be found compensations. A helpful spirit rules those who live in isolation. Good things and evil things that befall individuals are shared, and much joy is to be got from trifles. There is a deep sense of comradeship, and always there is somebody who can see the funny side of things. Among Quebec's early settlers one of the best loved was a happy Ursuline nun whom people learned to call the "laughing nun." There were priests who could share the amusement of those who watched them learning to use snowshoes. There were many nuns who could smile with friends or patients whose interest was caught by the many and varied patches that were spread over worn habits and made it hard to pick out the original cloth.

Perhaps the greatest compensations were those of being able to adjust more and more quickly to changing circumstance, of inventing, and of seeing the fruits of labor and thought ripen. In pioneer America Europeans had to learn his languages if they were to gain headway with the Indian. Cherished class distinctions tended to disappear. Clothing had to be adapted to new types of weather, food became necessarily coarse and extremely simple. There were times when money was all but gone and new ways of providing sustenance had to be found. White habits of nuns became brown when the former proved themselves unsuited to conditions; coarse but beautiful weaves in cloth replaced the fine ones of old lands. Indian moccasins were often substituted for shoes. Indian squaws taught herbal medical lore. Slowly, surely, progress was made. Tents and wooden buildings were replaced by stone ones, farms supplanted forests. Schools, churches, towns began to grow, and social gaiety was more frequent.

Two colonial ambitions met early fulfillment. Wealth flowed homeward to France through the trading companies, and missions were established among the Indians. So far, however, there had been only slow growth of population. The country must, in some way, be permanently settled. Men emigrated to follow the fur trade as it developed in New France. "Coureurs de bois," she called them, and they became used to a half-wild, carefree life in the woods. They did not promise to develop into the substantial type of citizen upon which a country could depend. The question of increasing the population in her colony became a serious one to France. It was obvious that if it was to develop there must be more men who would farm the land and women who would help them to build permanent homes and rear children. Indian girls educated by the Ursuline nuns sometimes fulfilled expectation by marrying a French settler but oftener reverted to native life. The idea of one husband who could not be divorced was foreign to them, and not pleasing.

MARRIAGE MART. The year 1654 saw the first of a series of importation from France of young girls who had agreed to become the wives of French colonists. Some of these girls had been brought up in orphan asylums, some were convent bred. All were carefully selected on the basis of character. Experience proved the most satisfactory group came from the farm homes of France. On the voyage across the Atlantic they were accompanied by a nun or a paid matron. Upon landing in Canada they were under the protection of the Ursulines. To the convent came prospective husbands with whom the girls were free to converse and interchange questions. Some girls were slow in making the great decision, some were difficult to please. They might turn down suitors but, until safely married, they stayed with the nuns. At the end of twenty years nearly one thousand new homes had been created through their cooperation. Royal dowries often went with them, and bounties might be offered for children. Colonial families seldom numbered less than ten.

LOUISIANA

Within the next hundred years France was busy acquiring land, building up her fur trade, and establishing outposts in settlements along the St. Lawrence and Mississippi waterways. Another French colony had developed around the mouth of the Mississippi and needed teachers and nurses. New Orleans was the front door to territory bordering the great river and called "Louisiana" in honor of France's king, whose "home town" also had been remembered in naming the infant capital city. Six or seven Ursuline nuns answered the call and left France in 1727. Their passage was an adventurous one, dragged out for five months. Storms beset them, they were chased by pirates, and finally landed in the harbor of Belize on the coast of Honduras. Another hazardous week was spent on two little freight boats that took them across the Gulf of Mexico to New Orleans. Here they fared somewhat better than the nuns of Quebec. Their new home was ready, and slavery provided helpers. Colonial life was less primitive here, and the site of their future labor was a fruitful land in contrast to rocky Quebec, but the mosquito produced a new enemy in yellow fever. Many epidemics of this disease, of cholera, and of smallpox had to be met. Political disturbances brought war dangers. It was under stress of many difficulties that the little house developed slowly into the present great Charity Hospital of New Orleans. A convent school, which probably had first place in Ursuline objective, was established too.

NEW ENGLAND

The Spanish were well established in Mexico, and the French claimed the region around the mouth of the St. Lawrence, before English seamen of Queen Elizabeth followed along as pirates who stole the treasure that ships of Spain were busy carrying home. Other British subjects became explorers, and one sailed around the world. Thus another people was being stirred by that restlessness which has kept the human race ever on the move, adding to its experience, seeking new knowledge and steadily spreading over the earth better ways of living. In 1584 England laid claim to a portion of the Atlantic coast lying between the claims already staked by Spain and France, and the area was named "Virginia" in honor of her virgin queen, Elizabeth.

In 1607 a colony called "Jamestown," for Elizabeth's royal successor, was planted at the mouth of a river called the "James." Its growth was impeded by the disappointment of men who came to carry away gold and found none. They could not believe that life in Jamestown was worthwhile, saw no way of making a living and completely failed to adjust. Many of them starved to death. The colony's spirit was changed and its destiny saved by constructive *Captain John Smith* who declared against unwillingness to work, brought out men of proved stability of character and manual skill, built cabins for permanent settlers, and set up trade with the Indians. A few years later the industry of raising tobacco was introduced, the privilege of individual ownership of land was granted colonists, and real progress began. An era of great estates and fortune-making followed. Tobacco ultimately proved to be a substitute for gold and as lucrative as the furs which had been the solace of France.

Before any of this came about, however, the colony had a miserable history of hardship and Indian massacre, sickness and heavy mortality. Its members were adventurers, frequently dashing young cavaliers belonging to noble families. The lure was sudden wealth which they meant to take home. No one understood sanitation necessary in camp life. Medical care was lacking, for doctors appointed by the colonization company would not stay. There was little that could be called nursing, and homesickness was depressing. Women do not appear in the picture until 1619 when a shipload arrived at Jamestown to be auctioned off as wives. The problems of instability and income having been solved, the settlement improved like an infant victim of malnutrition for whom the proper food at last has been found. Immigrants flocked to it.

Northern colonization had difficulties peculiarly its own, and the group of about one hundred men and women who undertook it in 1620 experienced hardship too. The little ship, "Mayflower," in which they chose to make their pilgrimage to America acquainted them with danger, seasickness, and scurvy. It landed them on a rocky wooded coast in the middle of winter. The pitiful little huts they were able to build were wholly inadequate as homes and even when the frost disappeared and they were able to clear the land, it made stony, unfruitful farms. In the meantime, one half of the colonists had died.

The survivors succeeded ultimately in their determination to make permanent homes, develop orderly government, and worship in their chosen way. The Indians proved friendly and, although missionary effort among them was limited, there was an attempt to be kind and just with them. Other settlers followed, and other colonies were developed. America was roomy enough to afford separate homes for all of those groups into which Christians were dividing themselves as they broke away from the one church in which, for fifteen hundred years, they had worshiped together one God.

Provision for medical care of settlers remained inadequate, as it had been in Jamestown. *Samuel Fuller,* a deacon of the church who arrived on the Mayflower, acted as physician to fellow colonists in New England for thirteen years, and the precedent was followed for long years after. Prayer was a large part of treatment, for patients expected it, and men like Fuller considered it a part of their duty to the sick. No degree was required, and any educated man among the colonists — clergyman, governor, or schoolteacher — was held equipped to essay the role of doctor. The ignorant quack throve and Indian folklore soon clouded the outlook further.

English pioneers lacked the organized service of the mission or the convent and the institutional experience of nun and priest. Women were scarce, although the wives of Englishmen accompanied their husbands more frequently than did those of the Spaniards or the French. The wife of Samuel Fuller was brave enough to assume the busy function of colonial midwife, and there were always some who followed this occupation or helped families during illness. When the doctor, in the midst of his long round of widely separated visits, found someone whose recovery depended on close supervision, he took him to his own home. Out of these repetitions of primitive hospitality, the hospital would take shape but, unlike the Spanish or the French, these early English builders of America took considerable time to get around to introducing it.

The missionary spirit of New England colonists demonstrated itself in the preparation of religious tracts for the Indian, and in establishment in 1638 of Harvard College and in 1750 of Dartmouth College, where he might be prepared along with the sons of colonists for the ministry. Their conception of care in illness is shown in two groups of selected quotations, the first the work of a biographer of *Cotton Mather* (1663–1728), the second taken from the diary of *Samuel Sewall* (1652–1730). Both were Puritan ministers of Massachusetts, men of public spirit, graduates of Harvard, and both shared the belief of their time in witchcraft. Cotton Mather was interested in medicine and, to some extent, used his knowledge. It did not prevent him, however, from prosecuting witchcraft trials in which his friend Mr. Sewall, in the capacity of Chief Justice, was forced to take the responsibility of endorsing a legal decision. That the latter's faith in witches wavered as a result of weighing popular testimony against them is evidenced by the fact that later he arose in his pew at the old South Meeting House, in Boston, to acknowledge publicly that he deplored his part in a judgment of human beings which gave their fellow creatures authority to hang them.

"At this time medicine had far to go. Men were credulous in this as in all scientific fields. Mermaids and mermen were accredited facts. A sailor on the boat that in 1686 brought the bookseller Dutton to Boston had seen both on voyages to the East Indies."

"Deformities were ascribed to witchcraft. Cotton Mather's own first son, born in 1693, lacked an anus, and in spite of efforts to relieve him, died in three days. Mather more than suspected witchcraft, his wife having been frightened some few weeks before by a *Spectre*."

"He was sure that he could confer one benefit upon Boston—he had never forgotten his medical interest—by spreading the news of inoculation, a treatment he had learned from a publication of the Royal Society lent him by Dr. William Douglas, the only physician in Boston with a medical degree and the one most inhospitable to the new idea. This was not vaccination in the modern method, but inoculation which induced a mild form of the disease. Though it had never been tried in America, Mather felt sure that many lives could be saved by it. Therefore he prepared a statement for the Boston physicians embodying a summary of the Royal Society publications."[2]

"N.B. Tuesday, Dec. 22, 1675, about the time of the Eclips Sister Sewall was delivered in my chamber of a daughter, Goodwife Brown being Midwife."

"This night Eliza Damon, servant to Nash the Currier, dyes about midnight of the small pocks, to our great startling, lest it should spread as in 1678. Had hop'd the Town was clear of it."

"About one at night, Jane comes up with an unusual Gate, and gives us an account of Mothers Illness. . . I went to Capt. Daviss and fetched some Trecle Water and Syrup of Saffron; Dame Ellis made a Cake of Herbs to try to strengthen Mothers Stomach. In the morn Roger Judd is sent to Cambridge for Dr. Oliver. . . . When he comes he advises to a Plaister for the Stomach, which is aplied; and a Potion made of Bexar (Bezoar) to be taken in Syrup of Saffron and Treacle water; of which took once or twice. About 8. or 9. I call'd Mr. Willard at her desire, who prays with her."[3]

First Hospitals. The growth of hospitals was slow. In over one hundred and fifty years before the American Revolution (1775–1783), only five hospitals appear to have been founded in the English colonies outside of Canada. Two were located in what is now New York City, two others in Philadelphia, and a special hospital for the mentally ill was founded at Williamsburg, Virginia. In only two of these did the quality of nursing improve beyond that which we have seen to be characteristic of city hospitals in the homeland.

---

[2]Boas and Boas: Cotton Mather, 1928, pp. 40, 42, 170, 226. By permission of Harper and Brothers, New York and London, publishers.

[3]Samuel Sewall's Diary, edited by Mark Van Doren, Macy-Masius, New York, 1927, pp. 8, 42, 123.

When Dutch New Amsterdam on Manhattan island was taken over by England, it already boasted more in the way of institutionalized charity than existed in English colonies. There was a home for the poor financed by the church, and a small hospital built in 1658 was maintained by the Dutch West India Company. This hospital, about which information is limited, was probably nothing more than an emergency shelter for homeless sick people.

New Amsterdam became New York, and there arose as adjunct to its hospital a *Publick Workhouse and House of Correction,* an institution lately devised in England where hard work was being used as a cure for crime and indigency. Criminal and pauper from now on staffed the hospital. Buildings were changed according to need, the city assumed a share of the expense of charity and, in time, these small beginnings of the present great *Bellevue Hospital* of modern New York were concentrated on the bank of the East River.

The *Philadelphia General Hospital,* or, as it was then called, "Blockley Hospital," originated in 1731, also with an almshouse as its background. Both Bellevue and Blockley, like St. Thomas' and St. Bartholomew's of London, were in their early days comparable to the xenodochia of ancient times. They cared for the destitute, the insane, the vagrant, or the homeless. Both, however, looked not to the church but among their inmates for workers, and for nurses too. Their management was complicated by frequent epidemics and conditions of increasing poverty due, in part, to individual difficulties of immigrant adjustment, in part to the influence of the Industrial Revolution. The penniless of Britain were moving to America. Under this new pressure, and lacking, as they undoubtedly did, the public interest, these institutions became neither better nor worse than institutions of their type and time abroad.

Treatment of the mentally ill was modeled on that of Newgate and places like it. Men and women victims of smallpox might lie in the same ward, the dead might be left on the floor, undisciplined attendants devoid of training might allow filth to accumulate, or run away from yellow fever or typhus. When nurses were sought by hire, only the roughest element among women and men could be procured. Drunkenness among them was common. Even those nurses who might be of more motherly quality lacked education and worked under disadvantages which are difficult for us to understand. There were no thermometers, no conscious application of hygienic principles, no knowledge of asepsis or antisepsis. Surgery was done without anesthesia by surgeons whose frock coats gained distinction as they accumulated dirt and bloodstains, who used unboiled instruments and unsterilized sea sponges for mopping blood, and who were content to stick needles and thread into velvet pin cushions.

It was all a part of Old World conditions. Bellevue and Blockley only followed the current model in city hospitals. The public responsible for New World institutions was in the position of the nurse who knows the ways of only one hospital. What they had to give was limited by a narrow experience. Doctors were protesting, and the fame of the well trained Sisters of Charity, who heralded nursing reform in France, was so great as to cause reforming spirits to seek to introduce some corresponding groups of nurses to America.

The *Pennsylvania Hospital* founded in 1751 and the *New York Hospital* founded in 1771 were the next two hospitals to be developed. They both departed from the xenodochial type in limiting admission to the sick only, and from the city hospital tradition by depending for support on privately donated funds which, for the Pennsylvania Hospital, were raised by Benjamin Franklin. Both were unique in the care given to selection of the women who were to nurse their patients, and both initiated methods of training them for their work. Physicians of the Pennsylvania Hospital taught simple procedures in nursing, and *Dr. Valentine Seaman* of the New York Hospital augmented similar teaching by lectures on anatomy, physiology, maternal nursing, and care of children. *He is the first doctor known to have lectured to nurses in America.* In 1775 war intervened to complicate nursing difficulties and suspend any other possible progress.

AMERICAN REVOLUTION (1775–1783)

The war of the American Revolution involved all the English colonies scattered along the Atlantic coast. Some wanted to be free to develop in their own way; others wished to remain with England. England's colonial children found themselves badly prepared to assume the burdens of expense and organization necessary to wage a conflict on their own account. Their hastily mobilized army had no medical corps, no Red Cross, no trained nurses. The only organized units of nurses in the country were the nuns of the Catholic Church. They nursed wounded soldiers in their hospitals, as well as those who fell victims to epidemic disease, for there were scarlet fever and dysentery, and smallpox broke out in spite of the fact that the new variolation was used on fighting men.

Loyalty to a cause, to some degree, made up for lack of system and experience, but much makeshift appears. Soldiers often got poor or meager rations. There were times when shoes and clothing wore out, and they marched barefoot and in tatters. There were women who followed their husbands to the battlefield and, under the greatest difficulties, nursed them through serious illnesses. Other women made clothing and bandages, and parted with precious pewter that it might be made into bullets. Homes were turned into hospitals, and so were barns. One farmwoman, at least, baked huge batches of bread, day after day, and served it by the roadside to hungry soldiers. Many tales are told of such resourcefulness. In heroism, woman did not fall behind her male relatives.

The war descended on the colonies just as they were getting a financial start. It left the usual poverty behind, with invalids who needed care, cripples for whom there were no rehabilitation centers, and none of the modern highly organized social services. Among these poor and sick people were many who never in their lives had asked for public help but now were unable to get along without it.

PHILADELPHIA DISPENSARY

Out of a deep social distress came a new type of institution which was the forerunner of today's clinic or outpatient department of the hospital. This institution, like the Pennsylvania Hospital, owed its origin to the social spirit of Quakers in a Quaker city. In 1786 the *Philadelphia Dispensary* was established. Independent of any hospital, the dispensary finances were met by appealing to public sympathy through a new plan of public service, the advantages of which were set forth by its sponsors somewhat as follows: Large numbers of persons needing treatment were not sick enough to be hospitalized, and the expense of their care in the hospital was unnecessary. A staff of volunteer physicians would treat both groups without charge and make visits in patients' homes when necessary.

The Philadelphia Dispensary was a success, and the idea spread to other cities. Pending establishment of city or state health departments, a dispensary came to be looked to as a means of controlling disease. Vaccination against smallpox was one of the earliest preventive treatments which it made widely possible. Dispensary physicians knew those streets from which epidemics commonly derived and, when one appeared, the hospital would supply the physicians with addresses of patients. After verification of the suspected source, newspaper publicity informed citizens of the hidden menace to their health and roused sentiment in favor of abolishing it. The next thing was a health law.

Later history shows the dispensary, which began with so much promise sinking into neglect and obscurity until its main functions are a badly managed first-aid service and the issuance of medicine free, or at cost. Comparatively recently, as the outpatient clinic, it has been revitalized and has recovered its dignity as the portal of entry to the hospital, an indispensable factor in modern preventive medicine and a radiating center for much of our community, health, and social work.

NURSE SOCIETY OF PHILADELPHIA

One of the physicians who gave his time to the Philadelphia Dispensary was keenly impressed by conditions surrounding the confinement of poverty-stricken young mothers. He hoped to get a hospital for them and a school in which to prepare nurses, but was forced to content himself with the *Nurse Society of Philadelphia,* established in 1839.

This was an organization of women who undertook to supply a maternity service in homes.

The Nurse Society of Philadelphia chose its nurses from applicants who had stability of character and experience as heads of families. These were given instruction in obstetrics in common with medical apprentices, and in the form of lectures and practice on a manikin. *Dr. Joseph Warrington* taught these classes, and lady visitors from the society supervised practice in allotted districts. Further systematized instruction was arranged that included lessons in cooking and experience in homes for two weeks at a time. The Society paid the salary of the nurse. Certificates were awarded, and the English system of renting rooms in the mother school and providing calls for private duty was adopted. Another brave attempt had been made toward instructing and supervising nurses under secular auspices, helping to fill a need that grew always more urgent.

GROWTH OF HOSPITALS

After 1800 an evidence of growth was to be seen in a great development of hospitals and, as they were called, "asylums for the insane," the latter usually under the control of states or provinces. The tendency to specialize institutions appeared in establishment of a Lying-in Hospital in New York in 1798. The same tendency, following woman's entrance into the field of medicine and her more frequent presence on hospital boards, became apparent later in the development of separate hospitals for women and for children, or of hospitals combining these two groups. The following are a few out of many well-known institutions established up to 1860, chosen to emphasize variety and spread rather than priority:

> Massachusetts General Hospital, Boston, Massachusetts – 1811
> McLean Asylum, Somerville, Massachusetts (now in Waverly) – 1818
> Montreal General Hospital, Montreal, Canada – 1819
> Cincinnati General Hospital, Cincinnati, Ohio – 1821
> Knight Hospital (later New Haven Hospital), New Haven, Connecticut – 1826
> St. Louis Mullanphy Hospital, St. Louis, Missouri – 1828
> Mt. Sinai Hospital, New York, New York – 1852
> Buffalo General Hospital, Buffalo, New York – 1853
> Woman's Hospital, New York, New York – 1855
> Children's Hospital, Philadelphia, Pennsylvania – 1855
> General and Marine Hospital, St. Catherine's, Canada – 1855
> San Joaquin General Hospital, French Camp, California – 1857
> Halifax Hospital (now Victoria General), Halifax, Canada – 1859

Quite a number of institutions that still carry on public service originated during this period, and a steady increase in immigration made the hospital or the dispensary more and more necessary. Medical schools needed them for training ground. As the tide of settlement flowed westward, they went with it. From east to middle west, and thence to the west, hospitals accompanied the immigrant public until they stretched from coast to coast, the dispensary, in the course of passing years, losing individuality as it became a hospital adjunct.

At the same time some further improvement was made in nursing by introducing to America European sisterhoods, Protestant as well as Catholic. These nursed in homes, founded hospitals and, in time, organized schools for nurses. In 1809 *Mother Elizabeth Seton* founded, at Emmitsburg, Maryland, the Catholic Sisters of Charity. In 1843 the Catholic Sisters of Mercy came from Ireland to Pittsburgh, and four years later founded the hospital which bears their name. In 1845 the Protestant Nursing Sisters were organized in New Jersey through the efforts of *Reverend Muhlenberg*. In 1848 *Reverend William Passavant* established a hospital in Pittsburgh, which he staffed with deaconess nurses imported from a Protestant mission house at Kaiserswerth on the Rhine in Germany where, a short time later, Florence Nightingale was to glean some of the ideas that enabled her to set in motion a scheme for worldwide reform in nursing methods.

SUGGESTIONS FOR STUDY

1. By what three European countries, and in what general locations, were colonies developed in the Western Hemisphere?
2. Show how differences in religion affected early provision for medical and nursing care in the new world.
3. How did Spain go about the task of developing her new possessions and making sure that they would show allegiance to her?
4. (a) What do you know of the first hospital to be erected on this side of the Atlantic? (b) The first one in Canada? (c) The first one in the United States? (d) By whom was each sponsored? (e) How was nursing care provided in each?
5. Where, and under what circumstances, was instruction first given to those who would do nursing on the American continent?
6. Tell what you know of the life and work of the first lay nurse of Canada.
7. (a) What political upheaval greatly changed conditions surrounding the management of the Hôtel Dieu of Quebec and the Hôtel Dieu of Montreal? (b) What novel adjustment was made in one instance?
8. What is the story of the founding of the Charity Hospital of New Orleans?
9. (a) How did English colonists make provision for care of the sick? (b) How soon did their first hospitals appear? (c) What was their attitude toward the Indians?

10. (a) Name the first four hospitals to be established by English colonists. (b) Which two were comparable to xenodochia? (c) What type of nurse was to be found in each?

11. (a) In what hospital, by what physician, and on what subjects were lectures first given to nurses? (b) With what undertaking was Dr. Joseph Warrington associated and for what is he remembered?

12. How far had nursing developed in the English colonies at the time of the Revolutionary War?

13. To what groups could appeal be made for supplying nursing care to soldiers?

14. Compare activities of the Philadelphia Dispensary and the Nurse Society of Philadelphia.

15. (a) When did rapid growth of New England hospitals get under way? (b) Give names and locations of several of these early institutions.

16. Improvement in nursing service was made by the importation of what European nursing sisterhoods?

17. Tell something of the origin and history of the modern hospital clinic.

18. Collect data in regard to the founding of the hospital with which your school of nursing is associated.

REFERENCES

Abbott, Maude E.: History of Medicine in the Province of Quebec. Montreal, Canada, McGill University, 1931.

Atherton, William Henry: The Saintly Life of Jeanne Mance: First Lay Nurse in North America. St. Louis, Catholic Hospital Association of the United States and Canada, 1945.

Austin, Anne L.: History of Nursing Source Book. New York, G. P. Putnam's Sons, 1957, Chaps. 8 and 9.

Boas and Boas: Cotton Mather. New York and London, Harper & Brothers, 1928.

Denis, Alberta Johnston: Spanish Alta California. New York, The Macmillan Co., 1927.

Dexter, Elizabeth Anthony: Colonial Women of Affairs. Boston and New York, Houghton Mifflin Co., 1924, Chap. 4.

Foran, J. K.: Jeanne Mance or "The Angel of the Colony," Montreal, P. Q., The Herald Press, Ltd., 1931.

Gibbon, and Mathewson: Three Centuries of Canadian Nursing. New York, The Macmillan Co., 1947.

Lyman, George D.: John Marsh: Pioneer (first doctor in California). New York, Charles Scribner's Sons, 1930.

Repplier, Agnes: Mère Marie of the Ursulines. New York, Doubleday, Doran & Co., 1931.

Sigerist, Dr. Henry E.: American Medicine. New York, W. W. Norton & Co., Inc., 1934.

Starkey, Marion L.: The Devil in Massachusetts. New York, Alfred Knopf, Inc., 1949. (Historical novel about Salem witchcraft.)

Van Doren, Mark (Editor): Samuel Sewall's Diary. New York, Macy-Masius, 1927.

Chapter 9

SOCIAL REFORM MOVEMENTS

Social conditions in Europe, such as have been described, were undoubtedly the direct results of the religious, industrial, and political revolutions which threatened to destroy any social recovery accomplished up to this time. Antagonism and ambition had replaced human sympathy in the emotions of upper and middle classes, and the intellectual revolution had given them an attitude of cold skepticism and the distraction of new interests. While the upper classes strove for wealth, leisure, and power, the masses huddled into slums where they sank deep into the mire of poverty, immorality, and brutality. War, famine, industrial abuses, and pestilence made the inadequacy of nursing care ever more obvious but here or there, in the darkness of social desolation, shone the light of a constructive idea.

CATHOLIC SOCIAL REFORM

Social Service Established.   The first to forward substantially a new type of adjustment was *St. Vincent de Paul* (1576–1660), an unassuming French Catholic priest whose experiences included parish work, missionary work among galley slaves, and travel and captivity in a foreign land where he picked up some knowledge of medicine before he reached Paris, the scene of his real achievement. Here he lived close to a hospital where many rich and influential citizens were giving volunteer service as nurses to help out the overworked Brothers of St. John of God. St. Vincent joined them and proved his usefulness by doing surgical dressings and otherwise assisting with care of patients.

St. Vincent came to believe that it was possible to prevent some of those evils in poverty which arise from a broken human spirit. Everywhere the social virus of professional begging was present. The young, the healthy, and the strong were dependent on almsgiving as well as the old, the sick, and the mentally retarded. Five years of work resulted in many changes. Many tramps were taken off the highways and given supervision by establishment of public night refuges; trade workshops were organized for teaching manual arts to idle youth; and jobs were hunted up for ablebodied adults. St. Vincent de Paul had organized the beginning of a system of *social service* which today is carried on by a large group of professional workers employed by public and private agencies. Research is carried on to determine the causes of economic and social conditions leading to dependency, and federal legislation has provided assistance through Social Security programs.

Order of Sisters of Charity Founded. St. Vincent de Paul had still another famous piece of work to do. While he was in Paris, a friend sent to him a pious widow of noble family who wished to be guided into a life of good works. She had already had experience in visiting nursing with a group of volunteer women working near her own home. *Saint Louise de Marillac,* as she is now known, had longed as a young girl to become a nun. Friends dissuaded her because of her delicate health and she

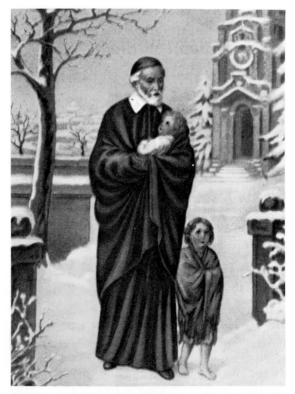

Figure 41. St. Vincent de Paul. (From "Miniature Stories of the Saints," Book One, by Rev. Daniel A. Lord, S.J. [Catholic publications].)

married into the Court circle. Louise de Marillac, however, avoided society, devoting all her leisure time to that work among the poor which now, after her husband's death, she urged St. Vincent to help her to continue.

Several years of training followed in which Louise de Marillac gained the reformer's viewpoint of a new and flexible type of human service. She then formed a plan of making her own house a home and a training school for peasant pupils. In 1633 the community of the *Sisters of Charity* was established, its object the service of the poor in different parts of Paris, its guiding motto "Caritas Christi urget nos" ("The Charity of Christ Presseth Us"). They are words that prove the intensity and sincerity of purpose that drove its two founders and their followers on and on to ever greater service, down to the present time.

A little over a year after the community was formed, on March 25, 1634, Saint Louise set an example by formally taking a vow and becoming the first Sister of Charity of St. Vincent de Paul. The date later became the annual one on which the sisters rededicate themselves to their work. If they do not wish to renew the vow, they are free to marry or to choose some other form of occupation outside the community. A few rules on which to base selection of these peasant girls were formulated. They must be of good family and good character. They were not allowed to enter without the consent of a male relative.

UNIFORM DRESS. The first members brought with them the peasant costume which they had worn at home and which now became the dress they wore as they went about their duties. It was not long before the gray-blue gown of rough woolen cloth with blue apron and spreading white headdress became the conspicuous reminder of humility and kindly human service which we still recognize in it. The period of training lasted five years and instruction included a basic education enabling them to read, write, and make some use of arithmetic. At the same time they were taught by Saint Louise all that she herself knew. The unavoidable limitation of this knowledge is dramatically apparent when we learn that one of the earliest of her graduates was a sacrifice to the then prevalent ignorance of means of preventing infection. Coming across a patient sick with plague on the highway, the sister took her to her lodgings and put her in her own bed. Patient and Sister of Charity both died.

St. Vincent was always aware of the danger of losing his new order to the monastery. The young girls and their friends were accustomed to associate religion and good works with monastic life in which care of the personal soul was of prime importance. It was necessary to build up in their minds, as he had in the mind of Louise de Marillac, the idea of a Sister of Charity doing her work where she found it, often far removed from institutional protection. Sisters must learn how to protect themselves, and their relatives sometimes were fearful.

St. Vincent made it plain that, in nursing, the patient's needs came before religious offices. He emphasized strict obedience to the orders of the physician as essential to the welfare of the sick, urged the sisters to observe all procedures so that they might be more efficient as medical assistants. At the same time he made it possible for them to harmonize these aims with a thoroughly religious life and spirit. Their motto, so happily chosen, became the inspiration for a long line of servants of the poor reaching down to our own time and into far places.

The Sisters of Charity, at the time they were founded, were a product of Catholic reform. Their first service outside of France was, naturally, in countries adhering to the Catholic Church. Increasing religious toler- ance and their own high reputation gradually extended these limits. In 1809 *Mother Elizabeth Seton* introduced Sisters of Charity into America. The rule of the motherhouse in France was obtained and a community established at Emmitsburg, Maryland. In spite of its proximity to France and its dominant Catholicism, Ireland lacked the benefit of the Sisters' work until 1815 when *Mother Mary Aikenhead* organized a community in Dublin.

During the Crimean War it was their efficient service to the soldiers of France that inflamed neglected British soldiers to a discontent that aroused England to action and sent Florence Nightingale to Scutari. In this twentieth century, they may be found all over the world, nursing, teaching, doing social work, guarding the orphaned and the foundling, the aged, the leper, any who need their friendship anywhere.

Seen in summary, the accomplishment of Saint Vincent de Paul and Saint Louise de Marillac attains deserved importance as a reform in nursing. The organization they founded was based on study and knowl- edge of existing conditions. The order reached the poor in their homes and also provided partial or complete nursing service for hospitals. In arranging the latter service, the legal contract was used to prevent exploitation and preserve identity of the order.

PROTESTANT SOCIAL REFORM

While the Catholic Church was thus busy adjusting its social service to accord with new conditions, Protestants in Germany, England and the Netherlands were making an effort to replace the lost nun with the deaconess. With organization and instruction both lacking, leadership proved too weak for the status of a movement to be realized. Scattered bands of Sisters of Charity had alleviated some phases of social mis- management, but many institutions, including hospitals for the mentally ill, lazarettos, prisons, workhouses, orphanages, factories, and their slums remained to grow into magnets for the reformer.

The general condition of hospitals has already been described. The English model was being copied with unfortunate faithfulness in New England, while the continental European model influenced New Spain and New France. Bethlehem Hospital or "Bedlam" in London and the "Lunatics' Tower" in Vienna were typical of institutions to which the "sane" bought admission tickets and repaired with their friends when they wanted amusement.

In prisons everywhere were great numbers of citizens, put there often for minor offenses. Gaolers could demand fees, prisoners often could not pay, and then the great gates did not open even if the law had granted acquittal. Two hundred and fifty different crimes were considered serious enough to merit death. The fact that the close of this period saw this number reduced to three illustrates the injustice that had crept into old Roman and Anglo-Saxon law.

A new type of institution was developed in England with a system of "workhouses" in which paupers and minor offenders against the law were detained and given work to do that brought no personal profit. Institutional upkeep was purposely made cheap, and harsh treatment was countenanced. The workhouse became the dread of the poor, while it protected the rest of society from offending sights that might have brought about earlier reforms. Hardly less humane than the workhouse were the numerous orphanages built to house the abandoned children and orphans whose numbers increased with war, immorality, and epidemics of disease.

Other social problems were arising to disturb England. It was here that the capitalist first replaced the feudal lord in control of the worker. None of the old paternal attitude went over into the new system which, in fact, was at first unconscious of any responsibility beyond profit making. After 1750 huge factories were built by builders who knew nothing of sanitary requirements. They were surrounded by equally unsanitary and carelessly erected homes for the workers, and slums developed. The public health in these neighborhoods was doomed. Epidemic disease was rife and uncontrolled. Factory machinery was put into the hands of operatives without adequate instruction. Accidents were many, and industrial insurance or any form of industrial compensation was as yet undeveloped. The lowest possible wages were paid. The problem of overproduction was solved by shutdowns which threw great numbers of men, women, and children out of employment.

Little children had to work with their parents to make enough to support the family, although this was not new, for they had always done so. Now the conditions were more difficult and all the evils of a lost family life became apparent. The first Factory Act to legally control industry did not come until 1819. Hours for adults had risen by that time to as high as eighteen a day and even children often began at three in the morning and worked until nine in the evening. Hours of women and children were now limited to twelve a day, and children under nine years of age were not allowed to work.

Fortunately, time had permitted the new group of Christians to settle differences of opinion and arrange themselves in various sects — Baptists,

Quakers, Methodists, Presbyterians, Unitarians, and others. Protestantism had reached a point where it was ready to give its own expression to the real work of Christianity, the practice of Christian love. The missionary spirit was apparent in its ranks, and the plight of victims of society's disruption was an increasing source of anxiety to the thoughtful or humane.

PRISON REFORM

John Howard. One of the early exponents of reform was *John Howard* (1727–1789), an English grocer's apprentice, to whom a legacy gave opportunity for travel abroad. A twist of fate made him a prisoner of war in France, and that unlooked-for experience gave him a lifework far removed from the grocery business. After regaining his freedom, Howard began to look around through other prisons to see if they were all as bad as the one he had occupied. He made seven continental tours and managed to find his way into places about which many people had never heard.

Allowing himself no more than six hours of sleep, he spent the time when he was not investigating filthy jails and foul, dark dungeons in writing up his observations. These he had the courage to publish or to present directly to rulers of different nations. The whole story of the degradation of often forgotten human beings was laid before the public, and many changes rewarded his courage and initiative. To Howard, whose primary interest was in prisons, there was some connection between the care of patients, as he had seen it there, and those institutions designed for disease segregation. He visited many hospitals incidentally and wrote a book on "Hospitals and Lazarettos." His comments were to the point, his observation critical and not biased by his faith as a Calvinist. The work of the nuns in Catholic countries impressed him, and he spoke favorably of the Beguines and the Sisters of Charity.

Elizabeth Fry. Howard died in 1789 and about twenty-five years passed before the next step in the history of prison reform was taken through the work of an Englishwoman, *Elizabeth Gurney Fry* (1780–1845), a member of the Society of Friends, or Quakers. About 1811 *Stephen Grellet,* a young French-American among her friends, had begun a round of English prisons, his primary interest being military prisoners from France. Finally he came to London's Newgate, most celebrated of all. It had been destroyed by rioters a few years before and rebuilt. The new exterior was beautiful, but windowless. Conditions within the walls may be gathered from a description which the visitor wrote after seeing the women's quarters to which interest and curiosity had led him:

"They occupied two long rooms, where they slept in three tiers, some on the floor and two tiers of hammocks over one another. . . . When I first entered, the foulness of the air was almost insupportable; and everything that is base and depraved was so strongly depicted on the faces of the women who stood crowded before me with looks of effrontery, boldness and wantonness of expression that for a while my soul was greatly dismayed."[1]

When the same visitor saw the infirmary, he was moved to write:

"On going up, I was astonished beyond description at the mass of woe and misery I beheld. I found many very sick, lying on the bare floor or on some old straw, having very scanty covering over them, though it was quite cold; and there were several children born in the prison among them, almost naked."[2]

It was to help the babies that Grellet hastened to seek out his friend, Elizabeth Fry, a woman on whom he could rely for action. She immediately bought flannel, gathered together a group of women to help with the sewing, and next day took a bundle of clothing to the prison. The sights which met her were strange and harrowing to one who never before had entered this type of institution. She saw sick prisoners lying on filthy straw that could not be changed because no funds had been provided for this necessity, and the prisoners had no money of their own with which to buy it from their gaolers. Adults as well as children were in obvious need of clothing, and all were ill-nourished. All were in need of occupation and diversion.

The outcome was that a school for children was started in Newgate Prison. After this was done, Mrs. Fry contrived to find books and materials for the women who wanted to learn to read and to sew. Already interested in the monitor system which lately had been introduced into English schools, she tried the experiment. Dividing the women into groups, she allowed them to choose their own monitors, and the system worked. She started the women prisoners on the making of gay patchwork and layettes, wisely bringing both color and a ready interest into drab lives. Her next idea was that of producing goods which could be sold outside the prison, the income from which would go to the worker. Soon there was a prison shop where the inmates could purchase simple food and the tea dear to all Englishmen. Elizabeth Fry and her reform of one of the worst prisons in the world earned a fame that spread far beyond England and influenced the steady, slow upward trend of circumstances bearing on the life of the prisoner.

Mrs. Fry thus added her share of stimulus to the movement toward development of social consciousness. Her work, in reality, was but one side of a greater movement progressing throughout England. Distraction of war prevented a corresponding advance on the continent.

---

[1]Whitney, Janet: Elizabeth Fry. Boston, Little, Brown & Co., 1936, p. 193.
[2]*Ibid.,* p. 184.

REFORM IN CARE OF THE MENTALLY ILL

Dorothea Lynde Dix. The next great figure on the stage of social reform came on the scene in America. *Dorothea Lynde Dix* (1802–1887) had been born into the New World just in time to focus her much-needed activities on two inescapable problems, care of the criminal and the mentally ill — problems which her country was then meeting with outworn Old World measures. Miss Dix was thirty nine years of age when she began the work that earned for her the title, "The John Howard of America." For years she had run a private school in Massachusetts for children of the well-to-do, a responsibility to which her social spirit prompted her to add separate classes for the instruction of children of the poor. Overwork and development of the popular public school finished this career and brought on a physical breakdown. Fortunately, she was able to arrange a sea trip which took her to Liverpool, England. The returning ship left behind an invalid who found refuge in a hotel. An influential American friend, however, had paved the way for her social reception by an influential resident of Liverpool, and William Rathbone sought her out.

We shall meet Mr. Rathbone later, as a philanthropist pioneering public health nursing, but now, for more than a year, he and his family undertook the care of Miss Dix. At their beautiful suburban home she not only regained health but experienced keen pleasure from her contacts with people whose interests spread over the field of social betterment. Industrial revolution had but lately embroiled Liverpool in its usual complications of crowding, poor housing, poverty, spells of unemployment, and disease. Miss Dix could lend both sympathy and interest to reformers, for she had seen much the same sort of thing in the mill towns of New England. With broadening social outlook she listened to the experiences and the plans of humanitarians, among whom were those who pushed improvement in prisons and asylums.

Returning to America after a year and a half, Miss Dix found adjustment difficult. Health and circumstances forbade her to resume teaching as a vocation; an inheritance had relieved her of the necessity of earning a livelihood. New interests drew her toward social work, but she had little contact with that considerable group of Americans who were dissatisfied with existing social institutions. People in New England especially, where industry and new facilities for travel were bringing wealth, leisure, and culture, were reading and writing and lecturing as they planned social experiments concerned with abolition of slavery, temperate drinking, better educational methods, better care of mothers.

Miss Dorothea Dix eventually became interested in care of the mentally ill and determined to study the problem from a state-wide point of view. Beginning in Massachusetts, she was able, through systematic investigation, to prepare such a careful record of observations that it could be presented to a legislature and influence its action. On the whole, conditions had been found to be little better than those observed by Elizabeth Fry and Stephen Grellet in England. Until 1839, when the Boston Lunatic Asylum was opened, the city kept its mentally ill in the almshouse, the jails, the House of Industry and the state hospital. Enlargement of the state hospital crowned this earliest work of Miss Dix with success. Thereupon she extended her work to other states, south, as far west as the Mississippi, then into Canada.

The whole present system of mental hospitals under government control gradually came into being as a result of twenty years of effort on the part of Miss Dix. Their foundation principles of expertness of supervision, legal commitment based on medical diagnosis, and abolition of restraint were advocated by one who knew from observation and experience the value of such a program. Success enabled her to carry this experience effectively into Britain and the countries of Europe.

PREVAILING NURSING METHODS EXPOSED

Charles Dickens. The social awakening which Vincent de Paul had stimulated two hundred years before by changing beggars into skilled workers, interesting women in better nursing service, and calling attention to the need of the foundling, John Howard and Elizabeth Fry had hastened through their efforts to reform prisons, and Dorothea Dix, by influencing legislatures to improve care for the mentally ill. *Charles Dickens* (1812–1870) added his weight to the movement by writing humorous, pointed descriptions of evils that he saw. Success enabled him to enlarge his audience by offering cheap editions of his works, and his influence spread over two continents. A lecture tour of America brought the further opportunity of observing and depicting evils there.

Of the middle class himself, Dickens found material for his satire in middle class manners and actions. Always in touch with the very poor lower class, his sympathy with their misery was deepened by an intimate, forced association with them in childhood. Dickens' father had been locked up in a debtors' prison, and there the entire family had resided until freed by a fortunate legacy. His descriptions in "David Copperfield" are the story of personal experience. England's indifference to housing and unsanitary conditions under which her slum dwellers were forced to live were never lost sight of by Dickens. The institutions which society tolerated were also subject to analysis. In "Oliver Twist" he was occupied with the workhouse and its education of children in the ways of crime. The harm wrought by cheap schoolmasters and poor educational method he made known through "Nicholas Nickleby"; the sad lot of the foundling found its way to the reader's heart in "Cricket on the Hearth."

"Martin Chuzzlewit" is a study of selfishness, the outstanding vice of a period when social consciousness lay half dormant. In his study appear two characters of especial interest in our story of trends in nursing. *Betsy*

Prig exemplifies the type of nurse employed as "night watcher" by the important London Hospital of St. Bartholomew. Her friend, *Sairey Gamp,* is the prevailing type to be found in private work. Both are tricking their employers and trying to eke out a better living by accepting double responsibility. Mrs. Gamp accepts a day case while on night duty with the delirious patient whose care she shares with Mrs. Prig as day nurse. A conversation passing between the nurses as they change places in the evening is only one of many disclosures:

" 'I began to think you warn't a coming!' Mrs. Prig observed, in some displeasure.
" 'It shall be made good to-morrow night,' said Mrs. Gamp, 'honorable. I had to go and fetch my things.' She had begun to make signs of inquiry in reference to the position of the patient and his overhearing them—for there was a screen before the door—when Mrs. Prig settled that point easily.
" 'Oh!' she said aloud, 'he's quiet, but his wits is gone. It an't no matter wot you say.'
" 'Anythin' to tell afore you goes, my dear?' asked Mrs. Gamp, setting her bundle down inside the door, and looking affectionately at her partner.
" 'The pickled salmon,' Mrs. Prig replied, 'is quite delicious. I can partick'ler recommend it. Don't have nothink to say to the cold meat, for it tastes of the stable. The drinks is all good.'
"Mrs. Gamp expressed herself much gratified.
" 'The physic and them things is on the drawers and mankleshelf,' said Mrs. Prig, cursorily. 'He took his last slime draught at seven. The easy-chair an't soft enough. You'll want his piller.' "

And yet Dickens, assigning his ideal of a good nurse to a poor one so that the ridiculous may emphasize the contrast, makes this same Sairey Gamp exclaim:

"What a blessed thing it is to make sick people happy in their bed, and never mind one's self as long as one can do a service! I don't believe a finer cowcumber was ever growed. I am sure I never see one![3]

Nevertheless, the dream of good nursing as an expression of Christian service was already on the way to realization, for a Protestant pastor in a tiny German village on the Rhine was busy blazing the trail that would help the nursing situation in Protestant countries, as St. Vincent de Paul's Sisters of Charity had been changing it in Catholic countries.

ORDER OF MODERN DEACONESSES FOUNDED

In the early days of the nineteenth century, in Kaiserwerth, a little town near Düsseldorf on the Rhine River in Germany, Theodor Fliedner, pastor of the local Lutheran church, and Friederike Fliedner, his bride,

---

[3]Dickens, Charles: Martin Chuzzlewit. New York, Charles Scribner's Sons, 1911.

embarked on a project that gave to Protestants a model social substitute for the lost monastery and changed the concept of nursing far beyond the borders of Germany. Behind the success that attended the Kaiserswerth Institution lay a long trail of attempts at organized nursing through Protestant sisterhoods, or through the restoration of the old church order of deaconesses. Much loyal service was given, as it always had been, by individual women.

Pastor Fliedner arrived at Kaiserswerth in 1821 to find himself head of a congregation that was learning the meaning of financial depression. The silk mills, which gave its members their daily bread, closed down a few weeks later. There was no chance of paying the new minister's salary. An offer of another church tempted him, but the young preacher in his earnestness wanted to be "a true shepherd, not an hireling." Faithful to an ideal in faithfulness to his flock, he set out to solicit abroad the funds which could not be found at home. He journeyed through Holland and England and obtained the money. Moreover, he met a great many people of influence, among them Elizabeth Fry whose work in Newgate prison made a deep impression on him. He inspected public institutions, schools, almshouses, hospitals, and prisons, and in Holland he observed the work of deaconesses. He returned to little Kaiserswerth with great eagerness to bring prison reform into Germany and to train deaconesses who would take hold of its problems of education, poor relief, and nursing. He and Friederike, both able organizers, entered upon a difficult path that eventually led them to fame.

Pastor Fliedner succeeded in starting a German Prison Association, but when he tried to interest women in prison work he met discouragement, for popular sentiment condemned the association of good women with degraded wrongdoers and decreed that all decent women stay at home. One day a homeless girl, who was an ex-convict, came to beg shelter of the Fliedners. Gladly, but with some misgiving, they installed her in a little one-room house that stood in their garden. *Minna* became a loyal friend, and the little house became a prisoner's refuge which grew and grew as it succeeded in bringing about the better adjustment of criminals to society.

The next unit was a hospital, a responsibility assumed to provide care of the sick and a field for the instruction of deaconesses. By this time, his observations and friendships at home and abroad had acquainted Pastor Fliedner with the general lack of good nurses. The deaconess seemed to him and his wife an ideal solution to the problem. Friederike's own experience as Kaiserswerth's first deaconess led her to believe that it was useless to try to revive the old-time order without due consideration of changed times and an altered outlook in young women. Both realized that it was an idea that would cost money to put into effect.

Faith in a divine goodness that had given them means to carry on their work up to this time led this pious pair to promise to pay for the best house in town, which stood empty. Their faith was justified, for when the time to pay arrived, they were able to do so. There was enough furniture in the house to begin work, and the first patient was admitted on October 16, 1836. The first probationer arrived shortly afterwards. She was *Gertrud Reichardt,* a doctor's daughter who had helped her father with his patients. Notwithstanding her old friendship with the Fliedners and her resolve to become a deaconess, Gertrud found staying difficult. The hospital looked very bare after her comfortable home, and there seemed so little to work with that she was moved to doubt God's favor toward the whole undertaking. " 'No I cannot work here,' she said, 'God cannot be with you, or He would at least provide you with necessaries.' She was about to put on her cloak when the rumbling of a heavily laden wagon was heard, and a gruff voice called out: 'Does Pastor Fliedner live here?' As the driver unloaded the precious freight of hospital necessaries, Gertrud Reichardt was convinced that God was indeed with Theodor Fliedner."[4] Under the leadership of Friederike Fliedner, Gertrud Reichardt served for seventeen years. During the first year of her training six other young women arrived who aspired to become deaconesses too.

The burden of organizing the work of the hospital, of selecting the right women to become deaconesses, of instructing them and assigning their work, all fell upon Mrs. Fliedner. How well fitted she was for the responsibility is clear from the systematic way in which she arranged things from the beginning. There were wards for men, women, and children, with a deaconess in each, and an orderly nursed the men under her direction. House cleaning, cooking, washing, and the care of linen fell in turn on the deaconesses. The garden which supplied vegetables and fruits was also theirs to care for, and one of them regularly spent her summer there.

An interested physician, with the help of a manual in use at the Charity Hospital in Berlin, gave clinical and theoretical instruction in the art of nursing. Students had opportunity, too, to study pharmacy and took the state examination for pharmacists. All of this looks simple, perhaps, to those accustomed to routinized procedure, but to Friederike Fliedner it was pioneer work that grew rapidly and had to be accomplished with minimum funds. There were inescapable family duties besides. Nine babies of her own came to her, so her personal household was large in spite of the fact that four died at birth. Nevertheless, her beloved hospital and school for deaconesses soon came to be known beyond Kaiserswerth and Germany, and Elizabeth Fry journeyed from England to see them. Her story brought Florence Nightingale, and there were many others interested in humanitarian and health problems who made similar pilgrimage. Kaiserswerth was generous in sharing experience and achievement, and visitors were made welcome.

---

[4]Gallison, Marie: The Ministry of Women: One Hundred Years of Women's Work at Kaiserswerth, 1836–1936 (a pamphlet). The Lutterworth Press, London.

The work of the Kaiserswerth Deaconess Institution profited, no doubt, by the example of St. Vincent de Paul, whose Sisters of Charity had proved the superiority of their preparation for nursing during two hundred years in which they had earned a world's affection. Its prime purpose was to instruct women of such religious bent that they wished to be admitted to the ancient church office of deaconess and participate in its social service. The training of the deaconess was designed to fit her for *teaching* or *nursing,* but with these vocations it combined the study of relief work among the poor, prison work, and rescue work. A simple vow was taken to work for the love of Christ and to follow Him in caring for the poor, the sick or those in need of any help.

One of the most amazing things about Kaiserswerth in its early stages of growth is the amount of work accomplished under conditions close to poverty. Donations are never a reliable source of income, and times were hard, but Father Fliedner's faith was great, and sometimes its reward savored of the miraculous. A framework of organization was developed with passing years which proved worthy to become a model for deaconess institutions wherever they were established. Around the original home of the pastor and his garden house there eventually clustered the following units offering facilities for the instruction of his deaconesses:

A hospital of one hundred and twenty beds
A "Lunatic Asylum" for female patients
An Infant School for forty children of all creeds
An Orphan Asylum for Protestant girls
A Day School for girls which was also attended by the orphans
A Normal School with grades for practice teaching in preparation
  for school and governess work
An asylum for released female prisoners and "Magdalenes"

All deaconesses were assigned, in turn, to definite stations, and teaching deaconesses were given a term of service in the care of sick children. Those deaconesses who would devote themselves particularly to nursing served in separate wards for men, women, and children, as well as in units for communicable disease, for convalescents, and for sick deaconesses. Additional stations included the apothecary's room, kitchen, laundry, sewing room, and garden.

A glance at the system regulating school organization and acceptance of students makes more obvious the relationship existing between Kaiserswerth methods and those of the specialized, secular school of nursing which later owed some inspiration to this source:

Three years' course
Eighteen years as minimum age for admission

Letters from clergyman and physician in certification of good character and health

Probationary period of three months to a year

Allowance of pocket money (about twenty-five dollars a year)

Instruction by class and lecture

Rotation of practice in departments of hospital and institution

Division of students into junior, senior, and head sister groups

Uniform dress

Student deaconesses at Kaiserswerth came from no one group in society, and their days were passed under most democratic conditions. Princesses and peasants alike got up at five o'clock in the morning and worked and studied side by side until nine o'clock at night. Night duty was covered by day nurses in turn. About once a week, instead of going off duty at nine o'clock, a day nurse would stay on until midnight. The night nurse who relieved her was one who had retired on leaving the wards at nine o'clock, and arose at midnight to begin a day that would end twenty-one hours later. The uniform dress is described as of dark blue material for workdays, with plain black for Sundays. A bibbed apron was worn with the blue dress, while a hoodlike cap with ruffle about the

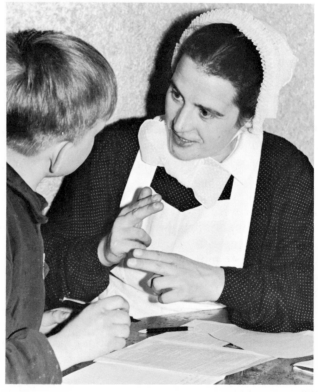

Figure 42. A Kaiserswerth Deaconess teaching the Handicapped. (Photograph by Hans Lachmann.)

face had broad strings to tie becomingly in a perky bow under young chins, a picture further enhanced by a becoming white collar. A black bonnet in the fashion of the day, and likewise held fast by white strings, covered the head for street wear.

Both Pastor Fliedner and his wife instilled ethics into their pupils and taught them the necessity of loyal cooperation with the physician for the benefit of his patient. However, the Fliedners made some mistakes. The placing of education in institutions dependent on voluntary subscription made their economic position hazardous. There was a temptation to keep deaconess nurses on cases in private homes and thereby increase the institutional income. Long hours of work and a rest period depending on conscience, were dangerous advantages to set before more commercial souls than those possessed by Theodor and Friederike Fliedner. Sooner or later, the tradition of no paid help would become firm as it was elsewhere in nursing institutions, and the loophole made for noneducational duties would show itself to be very elastic.

The *motherhouse system,* however, made up in some measure for abuses that were sure to come. It offered deaconesses a certain amount of security in providing for them a permanent home. They were children of Kaiserswerth, and from this home they were sent to district, hospital, and private duty assignment, and often to distant mission fields, but always they were under the direction and protection of the Institution. Always, they knew that in Kaiserswerth there was a place for them when their work was over. Obviously, the motherhouse system was an offspring of the old monastic system.

So honorable a reputation did the deaconess earn in society that Pastor Fliedner finally had to give up his pastorate and give exclusive attention to establishing branch Deaconess Houses, to assignment of graduates to teaching, prison or relief positions, and to the introduction of nursing staffs in hospitals. His work took on the proportions of a movement, and other pastors followed his lead by establishing schools, not all of which were as good as Kaiserswerth. Kaiserswerth deaconesses soon found themselves established at Jerusalem, Smyrna, Beyrouth, Constantinople, Alexandria, Cairo, Bucharest, and Budapest. In 1850 Father Fliedner took several of them to Pittsburgh in America where, at the request of Pastor Passavant, they staffed his hospital, still known as the "Passavant Hospital." About the same time a Deaconess Home and Hospital was founded at Milwaukee, young city in a great Middle West. When Father Fliedner passed away in 1864 there were nearly five hundred deaconesses scattered in small groups over four continents.

Friederike Fliedner, ambitious and energetic cofounder of Kaiserswerth, had died over twenty years before. To her the movement owed a primary stimulus, unmeasurable perhaps, but unforgettable. She was one of those first women who insisted on emerging from the retirement into which medieval conditions forced women, and who dared to combine family with public duty. Her capacity in both fields is acknowledged. On her shoulders rested the main burden of devising those details of general management, of curriculum, and of student practice which were the basis of the Deaconess Institution's success.

After the death of Friederike, Pastor Fliedner had been blessed further in finding a worthy successor to sustain his family life and his deaconess project. *Caroline Bertheau,* former pupil of Amalie Sieveking (founder of a home-visiting association. "The Friends of the Poor"), was in charge of the nursing at the Hamburg Hospital when Fliedner met her. She brought both experience and devotion to the Kaiserswerth institution. She was a good mother to Friederike's children, bore eight children of her own, and directed Kaiserswerth for twenty years after Pastor Fliedner died.

One immediate result of the experiment at Kaiserswerth was the establishment in England of an Institute of Nursing Sisters. Here, in 1840, Elizabeth Fry undertook to interpret her appreciation of Pastor Fliedner's work by gathering together in this home a selected group of women. They were known as *"Protestant Nursing Sisters,"* wore an attractive uniform and did district and private nursing among the poor. The only training was a short term of experience in Guy's Hospital, London, but this and their superior character unexpectedly led to Sisters being carried off into the private duty field.

The strongest church influence in England at this time was the national, or established, church, which deviated in considerably less degree from the old church than did the numerous sects grouped as "non-conformists." What followed was natural. A series of Sisterhoods under this English church made their appearance, beginning with the Protestant *Order of Mercy* in 1845. Three years later there came into being the *Sisterhood of St. John's House,* the name derived from its location in the district of St. John the Evangelist in London. *Sisters of St. John, first Protestant religious order devoting itself wholly to nursing, took a place beside the Augustinians, oldest nursing order of the Catholic Church.* Just as the latter had entered the hospital field through the Hôtel Dieu of Paris, so the nurses of St. John staffed the King's College Hospital in London and before long supplied improved nursing staffs for a number of other English institutions. Wherever they took over a hospital service, however, the Sisters of St. John's House established a new precedent of reserving to the Sisterhood the right to control the nursing activities.

In 1851 the *Sisterhood of All Saints* was established and, in 1854, that of *St. Margaret.* Other communities followed these, and there was a nursing fraternity known as the *Cowley Brothers.* The main accomplishment during these years of English experiment was the introduction of a minor group of more or less poorly prepared better-class women into district and private nursing.

Although they gave abundantly, and some of them still function, the new orders were not adequate to fill public needs, and the public mind was divided on the question of religious motive as a requisite for good nursing. In the main the orders themselves held nursing a secondary interest to spiritual self-development and missionary work. Ancient tradition set nursing aside as a service inspired by religion, free, and accompanied by self-sacrifice. People like Mrs. Fry, who felt that good women might do good nursing in secular groups and for remuneration, were "moderns."

Various proposals were forthcoming, and there were hints of plans for more substantial nurse training, but up to 1860 no great change came. Rich private patients and a limited group of the very poor reaped the advantage of any improvement made. England was not ready to use the principles of nurse preparation being demonstrated at Kaiserswerth. America made limited use of them, but continental Europe profited most, for here the deaconess throve side by side with the Beguines and the Sisters of Charity. Some of the filth of hospitals of this dark period was cleaned up; some patients received better care; but the majority of institutions remained unchanged. At the same time, more and more influential people were learning to appreciate the personal advantage of having cultured women take care of them and their families during illness.

FLORENCE NIGHTINGALE: REFORMER OF HOSPITALS AND NURSING

EARLY LIFE

Florence Nightingale belonged to the layer of English society which included those businessmen who had grown well-to-do through development of the natural resources of their country or through trade. Lead mining, marble works, and grocery stores in the capable hands of relatives had bestowed upon her parents, by inheritance, financial freedom and the privilege of collecting rents. In youth, both parents had been subject to the best influences of their time. Their lives were set in a milieu of people who shared with them the pleasures of what is known as "good society," but who, like them, enjoyed the privilege of friendships among the aristocracy. Politicians, literary men, artists, and some who merely played, were in their "set." Their religious affiliation, somewhat unique at that time, was Unitarian. Florence's beautiful mother appears to have been a woman of conservative tastes, thoroughly Victorian in her outlook, the daughter of a member of Parliament. Her father had more elasticity in his nature and took gentle pleasure in literature and art. He was a college graduate, knew mathematics, was a master of foreign languages, and read in the classics, natural science, history, and philosophy.

Travel at that time was difficult, but Mr. Nightingale was interested enough to overlook difficulties, and it was in Italy that his two daughters were born, Parthenope in Naples, and Florence, on May 12, 1820, in the beautiful cultural and intellectual center from which she received her name. It was a name which the fame of this distinguished owner made popular for girl babies of generations who followed this little Florence of the Nightingales. When the family returned to England, a comfortable new home was built at Embley Park, not far from Romsey. Here "Parthe" and "Flo" spent happy years amid the trees and flowers and birds of a southern English garden.

The monotony of country life was varied by an annual carriage drive to London and a visit to a northern home called "Lea Hurst," situated in Derbyshire, near the Derwent River and the lead mines of a chill area, the barrenness of which industry had made more forbidding. Long visits were made in both places, and governesses became part of the household. Mr. Nightingale himself took particular pleasure in teaching Latin and Greek to Florence along with mathematics, science, and languages, and in educating her to enjoyment of his books. These two became good friends as they read and talked and, when separated in after years, carried on lengthy correspondence. Mrs. Nightingale leaned toward the older and less original sister and found Florence somewhat difficult to understand.

At seventeen, Miss Nightingale, the young lady, finished her education in continental Europe. This time the family traveled for a year and a half in France, Italy, and Switzerland, enjoying scenery, art, and society. It was on this trip that Florence was introduced to one of the great salons where she met some of the most distinguished men of France and, incidentally, learned of some of the social activities of distinguished Frenchwomen. It was a time when the talk of liberty and war for liberty was stirring Italy as it had shortly before stirred France. She was interested in politics and people, but charitable institutions strangely intrigued her. Everywhere she went she tried to acquaint herself with social conditions for the conviction had come to her that some day God would appoint her to fulfill a mission of mercy for Him. She must be ready when the time came. Years after she explained this as she wrote.

"Thoughts and feelings that I have now I can remember since I was six years old. It was not I that made them. A profession, a trade, a necessary occupation, something to fill and employ all my faculties, I have always felt essential to me, I have always longed for, consciously or not. ... The first thought I can remember and the last, was nursing work; and in the absence of this, education work, but more the education of the bad than of the young. But for this I had had no education myself."[5]

[5]Cooke, Sir Edward: A Short Life of Florence Nightingale, 1925, p. 40. By permission of The Macmillan Company, publishers.

Meantime, Miss Nightingale went on doing what she could toward self-education, and she was always especially happy when helping someone. At home, she found opportunity in the industrial village beyond the trees of Lea Hurst for observing at close range the life of the poor, and for doing something toward relief of the sick.

"One sees in every cottage some trouble that defies sympathy."
"All that poets sing of the glories of this world appears to me untrue; all the people I see are eaten up with care or poverty or disease."
"To find out what we can do, one's individual place, as well as the general end, is Man's task."[6]

Diary writing, a current fashion in which men as well as women indulged, was not an altogether satisfactory outlet for this young dreamer, but it helped her to come to a decision as to the kind of work she would choose to do if choice were before her. As she wrote up her daily doings, she was reminded of unsatisfactory nursing conditions in hospitals and of a need for sisters in England like the Sisters of Charity of St. Vincent de Paul. Nursing would be just the work she would like best to do. She would be a nurse. To her orthodox mother, useful occupation was not an impossible thing for a daughter of hers, but the acquisition of a husband was of first importance. A married woman, under protection of a husband and his name, could do things that Victorian ideas of propriety did not permit an unmarried woman to do. An Elizabeth Gurney Fry might visit those terrible people in Newgate, but an Elizabeth Gurney! No, certainly not! She would try to make Florence forget a foolish, youthful notion.

In her own home, however, Florence was meeting people whose interests lay in many kinds of social work and reform — women and men who were free to carry on prison work, educational reform, and workhouse reform. Among them was a leading physician of the town of Salisbury in the neighboring shire. She thought it would be nice to go to the hospital in that town to learn nursing by doing it and to pick up what knowledge she might by observation. The big drawing room at home, she said, made her wonder how it could be made over into a hospital ward. She knew friends who were doing things away off in America, too. When Julia Ward Howe and Dr. Howe visited her home, she asked him if it would be a very terrible thing to devote her life to nursing. Indeed, it was not long before all sympathetic listeners came to know that young Florence Nightingale wanted to be a nurse, and that she was restrained from this thoroughly useful occupation only by parental unwillingness.

Accepting the parental dictum as best she could, Miss Nightingale turned to the study of the new sanitation that her friend, *Sir Edwin Chadwick,* was succeeding in bringing before the public. Friends abroad

---

[6]*Ibid.,* pp. 12, 14, 15. By permission of The Macmillan Company, publishers.

sent her what they could in the way of information regarding the Fliedner undertaking of which she had heard from Mrs. Fry. She continued to cherish her dream of becoming a nurse and, perhaps, of forming some day a Sisterhood of educated women who would be proficient nurses. In 1847 came an opportunity to visit the continent again, and in Rome she turned from the study of art to the study of a community of nuns. The Sister Superior found kinship in the attractive stranger and permitted her to stay in the convent during ten days of retreat. Miss Nightingale was privileged to listen to the addresses that she gave to nuns and novices and to study their mode of life. Systematic person that she was, she made notes of her observations for use when the longed-for opportunity to improve the nurses and the nursing of England should be hers. In Rome, too, she had the pleasure of meeting Mrs. Herbert and Sir Sidney Herbert, the man in whose hands fate, unknown to all of them, was preparing to place the key to this opportunity.

Other opportunities for gaining social understanding came to this girl who wanted to study nursing and could find no way of doing so. Inevitably she ran into the ever-recurring question of marriage. Indeed, one of her admirers proved so attractive that Florence found it hard to refuse him, and only after considerable deliberation made a decision disappointing to him and equally so to a mother who wanted to see her daughter "settled." The old desire for soul-filling work stood in the way. Florence Nightingale was one of those "new" women of the nineteenth century who wanted a career.

"I could be satisfied to spend a life with him combining our different powers in some great object. . . . Voluntarily to put it out of my power ever to be able to seize the chance of forming for myself a true and rich life would seem to me like suicide."[7]

Marriage without full community of interest looked impossible. She had only pity for the social-minded woman whom marriage thrusts into a little routine and compels to live apart from the larger life of the husband.

"Such a woman," she writes later when she had seen more of life, "longs for a profession . . . struggles to open to woman the paths of the school, the hospital, the penitentiary, the care of the young sick, the bad,—not as an amusement, to fill up odd times, to fancy they have done something when they have done nothing, to make a sham of visiting—but systematically, as a reality, an occupation, a 'profession.' . . . Without the right cultivation and employment of all the powers . . . there can be no repose, and with it repose may be found in a hell, in a hospital of wounds and pain and operations and death and remorse and tears and despair."[8]

---

[7]Cooke, Sir Edward: A Short Life of Florence Nightingale, 1925, p. 34. By permission of The Macmillan Company, publishers.

[8]*Ibid.*

In 1849, Miss Nightingale accompanied friends to Egypt. On the way home, she was to have a long promised visit with Theodor and Friederike Fliedner, the two persons who seemed to have realized an ideal that eluded her. Meantime, the city of Alexandria gave opportunity to learn intimately the work of the Sisters of Charity of St. Vincent de Paul. In Greece she met American missionaries and studied the school and orphanage which they were running. In Berlin she made the rounds of hospitals, and finally Kaiserswerth, her Mecca, was reached. For a happy two weeks in August, 1850, she observed what had been done and listened to the Fliedner plans and hopes. Then, more than ever impressed with the need of systematic training for that lifework toward which she groped, she returned home.

Not long afterwards, opportunity came. In 1851 her sister was advised to go to Carlsbad Mineral Springs for her health. The resort was in Germany and it was decided that while her mother and Parthenope remained there, the time was opportune for Florence to go into residence at Kaiserswerth. The visit was to be kept from the knowledge of friends, but the Sidney Herberts knew of it and came to see her and the institution. Three months spent at this time with the founders of the Deaconess Institution made a lasting impression and gave Miss Nightingale valued material to use later in the foundation of a profession that now seemed so remote.

After that, Miss Nightingale of Embley Park and Lea Hurst again sought satisfaction for the emptiness of life in writing. She was thirty-three before her mother, at last convinced of her determination to follow a "career," sent her abroad once more, this time to study the work of the Sisters of Charity in Paris. At the last moment the opportunity almost slipped away from her. Her father tried to keep her at home by offering her a little house to convert into an institution; her mother could not refrain from objecting; a sick relative needed her. In the end, however, she found herself installed in Paris with a public permit authorizing her to look over its hospitals, infirmaries, and religious houses.

FIRST POSITION

Every possible bit of printed information about methods of hospital management and nursing was meticulously written up. There were interruptions. Miss Nightingale got the measles while in Paris with the Sisters of Charity. She had to go home to nurse her grandmother in a fatal illness. Undaunted, she returned to the task to which she had set herself. Persistence and ambition were rewarded, at last, by news of a vacancy in the position of superintendent of the Establishment for Gentlewomen during Illness, a small institution at 1 Upper Harley Street in London, which offered shelter to homeless ladies and nursing care to sick governesses.

It is interesting to follow Miss Nightingale through the excitements of making formal application for a position and appearing before the Board of Managers for personal interview. She knew her own mind and succeeded in arranging for her share of authority without interference, as well as for conveniences like bells, hot water, and such an innovation as an elevator. The Board, in turn, would not act without assurance that her parents did not object. Finally all was settled, and Florence at the age of thirty-three entered upon the professional career for which she had been preparing herself since she was seventeen. Her ability was soon acknowledged, but her desire to organize a training school for nurses had to be curbed in deference to the ruling of a Board that could not understand it. Energy and imagination, however, led her to incorporate a degree of social work into her duties. Besides nursing her governesses, she characteristically undertook to find convalescent homes or jobs for them when they left her or, through her friend, Sir Sidney Herbert, to locate them in America through a placement society of his sponsoring.

CRIMEAN WAR SERVICE, 1854–1856

In a short time newspapers were full of complaints of neglect of English soldiers wounded in a war on the Crimean peninsula in the Black Sea where England and France were assisting Turkey in a war against Russia. Sisters of Charity were there nursing France's soldiers, and Sisters of Mercy were nursing those of Russia. "Why have we no Sisters of Charity?" someone asked in the London Times. Mr. and Mrs. Nightingale once more found themselves called upon to give parental sanction, and their daughter wrote to her friend Mrs. Herbert to tell her that she thought of accepting charge of a privately financed expedition of four nurses as an immediate answer to a public need. This plan was changed on receipt of a letter from Sir Sidney Herbert who, strangely enough, had already written Miss Nightingale to ask if she would consider going to the Crimea under appointment by the government. Their letters crossed and the young woman who one day was to write, "The Lord helps those who keep moving," was learning this truth. Always learning, always going ahead, she was ready for a great opportunity.

In his position of Secretary for War, Sir Sidney knew the situation thoroughly and understood the reluctance of army officials to introduce women to the service. He knew, too, that personality, knowledge, administrative capacity, and social prestige combined to make Miss Nightingale the "one person that I know of in England who would be capable of organizing and superintending such a scheme."[9] Five days later official

---

[9] Cooke, Sir Edward: A Short Life of Florence Nightingale, 1925, p. 74. By permission of The Macmillan Company, New York, publishers.

orders were put through, and Florence Nightingale began the work of preparation "as calm and composed in this furious haste as if she were going for a walk."[10]

It was with great difficulty that suitable nurses were found, but at last there was a unit numbering thirty eight in all, ten Roman Catholic Sisters, eight Sisters of Mercy and six Sisters of St. John's House, both orders of the English church, and fourteen practical nurses from hospital staffs. The government appointed Miss Nightingale as Superintendent of the Nursing Staff, or, as she came to be called, "Lady-in-Chief." On October 21, 1854, one week after she had written her letter to Mrs. Herbert, Miss Nightingale and the nurse corps were on their way. From London they traveled to the coast, crossed the English Channel to Boulogne, thence to Paris and on to Marseilles on the Mediterranean. There they boarded ship for Scutari, suburb of Constantinople and site of a hospital base opposite that city on the Straits of Bosporus. From the Crimean Peninsula on the other side of the Black Sea were coming the wounded, crowded into unsanitary ships, and without anything that could be called nursing care. Back in England Florence Nightingale, still a stranger to them, was already famous as the leader of a brave rescue. Public opinion was behind her, and soon the government as well.

On November 4, 1854, England's new nurses landed at Scutari and found, not one, but two hospitals filled and awaiting them. Ten members of the unit were assigned to the General Hospital, and the remainder quartered at the Barrack Hospital, a half-hour's walk distant. This had been a soldiers' barracks, and still was only partially adapted to housing of wounded men. A three-story building in the form of a square, it had wards opening off corridors, the total length of which was four miles. A tower arose from each corner, and the rooms in one of these towers became the nurses' quarters. In the cold hospital wards were nearly eighteen hundred patients, bedbug-ridden and lice-infested. Sanitary arrangements had proved inadequate. Ventilation was poor. Rats and mice ran free. Candles in bottles supplied illumination. Overflow patients lay on the floors, and all lacked adequate covering. Dysentery from a poor water supply and fever added their complications. Food was so poor that the men could not eat it, and besides, there were neither knives nor forks. "Not a basin, nor a towel, not a bit of soap nor a broom could be found."[11]

No time was to be lost for more wounded were even then being landed. What could be done toward feeding the sick in the wards and replacing dirty clothing was the first move. Miss Nightingale secured brushes and cloths, and when her group had done what they could toward cleaning up, she realized that a healthful hospital was still an impos-

---

[10]Cooke, Sir Edward: A Short Life of Florence Nightingale, 1925, p. 9. By permission of The Macmillan Company, New York, publishers.

[11]*Ibid.*, p. 96.

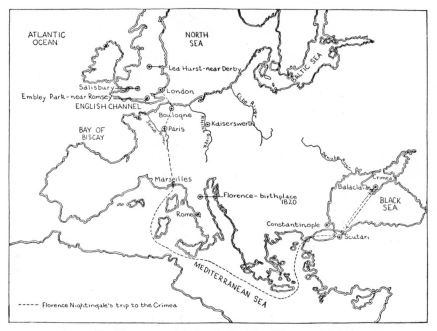

Figure 43. Places associated with the life of Florence Nightingale.

sibility unless water supply and sewer system were changed. These were things that must be reported to the government. An inadequate laundry service she remedied herself by renting a house in Scutari, having boilers installed, and paying soldiers' wives to do the washing. In the already crowded quarters of the nurses, in a central room on the first floor off which their bedrooms opened, space was made for a combined diet kitchen and storeroom, and a smaller room was used for an office.

In the three diet kitchens eventually opened the nurses cooked tempting, nourishing foods for the very sick. From the same storeroom which provided stoves and some of the food came other supplies which Miss Nightingale had had the foresight to bring with her, and which were issued on requisition signed by a medical officer. These supplemented army deficiencies or offset unbreakable "red tape." In a letter to Mrs. Herbert, Miss Nightingale described herself as a "kind of general dealer in socks, shirts, knives and forks, wooden spoons, tin baths, tables and forms, cabbages and carrots, operating tables, towels, soap, fine tooth combs, precipitate for destroying lice, scissors, bedpans and stump pillows."[12] In the first three months ten thousand shirts alone were given out. In order to provide necessary beds for eight hundred new patients, she even found it necessary to remodel unused wards at her own expense so as to have them ready in time for their occupants. The money thus spent was later refunded by Parliament.

---

[12]Official History of American Red Cross Nursing, 1922, p. 3. By permission of The Macmillan Company, New York, publishers.

The office became the seat of business and conference, and often, long after midnight, of a huge and personal correspondence that must all be done by hand. Social prestige made possible a direct confidential relationship between Miss Nightingale and people of political power. In other words, she had that useful possession now known as "pull." Comprehensive reports of sanitary conditions written by her aroused such concern among authorities in England that experts were sent to investigate. Changes made according to her suggestion, together with nursing care and dietary treatment, brought a drop in death rate from about 40 to 2 per cent. Graphic descriptions of surroundings and nursing brought large sums of money from individuals and groups who were eager to help. The following description of her personality was written while she was thus earning the gratitude of a people and the approbation of a Queen:

"In appearance, Miss Nightingale is just what you would expect in any other well-bred woman, who may have seen perhaps rather more than thirty years of life; her manner and countenance are prepossessing, and this without the possession of positive beauty; it is a face not easily forgotten, pleasing in its smile, with an eye betokening great self-possession, and giving, when she wishes, a quiet look of firm determination to every feature. Her general demeanour is quiet and rather reserved; still I am much mistaken if she is not gifted with a very lively sense of the ridiculous. In conversation, she speaks on matters of business with a grave earnestness one would not expect from her appearance.

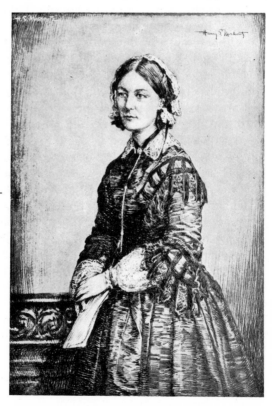

Figure 44. Florence Nightingale.

She has evidently a mind disciplined to restrain under the principles of the action of the moment every feeling which would interfere with it. She has trained herself to command, and learned the value of conciliation towards others and constraint over herself. I can conceive her to be a strict disciplinarian; she throws herself into a work as its head. As such she knows well how much success must depend upon literal obedience to her every order. . . . Miss Nightingale . . . in my opinion, is the one individual who in this whole unhappy war has shown more than any other what real energy guided by good sense can do to meet the calls of sudden emergency."[13]

Power, admiration, and respect gradually came to the young nurse who had longed for opportunity, but they were not won without opposition. There were medical officers and others who, mistaking her eager aggressiveness, looked upon her as a nuisance. There were those who went so far as to work against her, and there were patients who never knew the benefits of the care which her sister nurses offered but could give only when the doctor did not object. The hard-earned prestige was also threatened by bungling at home. Miss Nightingale had asked for more nurses, stipulating that they be given preliminary training in London hospitals. A group of forty six women arrived, but they were under a new and untrained head and knew almost nothing about nursing themselves. Their orders, moreover, assigned them, not to Miss Nightingale, but to the military officer in command. The complications resulting almost ended in her resignation but ultimately were straightened out and the young women distributed.

Other groups of nurses followed, and lady volunteers with neither training nor experience beyond home nursing. The number of women working under Florence Nightingale's direction gradually came to be one hundred and twenty five. Some returned home of their own accord or were sent back for misdemeanor or incompetence. Some became too ill to continue in the service, and nine died.

Two hospitals located at the front in the Crimea were staffed with nurses and equipped with diet kitchens like the three already set up in Scutari. Miss Nightingale crossed the Black Sea to take charge of the nursing in these hospitals at Balaclava. On horseback or in a carriage given her by the army, she covered the distances between them, ignoring darkness and loneliness, danger, storm, cold, and weariness. By special permission she went on the battlefield itself. It was in the midst of this strenuous work that she contracted Crimean fever. She was always indifferent to contagion, but it had caught up with her finally and now brought her very close to death. After her recovery part of her time was spent at Scutari and part at Balaclava.

Army nursing under Florence Nightingale gradually expanded into a health service, working hand in hand with the new sanitary science.

[13]Cooke, Sir Edward: A Short Life of Florence Nightingale, 1925, p. 134. By permission of The Macmillan Company, New York, publishers.

Drunkenness among the soldiery was lessened by setting up reading rooms, providing amusements and lectures, and establishing a canteen. She eased minds of sick men by writing letters for them, starting the allotment of their pay to needy families at home, and providing employment and care for those wives who accompanied their husbands to the scene of war. Always it was her custom to make rounds in the wards at night, stopping to observe the condition of the sickest patients. She was lighted along her way by a lantern or oil lamp, famous in the army long before Henry Wadsworth Longfellow endowed with immortality "Santa Filomena," the Lady of the Lamp.

While the soldiers of England were thus benefiting under the supervision and care of Florence Nightingale and her nurses, in the hospitals of the Russians, sick and wounded men were finding corresponding help and encouragement through the efforts of one of their countrywomen. The *Grand Duchess Pavlova*, having secured the enlistment of three hundred ladies of Moscow and St. Petersburg who were willing to give assistance, used them to staff Russian army hospitals of the Crimea. So much did she accomplish and so great was the appreciation of her group, known as "Sisters of Mercy," that it was said of them, "She provided them with

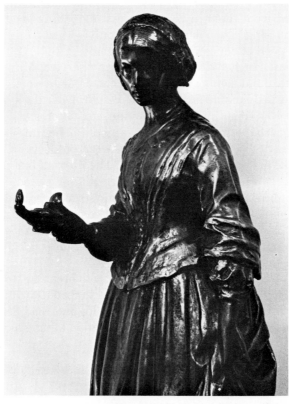

Figure 45. Statue of Florence Nightingale. From the Crimean Memorial that stands on the Thames embankment at Waterloo Place, London, England. (Photo by Paul Barbuto.)

everything necessary and these saintly women were blessed by thousands of soldiers."[14]

Professionally, some of the English nursing group proved to be excellent nurses, some very poor, and some gave a lot of trouble. As the army had not heretofore had the service of women nurses, they had no defined position in its organization, and a defined position is a sacred thing to military men. With little help from tradition, a method of discipline suitable to the circumstances of army life had to be worked out and established. Even under the advantage of accepted power of control, this was not easy among women of varying social status, varying education, varying religion, in times when people were highly conscious of class and sectarian barriers and anxious to maintain them.

It was Florence Nightingale's first real job of nursing supervision, for the Harley Street institution had been small. Her own broad views prevented discrimination between sect or church, and she asked only that the women work together in "a common brotherhood of love to God and man."[15] No one knew better than she what she owed to those women who stood by her loyally, adapting themselves to new and difficult circumstances, and giving the best that was in them to their patients. She learned to have an intense pride in their accomplishment and appreciated all she gained from them in regard to distinguishing good from bad in nurses and nursing. Their shortcomings only served to make her more aware of the need of education for all nurses.

Army Dress. In her dress while in army service, Miss Nightingale favored practical but sombre shades. She customarily wore gray or black, with the then fashionable simple white cap over her dark hair. A black handkerchief was sometimes tied over the cap. Often she added a rough apron which, perhaps, may be taken as symbolic of her intensely practical outlook. A heavy cloak and bonnet were worn outdoors in this country where the winters brought snow storms. The dress of her nurses was of corresponding sobriety. They wore dresses of grey tweed, wool jackets, and caps so unbecoming that at least one nurse declared she would never have come had she known about the head gear. A brownish linen scarf embroidered in red with the name "Scutari Hospital" was worn as a protection in going about the eastern port town. Short woolen capes completed the outfit.

The time finally drew near for the group to break up, to discard conventions of army life so harshly learned, and to readjust to civil life. They were tired out, just as was Miss Nightingale, and readjustment would be hard. Some among them would be fortunate in having a convent wait-

---

[14]From The Origin of the Red Cross ("Un Souvenir de Solferino") by Henri Dunant, translated from the French by Mrs. David H. Wright. The John C. Winston Co., 1911, pp. 80–81.

[15]Cooke, Sir Edward: A Short Life of Florence Nightingale, 1925, p. 80. By permission of The Macmillan Company, New York, publishers.

ing to enfold them in its sheltering peace, others would go back to luxurious homes, but there were also those who must go back to work. While they were still in service, London too was thinking of the nurses and considering the matter of employment for the professional among them. Miss Nightingale gave her assistance by sending careful and detailed reports of each.

In March, 1856, the war was over. The nurses, gradually detached from service, sailed off on different transports. It was August before the hospitals were evacuated and Santa Filomena herself could take ship for England. Before leaving Scutari she visited the cemetery where lay so many who might have been saved had men known more about what army medical service, army hygiene and sanitation, and army nursing could be. "While I live, I fight their cause," she pledged herself. It was a dedication that ultimately filled the days of her life.

POSTWAR ACTIVITIES

All England was waiting to honor Miss Nightingale when the ship that would bring her back should reach port, but the people's heroine slipped in unknown to them. Avoiding all well-meant publicity, her first thought was to see about sending off to Lea Hurst a collection of those mascots dear to all soldiers. The Nightingale family was called upon to make room for a one-legged sailor boy named "William," a little Russian orphan picked up on a battlefield, and a black pup called "Rousch" given her by the soldiers. Alone, the beloved Florence followed after, and no one met her at the little country railway station because no one knew when she would come. She walked home, seeking peace now behind those tall trees that had once seemed a barrier between her and the busy, unhappy world that she had wanted to help.

Miss Nightingale, however, had never been content in idleness and, in spite of periods of physical and mental exhaustion, knew that she must get back to work while public interest was keen. People would forget this war as they had forgotten others. The mail in far-off Scutari had brought her two letters that seemed keys to opportunity. One of these was from Queen Victoria who had expressed a desire to meet her on her return. With it had come the badge of honor that carried the Cross of St. George, England's royal emblem, done in red enamel, with the name "Crimea" and the Royal monogram surmounted by a crown of diamonds. Surrounding all were the words "Blessed are the merciful," and on the back was inscribed: "To Miss Florence Nightingale, as a mark of esteem and gratitude for her devotion to the Queen's brave soldiers. From Victoria R. 1855."

Nightingale Fund. The other letter had come from her old friend, Sir Sidney Herbert, thrilled to tell her of a great public meeting held in London on November 20, 1855. The purpose of this meeting had been to find some way of expressing the gratitude of the British people for the unselfish service that she had given. Important men and women had taken part and, unanimously, a resolution had been passed to raise a "Nightingale Fund" that she could use to make that old dream of hers come true by establishing a school in which a superior group of women might be taught the art of nursing and go thence to teach it to all the world. This answer to her years of longing meant a great deal to Miss Nightingale, but she knew that fulfillment must wait until she had done what she could toward improving the health protection of the army.

Army Sanitation.   Florence Nightingale must keep that vow given in the soldiers' cemetery at Scutari and to do this she had to bring influential men and conservative military officers to see what things should be different. It was, therefore, to the work of improving health conditions in the army that Miss Nightingale now gave herself. She rooted out statistics that showed the death rate among England's soldiers *in times of peace* to be double that among her civilians. This, as she pointed out, was obviously unnecessary. In the light of advances made in sanitation, it was criminal. Sympathizers gathered about her, a meeting was held at the home of the royal physician, and it was made possible for her to present her views to the Queen. She was requested to write her experiences and her suggestions for reform that they might be brought before the government; for direct parliamentary contact, like the suffrage, was not permitted to women of her day.

Political obstacles began to turn up in Miss Nightingale's path, but in six months she was ready with "Notes on the British Army." In 1857 the notes were printed at her expense and privately circulated. Their appearance marked a turning point in the history of military medicine. From this time curative measures became secondary in importance to preventive measures and reforms were outlined to make health possible. Even her enemies recognized the clarity of her thinking and the value of her contribution. She was requested to supplement this report with another on what she considered feasible in the way of army nursing by women. "Subsidiary Notes as to the Introduction of Female Nursing into Military Hospitals in Peace and War" was her answer.

A considerable portion of the next sixteen years was spent in behalf of the army. Miss Nightingale moved to London, found time and strength to extend her acquaintance with experts and, for a time, resumed her habit of hospital visiting. Many of her suggestions were followed in building a model military hospital, and other military hospitals and barracks were remodeled to provide what they had not had—good water, ventilation, light and heat. Their dietary and sanitary facilities were revolutionized. All of the practical experience and the knowledge that she had been collecting through the years was put to use.

Hospital and Nursing Reform.   In spite of ill health resulting from army experiences, Miss Nightingale also extended her exertions to include reform in civil as well as military hospitals. She began to write a long series of articles and books for publication. In 1859 "Notes on Hospitals" was published to spread the message of better care for the sick through better construction, better sanitation, and better management with more careful statistics, a new viewpoint on housekeeping, and changed ideas of nursing. That this book filled a great need was proved by its widespread circulation. In a time when such information was scant and hard to obtain, it became an authority for persons in many countries who wished to bring about an era of hospital reform. In the same year appeared "Notes on Nursing." This book immediately became a "best-seller." Not only was it popularly read in England for its novel approach to one of the great home problems, but it became a textbook for nurses in the school she founded later. America put out an edition, and it was translated into foreign languages. Even today reprints are available.

On hospital and nursing reform such as Miss Nightingale advocated was to depend the success of the concurrent development of medical science. Her personal friendship for health reformers, such as the great public sanitarian, Sir Edwin Chadwick, and the military hygienist, Sir Sidney Herbert, brought an unusual understanding of problems of health in the relation to the broader field of hospital environment, and the still broader one of national health. As a group they formed with her an advance guard, unknowingly clearing the way for *Louis Pasteur* who already was working along lines that would open up a great era of bacteriological science.

Sanitation in India. It was also in 1859 that Florence Nightingale began to work for the health of the English Army in India. Here was repeated the dramatic success in reduced death rate obtained in the Crimea and, later, at home. Again she turned from purely army problems to public health problems. This subject held her interest for over twenty years, during which time she did much to arouse official and civilian England to improve living conditions for the native population of India. Her plan for India's health reform was discussed with important Indian officials who visited London and with powerful English friends and, through their influence, it was initiated. When progress seemed slow, she wrote what she had to say, had it translated, and saw that it reached those educated leaders of rural India who could influence their backward brethren toward new ways of thinking.

Two other papers were written, one on "How People May Live and Not Die in India," and the other on "How Some People Have Lived and Not Died in India." Sanitary regulations gradually controlled health conditions created by great travel movements such as India's fairs and pilgrimages. Hospitals, prisons, and other institutions were improved. Great cities put in drainage systems, sewage disposal systems, and other means of sanitation that kept down the common epidemic diseases. India was helped to begin a huge task of cleaning up.

In a few years the heroine of the Crimea had arrived at the position of world consultant on matters pertaining to health measures for armies, institutions, and towns. Plans for hospitals poured in for her criticism and advice. She gathered around her experts on different phases of her many-sided work, but never again did she appear in public. The greatest accomplishment of a great woman's life now radiated from a simply furnished apartment at 10 South Street, London. Progressive, systematic, creative, wise, Florence Nightingale won the right to a place among the pioneers of those movements that have shown the early nineteenth century to be a period of exceeding growth in the humanitarian spirit. Sir Sidney Herbert was a mainstay in all that she attempted up to the time of his death in August, 1861. Personally, he gave her a wholehearted sympathy. His influence as Secretary for War, and later as Secretary of State, gave her political access. To both of them work was life, and life was work, and mankind owes much to an unusual friendship.

Suggestions for Study

1. (a) What points of resemblance do you find between the organization of the Catholic Sisters of Charity and that of schools of nursing of today? (b) Between the Protestant Order of Deaconesses and modern nursing schools?
2. Describe the effect of development of factories on family life in England.
3. Discuss the contribution toward social reform of each of the following:
    St. Vincent de Paul
    St. Louise de Marillac
    John Howard
    Stephen Grellet
    Elizabeth Fry
    Dorothea Lynde Dix
    Charles Dickens
4. Compare the spirit of the ethical principle stated by Sairey Gamp with that put into practice by Betsy Prig and herself.
5. What can you find in encyclopedias and elsewhere concerning the city of Florence, Italy, its intellectual and artistic life, its famous painters, and its history as center of the Renaissance movement?
6. Give an account of the early life of Florence Nightingale including the following: (a) Her family life; (b) Influences that led her to become interested in nursing; (c) Opportunities of her time for studying nursing; (d) Her means of becoming familiar with hospital methods; (e) Her first position; (f) Events that led to organization of a group of women for service in army hospitals of the Crimean War; (g) Her demonstration of the therapeutic power of nursing to save human lives; and (h) Her postwar activities.

7. What changes in ward management, introduced by Miss Nightingale at the Crimea, resulted in a greatly reduced death rate?
8. (a) Procure a copy of "Santa Filomena" for your notebook. (b) Who is its author?
9. Add new names to your map of the Eastern Hemisphere and show the route of Miss Nightingale's trip to the Crimea.

References

Abel-Smith, Brian: A History of the Nursing Profession in Great Britain. New York, Springer Publishing Co., Inc., 1960.

Andrews, Mary R. S.: A Lost Commander: Florence Nightingale. Garden City, New York, Doubleday, Doran & Co., Inc., 1933.

Austin, Anne L.: History of Nursing Source Book. New York, G. P. Putnam's Sons, 1957, Chaps. 5 and 6.

Bauman, Sister Mary Beats: Mother Mary Catherine McAuley's Contribution to Nursing. New York, Vantage Press, 1958.

Bishop and Goldie: A Bio-Bibliography of Florence Nightingale. Published by Dawsons of Pall Mall for the ICN. 16 Pall Mall, London S.W. 1.

Cooke, Sir Edward: A Short Life of Florence Nightingale. New York, The Macmillan Co., 1925.

Cooke, Sir Edward: The Life of Florence Nightingale. New York, The Macmillan Co., 1913.

De Barberey, Helene R. B.: Elizabeth Seton. New York, The Macmillan Co., 1931.

Gallison, Marie: The Ministry of Women: One Hundred Years of Women's Work at Kaiserswerth, 1836–1936. The Lutterworth Press, 4 Bouverie Street, London E.C. 4. (A pamphlet, price 6d. net.)

Marshall, Helen E.: Dorothea Dix. Univ. of North Carolina Press, 1937.

O'Malley: Florence Nightingale. Butterworth Publishing Co., England.

Pavey, Agnes E.: Story of the Growth of Nursing. Philadelphia, J. B. Lippincott Co., 1953.

Richards, Laura E.: Florence Nightingale: The Angel of the Crimea. New York and London, D. Appleton & Co., 1927.

Sellew and Ebel: A History of Nursing, 3rd edition. St. Louis, The C. V. Mosby Co., 1955.

Stowe, Lyman Beecher: Saints, Sinners, and Beechers. Indianapolis, Bobbs-Merrill Co., 1934.

Strachey, Lytton: Eminent Victorians. New York, G. P. Putnam's Sons, 1918.

Whitney, Janet: Elizabeth Fry, Boston, Little, Brown & Co., 1936.

Willis, Irene Cooper: Florence Nightingale. New York, A. L. Burt Co., 1931.

Woodham-Smith, Cecil: Florence Nightingale. New York, McGraw-Hill Book Co., 1951.

Chapter 10

DEVELOPMENT OF
SOCIAL AGENCIES

NONSECTARIAN NURSING REFORM

In 1860 Miss Nightingale began the reform of nursing through establishment of a model school in which the art of nursing might be taught. The Nightingale Fund, raised in her honor for this purpose by subscription of the grateful people of her country, now amounted to approximately fifty thousand English pounds. This represented a much greater sum at that time than it would today. St. Thomas' Hospital in London, with medical school connection, rich and influential, charitable and long-established, had been chosen as desirable for making what was then a radical experiment. The first need was to find someone to take charge of the school, for Miss Nightingale, although she had wished to do this herself, was not now in sufficiently good health. She would provide a plan, but another must carry it out under her direction. In the days when she had been trying to find nurses to accompany her to the Crimea, she had run across one matron apparently so able, and of so superior a personality, that she always remembered her. Mrs. *Sarah Elizabeth Wardroper* seemed to be just the one to undertake supervision of the Nightingale School. Her position of matron in St. Thomas' Hospital, where she had improved the nursing considerably, made her a particularly advantageous choice.

Mrs. Wardroper was willing to accept the additional responsibility, and the Nightingale Fund Committee appointed her to the position of matron of the school. Miss Nightingale unfolded her plan. Well bred young women, not less than twenty five years of age, and not over thirty five, were to have a course of class instruction and practical training in the hospital to prepare them to earn a living as efficient nurses. *This first modern school of nursing was to be an endowed school.* The Fund would pay the matron, ward sisters or head nurses, and medical lecturers for the time devoted to the school.

Basic principles underlying the general plan, in addition to selection of a general hospital offering broad experience, were that pupils must live in a comfortable, well-kept home under supervision and discipline such as would ensure character safeguarding and development, and learn nursing under the direction and instruction of a cultured matron, assisted by a selected group of teaching sisters, for a period of three or four years. This long training under nurses was an innovation for, up to this time, nurses had been taught a few simple procedures by doctors or their assistants who themselves took temperatures, gave hypodermic injections, and sometimes changed the sheets under those patients who were critically ill. The upper floor of a new wing at St. Thomas' was fitted up for residence. Separate bedrooms were arranged for students, with a sitting room to be used by them in common, and a suite for the sister deputed to take charge of this, their home.

The regulation of life in this home was necessarily outlined in accordance with the times, which had necessitated Miss Nightingale's being accompanied to the shores of the Mediterranean by an uncle and chaperoned throughout her whole Crimean experience by trusted friends of her parents. Its rules, unavoidably, belonged to the Victorian Age when women were just beginning to venture forth from the shelter of family life and were formulated, besides, under the influence of Kaiserswerth and the convent. A student, for instance, might not go out alone, but must have with her another student as companion. A chaplain must give two sermons a week. Every act was to be watched that no criticism might be brought on the school by unguarded use of unaccustomed freedom. Its founder knew well that it was on trial. The prejudices of "nice" families had to be overcome by promising protection to their gently reared daughters. The prejudices of those doctors and laymen who thought the old kind of nurse, with all her faults, good enough had to be overcome by providing a better nurse.

There would be two social grades represented among the women in the school, as there had been in the nursing group at the Crimean War. Educated probationers from the upper class would pay about thirty pounds a year for tuition. A nonpaying group, selected for fitness and character, would represent a less distinguished stratum of society. Probationers would enter on a trial period of one month, and a primary course of study for all was to cover one year.

The form of application blank to be filed with the matron contained some of the same questions that have been asked candidates for nursing schools down to the present day. One question, however, has been lost

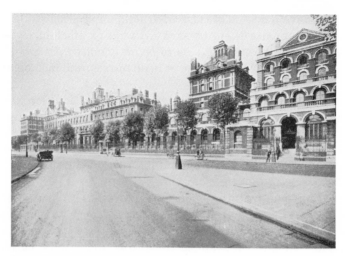

Figure 46.   Main entrance to St. Thomas' Hospital. (From bulletin of The Nightingale Training School for Nurses, St. Thomas' Hospital, London, England.)

by the way, and this loss is significant of another reform already begun, that of education for all women. The question was, "Can you read and write well?"

During the year of training, the probationers would serve as assistant nurses, and would be taught nursing procedures by the sisters in charge of wards. They were to be kept free from subsidiary work and provided with all conveniences possible to make nursing efficient. Instruction was to be given also by the resident medical officer of the hospital whom Miss Nightingale requested to prepare a form for what we would call a "Nursing Care Study"—written notes of observations of patients which students were to keep with the greatest care and hand in for examination. The hospital staff was asked to supplement this teaching by a systematic course of lectures and bedside clinics. Students were to receive board, lodging, laundry, and uniforms, with about ten pounds for incidental expenses.

When members of both student groups had finished studies of the first year, an examination was to be given and those who passed it were to be known as *Certified Nurses,* although it was decided to issue no printed certificates. Their classwork was finished, but there was to be a second part of their course requiring three years for the nonpaying pupil, two for the one who paid, and would be devoted wholly to ward practice, on salary, at St. Thomas' or another hospital chosen by the Nightingale Fund Committee. A record of each girl's service was to be sent to the Committee which would find her a suitable hospital position after completion of the entire course.

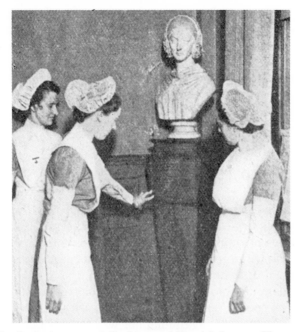

Figure 47. Student nurses at the Liverpool Royal Infirmary. They are inspecting a bust of Florence Nightingale which she presented to their school. (From *Nursing Times,* August, 1941.)

The latter arrangement helped to fix in the minds of all interested in her scheme the intention of the founder that graduates of the Nightingale School were not expected to enter the field of private duty which had been accustomed to absorb the best nurses, but were to spread over the hospital field throughout the world as nurse missionaries, teaching the art of nursing, hygiene, and health.

Newspaper advertisements brought applicants for interview, and fifteen of these were selected for the first class. *On June 24, 1860, these fifteen young women became probationers in the Nightingale School for Nurses, St. Thomas' Hospital, London, England.* The school was privileged to have the services of Mrs. Wardroper for more than twenty five years, and during this period five hundred nurses were graduated to take hospital positions in St. Thomas' and elsewhere. Fifty of this group belonged to the "paying pupil" group and became matrons or superintendents, some of them far away from the homeland and their school. *Modern nursing was founded.* As with all new ideas, this one met with considerable opposition from conservative hospitals and medical men. Its success, despite such opposition, proved the value of a definite plan of education for nursing and the idea spread throughout the world.

Florence Nightingale, deeply religious herself and living in days when a rabid sectarianism tore people apart, had found a way to end nursing's "Dark Period" by providing an efficient nursing service outside of the control of any religious group. Her success marks the beginning of a complete secularization of nursing. She provided a means to prepare for a useful, suitable occupation many women who were seeking to use their talents outside the home circle. The early nurses of the Nightingale School she was accustomed to refer to as her "daughters," and she prepared annual letters for them which have been gathered together in the book, "Florence Nightingale to Her Nurses." Her successors in every corner of the world acknowledge her the "Mother of Nursing."

DISTRICT NURSING ESTABLISHED

Experience had shown Miss Nightingale that there was a field for nurses' work lying neglected beyond the walls of hospitals. Home nursing had been always of supreme interest to her. In 1861 a rich resident of Liverpool, *William Rathbone*, had written of his desire to secure nurses from her new school to undertake this type of nursing among the poor of his city. He was coming to see her about it. The students of St. Thomas', however, had no special training for district work and, in any case, none of the new graduates were available, nor was there a nurse to be had at King's College Hospital where the Sisters of St. John's House did such excellent work. She suggested to him that it might be a good thing to start a school for nurses similar to the Nightingale School at the big Royal Infirmary of Liverpool.

Mr. Rathbone will be remembered as the kind friend who, with his wife, gave refuge and care to Miss Dorothea Lynde Dix, the American reformer, when she found herself alone and ill in England. Mrs. Rathbone had passed away in 1860 and her husband, during her last illness, learned to appreciate deeply the dependence of sick people on nursing. He wanted to use some of his wealth to make it available to those who needed it as she had and lacked means to pay for it. At his request *Mary Robinson*, an untrained but capable nurse who had cared for Mrs. Rathbone, gave up private nursing in order to nurse the sick poor in the great industrial and seaport city of Liverpool, and Mr. Rathbone paid her a salary. He supplied, too, the needed sickroom appliances and made arrangements for any special diets. Popularity soon brought her more work than she could do, and a search for other nurses to help showed that none were available. It was then that Miss Nightingale's welcome suggestion of a school offered its great possibilities.

By 1862 necessary school buildings, built and equipped by Mr. Rathbone, had been added to the Royal Infirmary. *Miss Merryweather*, a graduate of the Nightingale School, was secured for the position of superintendent of nurses. It was arranged to train student nurses on the Infirmary wards, after the manner of the School of St. Thomas' but in addition to this training they were to be sent to nurse in the homes of the poor. Liverpool was divided into eighteen districts, with a nurse in each to supervise the work of a group of volunteer lady visitors. Mr. Rathbone himself followed up the work closely and personally accompanied nurses on their visits to the sick.

London, too, developed a district nursing service, details of which were worked out by another Nightingale nurse, *Florence Lees*. A school for teaching home nursing as a specialty was part of this new organization. It was planned to build up gradually a national system of similar schools and homes for district nurses. Instead of a course which had really been a preparation for hospital work, the students of district nursing entered upon a course that included, with one year of hospital work, a six-months' period of special instruction in the district by teachers of home nursing.

This special type of instruction for a special kind of nursing was new. Another innovation was the limiting of admission to the course. Only ladies were permitted to become district nurses. This was a further step toward raising the general status of nursing. Englishwomen of this class had education in those days while few of the class below them enjoyed its privileges. It was a problem destined to vanish before the spread of educational facilities. Meanwhile, district nursing homes were developed throughout Great Britain and Ireland.

To William Rathbone and to Florence Nightingale is due the introduction of a new phase in nursing history, for out of her idea and his pioneering grew the modern schools for public health nursing.

WORKHOUSE INFIRMARY REFORM

Because he had unusually close contact with the poor, which district nursing work made possible, William Rathbone stumbled upon the Liverpool Workhouse and House of Correction, one of those institutions popular at the time, and combining in their functions a hospital for incurable and chronic cases among the destitute. Crowded into it were over a thousand patients cared for by inmates of the workhouse, who were rough, often drunken paupers, women and men. Officials of the institution, wearing kid gloves to keep their hands clean, made rounds by day, supposedly, to supervise. By night a policeman kept order in convalescent wards, but sick patients were locked in their rooms and left alone. Infirmary and patients, too, as might be expected, were dirty beyond present-day conception. Food was indeed poor. It seemed to Mr. Rathbone that Miss Nightingale was the very one to turn to again if this terrible place was to be made better. He went to London to suggest that he would maintain a staff of trained nurses for three years if she would find for him another superintendent of nurses.

The outcome of his visit and much correspondence was that in 1864 *Agnes Jones*, Nightingale nurse, and twelve other certified nurses from the same school essayed the task of organizing a better nursing service for the twelve hundred patients then confined to the Liverpool Workhouse Infirmary. Some pauper nurses had to be retained for a time, and eighteen probationers were secured for a first class. It was a meager staff, and certainly the work that confronted this young woman in her first executive position must have been discouraging.

Miss Jones found it difficult to stay in spite of the fact that Mr. Rathbone had provided her with a pleasant apartment to offset the wards in which she must spend so much of her day. It seemed almost impossible to cope with a situation where people and things were so filthy, and little sick children had to be piled seven or eight in a bed. It was all very unlike Kaiserswerth or the St. Thomas' Hospital, in both of which she had been trained. To encourage her Miss Nightingale had written that it was "Scutari all over again." She pulled herself together, and went on.

It was all so strenuous, however, that her physical resistance fell and, after three years, Agnes Jones, reformer of workhouse nursing, died of typhus fever contracted in her ward contacts. That short time proved the success of Mr. Rathbone's second experiment. London followed suit and, again under the sympathetic direction of Florence Nightingale, the nursing in forty workhouses was changed. By 1874 English workhouse infirmaries were changed places, and there were no longer any pauper nurses in them.

Once more the leadership of William Rathbone, the citizen, and of Florence Nightingale, the nurse educator, had changed the course of nursing history, this time by transforming the infirmaries of public workhouses.

BIRTH OF THE RED CROSS IN 1863

In 1859 Europeans were again at war. Italy was trying to free herself from Austrian rule, and France and Sardinia were helping her. In June of that year a great battle took place near the little town of Solferino, in northern Italy. About forty thousand men were killed or wounded. Both armies had trampled down fallen friends as well as foes. A traveler from Geneva in neighboring Switzerland, who had managed to get near enough to see what a battle was like, wrote this about it:

"In the burning midday heat still more furiously, the battle rages. . . . Drunk or mad with blood, the butchery goes on. Over the field of slaughter dashes the wild cavalry charge, the horses iron hoofs beating down the wretched men. . . . Back of dark, threatening clouds, the sun is lost. A tempest of wind and lightning arises; icy rain sweeps across the field. As the shadows of the night begin to fall the tumult of the battle dies away. Exhausted men sink down to sleep where they stand, or search for some missing comrade. The silent darkness is broken by the groans and cries for help of the wounded men."[1]

---

[1]Quoted in "Under the Red Cross Flag at Home and Abroad" by Mabel T. Boardman. Philadelphia, J. B. Lippincott Co., 1915, p. 33.

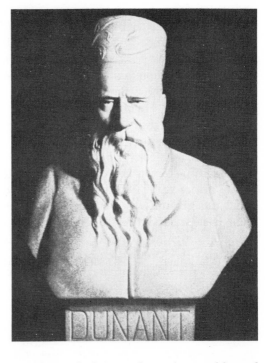

Figure 48. Henri Dunant. (Sculpture by Ernst Durig, in the National Headquarters of the American Red Cross, Washington, D.C.)

The stranger moved among them, helping where he could, and shaming cruelty in men who still went about killing enemies as they came across them. "We are all brothers," he cried. Preparation for care of the wounded soldier was as poor as it had been in the Crimea five years before. An inadequate medical service was again overwhelmed and something had to be done. Suffering men shouldn't be left lying on a freezing field. Springless village carts arrived to torture them still further as they jolted back toward neighboring villages. There churches, convents, soldiers' barracks, and private homes were being turned into makeshift hospitals. Verandas and streets had to take the overflow.

The traveler followed and, being a man of initiative, gathered together a group of volunteers among the women of one of the villages. Under his direction, they helped him to give what nursing care was possible. To wounded men of any nationality *Henri Dunant* and these women gave water to drink, or soup, put on warm covering or dressed wounds, or just comforted if that was all that they could do. Italian mothers took up his cry, "We are all brothers," and, as they worked, kept saying over and over, "Tutti fratelli." After the great emergency was over, Dunant wrote letters for survivors, bought little luxuries for them, sent money to their families from their pay, did all the little things which Florence Nightingale had found meant so much to wounded and homesick men.

In a town not far away were other thousands of wounded. Monsieur Dunant went to see what was being done for them, and witnessed operations being performed without anesthetics, although the use of both ether and chloroform had been demonstrated more than ten years before. More and more he realized how much could be done to improve conditions for soldiers wounded while fighting for the safety of those at home. He was aware of the very recent work of English nurses during war and, speaking in London years after, he referred to the work of Miss Florence Nightingale in the Crimea as the inspiration for his trip to Italy during the war of 1859. He determined to find a way to make war less horrible. With Solferino fresh in mind, Henri Dunant put the following question to his readers among the public: "Would it not be possible to found and organize in all civilized countries permanent societies of volunteers which in time of war could render succor to the wounded without distinction of nationality?"[2] This was the germ idea, born of his sad experience, which has given us all of our familiar Red Cross Societies, but its development consumed the rest of Dunant's life and used up all his funds. He wrote a pamphlet entitled "A Remembrance of Solferino" which awoke Europeans to a realization of the ugly truth that lay behind the glamour of glory with which the horror and cruelty of war had been veiled. This story was followed by visits to many countries where he enlisted the support of kings and influential citizens.

Treaty of Geneva.   After four years of work Henri Dunant had the satisfaction of seeing a National Congress gather at Geneva in 1863 to consider ways and means of raising volunteers to serve in the event of another war. What is known as the *International Committee of the Red Cross* was set up immediately and continues to function to the present time. The following year representatives of sixteen countries signed the *Treaty of Geneva* in which they agreed that military hospitals were to be respected by all armies as zones of safety, while their staffs of doctors and nurses were to be regarded as neutral and would serve the wounded of any nationality without prejudice. Suffering, in a very practical sense, was to make the whole world kin, "Tutti fratelli," as Henri Dunant had dreamed.

It was agreed also that each country would develop its own separate volunteer society but all would operate in accordance with the fundamental principles for which the Red Cross stands. Safeguarding these principles for all time was made the immediate responsibility of the International Committee, which is composed of a group of Swiss citizens. All societies would use the same design for their flag and set it up as a sign of neutrality over all hospitals in which they were called upon to serve during the war. It would indicate readiness to care for the wounded of all countries involved. Such a flag, in itself, would go a long way toward facilitating early treatment, for hitherto the injured who were able to walk had been compelled to search for a field hospital flying their own national flag. A field hospital under another flag would refuse to take them in.

---

[2]From The Origin of the Red Cross ("Un Souvenir de Solferino") by Henri Dunant, translated from the French by Mrs. David H. Wright. The John C. Winston Co., 1911, p. 78.

The design selected for the new common flag of the various national Societies was that of the flag of Switzerland with its colors reversed, a red cross on a white background, a gesture conferring public honor on both Henri Dunant and his native country. However, the symbol of the Red Cross has been modified by non-Christian nations, Moslems using a red crescent, Zoroastrians a red sun, and Israelis a red star of David. England signed the Treaty of Geneva in 1870 and, as time went on, other countries did the same. In line with its established policy of avoiding all foreign entanglement, the United States refrained from confirming it until 1882.

THE AMERICAN CIVIL WAR (1861–65)

When the next war came, only two years after the battle of Solferino, it was a civil war in the New World. By 1861, however, many of the people of the United States had learned of the work of Florence Nightingale, and probably a lesser number had heard of the efforts of Henri Dunant to form a neutral organization of volunteers to serve combatants of all armies at war. That they profited by adopting some of the ideas of both of these notable persons is evident from the system of relief which they developed. Although they did not form one of the Red Cross Societies advocated by Dunant, an organization similar to these grew out of a widespread development of women's circles or soldier's aid societies aiming to provide clothing or dressings for army use.

WORK OF THE SANITARY COMMISSION

It soon became evident that a central organization through which supplies might be distributed was desirable. New York sent a group of representatives to Washington from its women's societies and an association of local physicians. The government was asked to appoint a body to be known as a "Sanitary Commission," its aim set forth as "a simple desire and resolute determination to secure for the men who have enlisted in this war, that care which it is the duty of the nation to give them."[3] The usual opposition, governmental and military, was met but, in spite of it, the idea was put over and a *Sanitary Commission* was appointed.

The Commission thus became the center of relief activities and among its first undertakings was inspection of army camps in the vicinity of Washington. These were found to be lacking in drainage, in bathing facilities and in adequacy of space. Crowding, cold, and lack of ventilation forced the men to spend much of their time in foul air. Clothing and bed coverings were filthy. Food and cooking were poor, and rations lacked

[3]Boardman, Mabel T.: Under the Red Cross Flag at Home and Abroad. Philadelphia, J. B. Lippincott Co., 1915, p. 53.

fresh vegetables. Scurvy and dysentery were present. Troops arrived in these camps without rest and there was no place for them to clean up after a trip in ordinary freight cars that might have carried them all the way from the far west. On the basis of such findings recommendations were made, but the usual number of conservative souls in authority were satisfied with things as they were.

Then something happened, and government and army were jogged into action. The northern forces suffered defeat at the battle of Bull Run. An inquiry into the reason for this showed that it lay in conditions already exposed by the Sanitary Commission. The health of the men had not been conserved; they had gone into battle unfit. From now on preventive medicine readily held its own against the theory that physical endurance was produced by rough treatment. The interrelation between health and morale had been plain enough for all to see.

The activities of the Sanitary Commission continued to grow apace with the progress of war. It became a source of such volunteer assistance to the army as Dunant had been suggesting, an efficient agency of relief for the soldier. Supplies began to flow through central distributing offices. Enormous amounts of money were raised and deposited in its treasury. When shortages of vegetables resulted in scurvy, the Commission remedied the condition by enlisting the help of the only too-willing farmer. Great soup kettles, mounted on wheels and with a base so contrived as to permit carrying their own fire beneath, were moved to follow the battle lines. It was the Sanitary Commission, too, that arranged for fitting up hospital trains by installing swinging beds in freight cars and seeing that doctors and nurses were assigned to these traveling hospitals, which were to become a permanent feature of army equipment.

The Sanitary Commission established itself also as a connecting link between the individual soldier and his family. When the war ended, it provided temporary maintenance for thousands of discharged men, got their discharge papers for them, paid their way home. The sum of its activities and the spirit of neutrality which characterized the Commission gave it the character, without the name, of those Red Cross Societies that were being talked of abroad. Florence Nightingale, from London, kept in touch with its leaders, enthusiastically sharing with them her knowledge of European moves toward improved care of army health. In her sympathetic eagerness she offered to cross the Atlantic to give personal assistance, but was restrained from doing so by recurring illness.

As there was no Red Cross Society ready to step into relief and social work in 1861, so there was almost no organized nursing. What there was existed solely among Catholic and Protestant Sisterhoods, and the governments of both sides naturally turned to them for help. All of these women were disciplined to institutional life, and some of them devoted themselves wholly to care of the sick. As soon as the need for their services was known, the sisters led the way in nursing. Their established hospitals became crowded with patients, their convents were turned into emergency hospitals, the devoted sisters served at the front or were to be found on battlefields throughout the war.

VOLUNTEER NURSING

Everywhere throughout the country there were young girls who had thrilled to the story of Florence Nightingale and her nurses in the Crimea. There were thousands of Louisa M. Alcotts pining for "something to do," and war was offering to women in America the same opportunity for useful occupation that it had offered Florence Nightingale in the same dissatisfied state. They made dressings, rolled bandages, stitched uniforms, nursed.

The circles of northern women had their counterpart in the south. A centralized organization was lacking here, it is true, but the spirit of cooperation was notably strong. Hospitals were opened in homes and in tents. Southern women ploughed the fields and harvested the crops. Money became so scarce that even those who had been richest among them found their families nearing privation. Everywhere American women were leaving the home for a life in public, assuming civic responsibilities. As they did so, they inevitably passed beyond old ways of thinking and old satisfactions.

It was not long before there was a rush of womankind into nursing. In the great need, they were seldom refused but, as time went on, they were not always welcomed. Some gave splendid service throughout the war; but some talked inadvisedly, stirring up trouble. Among leaders in relief work were those who urged training for women who wanted to do this particular work. *Dr. Elizabeth Blackwell*, one of the earliest of the "new women" in America, as well as the first woman to receive the degree of Doctor of Medicine anywhere in the world, understood this need probably better than most. On terms of intimate personal friendship with Florence Nightingale, she had but recently made a visit to her and was very familiar with her views. Professional contact with New York's hospitals enabled her to arrive at further conclusions of her own.

Through the cooperation of Bellevue and other New York institutions a course of one month of practical experience in their wards was arranged for those wishing to enlist for war nursing. One hundred women took advantage of this preparation. Other women here and there throughout the country also fitted themselves for nursing by varying periods of hospital practice. The majority of volunteers, however, were like *Louisa M. Alcott*, who described graphically in "Hospital Sketches," her first successful book, the experiences of one who went to war without it:

"My three days' experience had begun with a death, and owing to the defalcation of another nurse, a somewhat abrupt plunge into the superintendence of a ward containing forty beds, where I spent my shining hours washing faces, serving rations, giving medicine, and sitting in a very hard chair, with pneumonia on one side, diphtheria on the other, two typhoids opposite, and a dozen dilapidated patriots, hopping, lying, and lounging about, all staring more or less at the new 'nuss,' who suffered untold agonies . . . and blundered through her trying labors with a Spartan firmness."[4]

All was "hurry and confusion," and an army nurse-in-the-making found her way to a great ward that once had been a gay hotel ballroom. Not knowing what to do, and filled with an unexpected longing to hide, she took stock from a sheltered corner.

"Round the stove was gathered the dreariest group I ever saw—ragged, gaunt, and pale, mud to the knees, with bloody bandages untouched since put on days before."[5]

Yearning to serve, but not knowing how, she stood in her refuge until somehow the ward machinery carried her on:

"Great trays of bread, meat, soup, and coffee appeared; and both nurse and attendants turned waiters, serving bountiful rations to all who could eat.[5]
"The amputations were reserved until tomorrow, and the merciful magic of ether was not thought necessary that day, so the poor souls had to bear their pains as best they might. . . . Their fortitude seemed contagious, and scarcely a cry escaped them, though I often longed to groan for them, when pride kept their white lips shut, while great drops stood upon their foreheads, and the bed shook with the irrepressible tremor of their tortured bodies."[5]

The work had not stopped since that dusky evening more than twenty-four hours ago, and Louisa M. Alcott had learned a few things about war nursing. No day would ever be so hard again, and a succession of days made it possible for her to express very beautifully for all nurses one of the satisfactions that few among them have missed:

"More flattering than the most gracefully turned compliment, more grateful than the most admiring glance, was the sight of those rows of faces, all strange to me a little while ago, now lighting up, with smiles of welcome, as I came among them, enjoying that moment heartily, with a womanly pride in their regard, a motherly affection for them all."[6]

Individual or local accomplishment has been lost sight of in the years that have passed since women made history by adapting meager but womanly knowledge to public service. Only a few stood out from the mass for conspicuous action. One who understood the hardships of adjustment vainly tried to establish a school for war nurses. One, at least, rode on to the field to rescue the wounded. Some braved official rules, as had Florence Nightingale, that the men dependent upon them might have what they needed. At night big-hearted, famous *Mother Mary Ann*

---

[4]Alcott, Louisa M.: Hospital Sketches. Boston, Roberts Brothers, 1885, p. 26.
[5]*Ibid.,* pp. 28, 33, 37.
[6]*Ibid.,* p. 41.

Bickerdyke searched the lines of the dead to make sure that none who might be living had been laid there by mistake. A daring free-lance by the name of *Clara Barton* went where she pleased, nursing friend and enemy, using her own resources to furnish necessities. After the wounding of a brother, *Walt Whitman* (1819–1882) served as a military nurse in army hospitals until the war ended about three years later, following which he wrote "The Wound Dresser," a poem included with *Leaves of Grass*. Northerner and southerner, white and black, man and woman, gathered to render service but, just as in the Crimea, of all the nurses of the Civil War a small proportion only could be gifted with outstanding qualities of leadership.

ORGANIZATION OF ARMY NURSING

It took only about six months of this uncertain type of nursing service to convince the authorities in Washington that it would be unwise to depend upon it too much. To organize army nursing, a woman was chosen whom the country adored for her unselfish public work toward reform of prisons, poor houses, and hospitals for the mentally ill. *Dorothea Lynde Dix* was a volunteer nurse herself, in Washington, when she was appointed "Superintendent of Female Nurses," and proceeded to gather together *the first nurse corps of the United States Army*.

The regulations which Miss Dix outlined were suggested by difficulties experienced by Miss Nightingale who, among many trials of similar nature, was once confronted by six of her nurses bent upon immediate marriage. No nurse was to be less than thirty years of age, and all must be as homely as possible. Hair dressing must be of the plainest style. Ribbons, jewelry, and the wearing of any ornament were forbidden. While no uniform dress was designated, sombre brown or black were the colors insisted upon, partly to sober charm, party as an acknowledgment of difficulties in matters of warmth and washing. An allowance of twelve dollars a month was arranged for accepted applicants, although Miss Dix herself served without remuneration throughout the war.

At no time, however, did these nurses enlisting directly through the governmental agency solve the whole problem of nursing during the Civil War, even in the north. Large numbers of men served as nurses, some as members of the army, others as auxiliary volunteers, and some as representatives of a society then rather new, the Young Men's Christian Association. Before the war ended there were thousands of women nurses throughout north and south, constituting a varied group with many differences in intelligence, diplomacy, daring, and experience. All levels of society were represented. The predominant spirit was one of great courage and self-sacrifice, while nursing methods savored mainly of the home and the Middle Ages, and often must have failed to achieve results.

When peace was made, the smaller, restricted group of women war workers with talents of leadership found other public tasks to which they turned. Dr. Elizabeth Blackwell, Dorothea Lynde Dix, Louisa M. Alcott and Clara Barton continue to stand out as progressives in feminine ranks. Dr. Blackwell bent her energies once more toward improving the opportunities for women in the field of medicine. Dorothea Lynde Dix, whose war service had been a sequel to years of effort to improve mental hospitals, took up that work again. Louisa M. Alcott resumed her literary career where she had left off and spent the rest of her life entertaining young America through her novels. Clara Barton, for the time being, applied herself to tracing missing soldiers, and with characteristic hard work and persistence ran down records of fully one quarter of many thousands of unaccounted for men. She remained the spectacular, isolated figure that she had been, destined to know great publicity and to win an international acknowledgment of the place of womanhood in public affairs.

AMERICAN NATIONAL RED CROSS

In 1870 the Franco-Prussian War broke out and Clara Barton went to work with the Red Cross Society which Germany had developed. As she helped in German hospitals she learned of the superior nursing done by deaconesses trained after the manner of Kaiserswerth, and of Red Cross nurses trained in the specialized Red Cross hospitals that were springing up everywhere along the trail of Henri Dunant. She burned with enthusiasm to start a Red Cross Society of the United States. However, the new country wanted to maintain its political isolation and was determined to take full advantage of a geographical location that put an ocean between it and Europe's squabbling kings. When Miss Barton came home full of her plan to push formation of an American Red Cross Society, her ardor was not dimmed by a warning that this was a project to leave alone.

By writing and talking about it, Miss Barton did her best to bring the idea of a Red Cross Society before a widening public audience. Several times she ventured personally to enlist presidential or congressional influence, but her country was convinced that there would be no more wars, and its leaders withheld their support. The usefulness of a Red Cross Society in other forms of disaster became her talking point.

"None is more liable than our country to great overmastering calamities. Seldom a year passes that the nation from sea to sea is not brought to utter consternation by the shock of some unforeseen disaster and stands shivering like a ship in the gale, powerless, horrified, despairing. Plagues, cholera, fires, floods, famine, all bear upon us with terrible force. . . . What have we in readiness to meet these emergencies save the good heart of the people and their impulsive gifts?—Certainly no organized system for collection, reception, distribution, no agents, no nurses."[7]

Finally, in 1882, the American National Red Cross became a reality, and Miss Barton its first president.

REFORM OF NURSING IN AMERICA

Shortly after the Civil War, representative citizens of New York—men and women who had taken part in relief activities—determined to find out through personal visits what kind of care was provided for the prisoner, the mentally ill, the poor, and the sick by tax-supported institutions in their state. Prevailing methods of hygiene and sanitation, of nursing and administration constituted the basis of their studies. The findings in Liverpool and in London of Elizabeth Fry, John Howard, William Rathbone, Dorothea Lynde Dix, and Florence Nightingale were repeated wherever they went.

Actual reform of nursing in America, however, began with a group of women which followed this first group and was known as the *New York State Charities Aid Association*. The majority of members had seen some kind of service during the Civil War. A committee was appointed to concentrate its investigation on Bellevue Hospital, New York City, and make report after a careful study of conditions there. The story was the same—inefficient management, bad nursing, and miserable, neglected patients. A soapless laundry in an institution admitting the dirtiest of city slum dwellers was indicative of conditions throughout. One of the new schools for nurses was recommended as the first and biggest step to be taken toward transforming the situation.

Meantime, the fame of the Nightingale system of preparing nurses had spread among medical men, who were meeting changes brought into their practice by the science of Pasteur, Koch, Lister, and others, as well as by the advent of the use of ether as a general anesthetic. They felt the need of better assistants in the care of their patients and, through the American Medical Association, advocated formation of modern schools throughout the United States. America was on the threshold of a period of pioneering in nurse education during which the Nightingale system would be the basis for development of new methods.

PRE-NIGHTINGALE REFORM

It was not America's first experience in training nurses for their work, for already two schools existed. As early as 1860 the *New England*

---

[7]Epler, Percy H.: The Life of Clara Barton, 1927, p. 231. By permission of The Macmillan Company, New York, publishers.

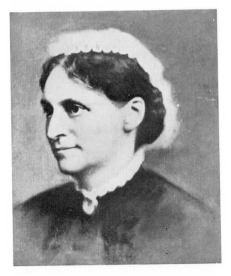

Figure 49. Linda Richards. (From a painting given to the New England Hospital for Women by its alumnae.)

Hospital for Women and Children in Boston, Massachusetts, had attempted the teaching of nurses, but had no success until it introduced the Kaiserswerth method. When this change was made, the first student to enroll was a young woman named *Linda Richards,* who was graduated in 1873 and ever after known as the "first trained nurse in America." According to her own account, her course of one year involved both patriotism and considerable physical endurance.

"My desire to become a nurse grew out of what I heard of the need of nurses in the Civil War."[8]

"We nurses did very different work from that done by pupil nurses nowadays. Our days were not eight hours; they were nearer twice eight. We rose at 5:30 A.M., and left the wards at 9 P.M. to go to our beds, which were in little rooms between the wards. Each nurse took care of her ward of six patients both day and night. Many a time I have got up nine times in the night; often I did not get to sleep before the next call came; but, being blessed with a sound body and a firm resolution to go through the training school, cost what it might, I maintained a cheerful spirit. We wore no uniforms, the only stipulation being that our dresses should be washable."[8]

In 1861, one month before the beginning of the Civil War, a group of Quaker ladies of Philadelphia established the *Woman's Hospital,* and announced their intention of opening a school for training of a superior type of young women. In 1864 their records show, "one thoroughly qualified nurse had left the institution to follow her profession in the community." In 1876 *Martha M. Waldron* was graduated. Both she and Miss Richards, neither of them Nightingale nurses, were yet trained in nursing and valuable as superintendents for some of the new schools. Side by side with them in the first attempts to implant ideals in Ameri-

[8]Richards, Linda: Reminiscences of America's First Trained Nurse. Boston, Whitcomb and Barrows, 1911, pp. 5 and 10.

can nursing, was *Sister Helen*, of the Protestant Sisterhood of All Saints of England and acquainted with the system at St. Thomas', who inaugurated the school at Bellevue Hospital. In addition, several Nightingale nurses were imported by Canada.

NIGHTINGALE REFORM

The urgent need for schools for nurses on the pattern of the renowned Nightingale School in London was shown by the Civil War, just as the Crimean War had exposed it to England and Europe. The following list of some among the early American schools based on the Nightingale system will serve to illustrate the rapidity with which the idea spread, the breadth of geographical area touched, and the scope of a social movement which envisioned service for all the people:

1873 – Bellevue Hospital Training School, New York
      Massachusetts General Hospital Training School, Boston
      Connecticut Training School, New Haven Hospital, New Haven
1874 – General Marine Hospital Training School, St. Catherines, Ontario, Canada. Later known as the "Mack Training School'
1875 – Montreal General Hospital Training School, Montreal
1879 – Spellman Seminary Training School for Colored Nurses, Atlanta, Georgia
1880 – Children's Hospital Training School, San Francisco
1881 – Toronto General Hospital Training School, Toronto
1884 – Blockley Hospital Training School, Philadelphia
1887 – Winnipeg General Hospital Training School, Winnipeg
      St. Luke's Hospital Training School, Denver
      California Hospital Training School, Los Angeles
1888 – Mills Training School for Men, Bellevue Hospital, New York
1889 – Johns Hopkins Hospital Training School, Baltimore
1890 – Royal Jubilee Hospital Training School, Victoria, British Columbia, Canada
      Good Samaritan Hospital Training School, Portland, Oregon
1891 – Harper Hospital Training School, Detroit, Michigan

Inevitably, the complete story of the development of nursing schools would show deviations from the original plan and be colored by national or economic circumstances springing from conditions of growth in young lands. Two Nightingale principles were always kept in view. Women, as expert in nursing as the times allowed, were placed in charge of the schools. Courses stressed continued practice in nursing over a long period of time. In the beginning one year of training was to be followed by one year of practice, supposedly supervised.

As it turned out, America tried and failed to make a successful adaptation of that system of apprenticeship known to the manual arts. It was unfortunate that in these days of imitation the importance of clinical and bedside instruction as stressed by Miss Nightingale was apt to be overlooked. There was a tendency, too, to a let-down in the matter

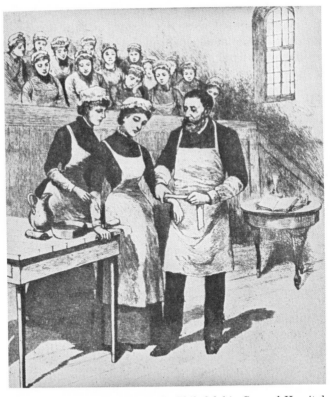

Figure 50. A class in bandaging at the Philadelphia General Hospital about 1890. (Courtesy of "The Nursing World," February, 1939.)

of care in selection of applicants. In the real apprenticeship system the apprentice learns under the personal direction and supervision of a master in an art. He is given time also to observe the master as he works in skilled fashion. In the face of an obvious lack of artists to teach nursing, this was difficult, and a crucial point in nurse education was soon lost. Student nurses in their second year often were given a major share of responsibility for instruction in nursing procedures of first-year students. Schools were organized as departments of hospitals and, naturally enough, became tools of the institution.

It did not take long, either, for these institutions to recognize the profit in a subsidiary organization that provided more efficient care for patients than had been procurable hitherto, and at surprisingly low cost. The graduate head nurses eventually placed in charge of wards accepted remuneration slightly above that allowance which Miss Nightingale had advised for the student. Students in their second year began also to take special duty cases in and out of the hospital, the hospital augmenting its own funds with the fee charged for their services. It is not strange that student nurses frequently did not complete their course but, as free-lance nurses, seized an opportunity for themselves in the remunerative field of private duty nursing. There were long days ahead when a price must be paid for the mistakes of these early days. The responsibility which nursing then was forced to shoulder was that of getting schools started in order that there might be even inadequate response to the sudden public demand for more and more of the new luxury — trained nurses.

Throughout the whole period from 1860 to 1893 the eyes of the world were focused on the Nightingale system of training women for nursing as exemplified in the Nightingale School. British possessions and Protestant countries first sought its help, then came Germany where the empress, a daughter of Queen Victoria, sponsored its reception. Holland followed, but in neither of these countries was there the same need for good nursing that existed in the others. They had deaconesses, Red Cross nurses, Beguines and others. Catholic countries were well supplied with nursing sisterhoods or brotherhoods. Probably the most extensive movement, and one which ran almost parallel with that in America, began in Australia in 1868.

When it is considered that the city of London alone started eight schools, that the first thought of all who wanted to share in this great reform was to get a Nightingale nurse to show the way, it is clear that the Nightingale School could not supply all the demands upon it. As soon as possible, therefore, the young schools sent forth a proportion of their own graduates to shoulder part of the burden of pioneering. This proved to be a most desirable way of meeting a problem which entailed not only development of schools, but very often demanded radical personal adjustments to people and surroundings.

In 1868 *Lucy Osborn* took to Sydney Hospital, Australia, a group of five nurses. A school was organized and, as the need grew for the services of nurses whom they trained there, these Nightingale nurses, with the help of a few more St. Thomas' graduates, raised a line of nursing schools throughout Australia and New Zealand. In Edinburgh, Scotland, *Miss Barclay* and a group of Nightingale nurses reorganized the nursing at the Royal Infirmary. In 1874 *Miss Money*, with the help of two nurses from Guy's Hospital in London, successfully organized the Mack Training School in St. Catharines, Canada, and in 1884 *Alice Fisher*, another Nightingale nurse, performed a task of conspicuous difficulty in the establishment of a school for nurses at Blockley Hospital, now the Philadelphia General Hospital.

Graduates of Bellevue Hospital Training School. The Bellevue Hospital school in New York was the first to establish itself as an outstanding exponent of the Nightingale plan in America and supplied many pioneers of reformed nursing on this continent. Some established schools which they served for many years; others assumed what was to them the more appealing role of traveling reformers who laid foundations for various schools. Outstanding among this brilliant group of Bellevue graduates was *Isabel Hampton*, who had been a young schoolteacher in

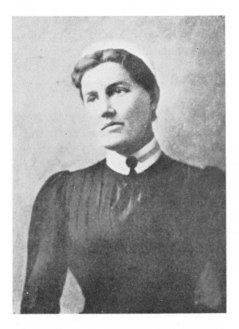

Figure 51. Isabel Hampton Robb. (League pamphlet, "Nursing Leaders.")

Canada when she decided to change her profession. She was only twenty-six years old when, in 1886, she was made superintendent of the Illinois Training School which supplied a nursing staff for Cook County Hospital, Chicago. In this difficult situation her constructive influence and educational insight brought into effect something that was quite new—a *graded system of theory and practice.* In 1888 she succeeded also in arranging for the first *affiliation* by which the course taken by her students could be rounded out to a desirable completeness through experience in care of private patients, while the abuse of special duty for students which had crept into this and other schools was no longer permitted.

In 1889 Miss Hampton left the Illinois Training School and went to Baltimore to organize a new school in connection with the Johns Hopkins Hospital. It was a thrilling opportunity, for the school, like the hospital, was planned to serve in America as a model for American institutions. It was to avoid those unfortunate deviations from the Nightingale plan which pressure so far had forced upon American nursing schools and was to assume a leadership in nurse education. Significantly, the title chosen for the head of such a school was *"principal,"* rather than *"superintendent."* During her years at Johns Hopkins Training School, Isabel Hampton arranged for a regular period of two hours of free time during a day which was limited to twelve hours, and which she would have liked to have limited to eight. Definite recreation periods, time allowance for meals, and even the limit placed on a day's work were innovations.

Miss Hampton strove to demonstrate nursing education as a balanced development, intellectual and manual. Women of mental ability

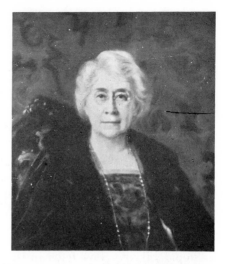

Figure 52. Mary Agnes Snively. (Courtesy of *The Trained Nurse and Hospital Review.*)

gathered around her as students and as head nurses. Recognizing the dearth of books written especially for nurses, she wrote one which came to be recognized as a standard text in American schools: "Nursing: Its Principles and Practice for Hospital and Private Use." Another text, "Nursing Ethics" followed after Miss Hampton had married Dr. Robb and had given up the project which she made so successful. By that time one of the pupils in her first class at Johns Hopkins was ready to assume her role in American nurse education through the medium of Johns Hopkins model school. This was *Mary Adelaide Nutting*, another young woman from Canada, who went on to establish a course of training preliminary to the actual ward practice. Miss Nutting also succeeded in reducing the student's day to eight hours, in a course lengthened to three years.

When Isabel Hampton was in her second year at Bellevue, another Canadian schoolteacher arrived to enter the school as a probationer. This was *Mary Agnes Snively*, who had grown up only a few miles from the home of Miss Hampton. In 1884, on completion of her course, Miss Snively returned to Canada to take charge of the training school for nurses which had been started two years before at the Toronto General Hospital. For twenty five years she guided the development of this school, from which she sent trained nurses wherever Canada needed them. At the same time, Miss Snively bore a large share of responsibility for the direction of Canadian nursing organization and the general advancement of its nursing education.

Another distinguished graduate of Bellevue in these early days was *Lavinia L. Dock*, who held executive positions in Bellevue, was assistant to Isabel Hampton at Johns Hopkins, and superintendent of the Illinois Training School. It was while she was night superintendent at Bellevue that Miss Dock made time to write a textbook on materia medica. Her whole professional life shows her to have been an adventurer, delighting to get off the beaten path, performing brilliant service in her own way. Not the least brilliant part was her joint authorship with Miss Nutting of a standard text on the history of nursing, in four volumes.

As early as 1890 the graduates of Bellevue had found their way to communities far from the home school, and *Emily L. Loveridge* had crossed a continent to establish the training school for nurses at Good Samaritan Hospital, Portland, Oregon. Upon arrival she found herself to be one of only three nurses in the city. Her first class consisted of five students, for whom she held classes in her room in the evening. For fifteen years Miss Loveridge served as head of this school and then for twenty five years longer as administrator of the hospital, leaving behind her an enviable record of achievement.

Jane A. Delano was another schoolteacher among Bellevue's nurses who leaned toward the excitement of emergency and the unknown. Miss Delano was graduated in 1886, saw service with the Red Cross in Florida's epidemic of yellow fever in 1888, and had charge of a mining hospital in Arizona before she settled down to nursing education work as superintendent of the nursing school at the University of Pennsylvania Hospital in Philadelphia. Later she served in similar capacity at her alma mater.

Graduates of New York Hospital Training School.   There was another school in the city of New York which was sending out an almost parallel group of graduates who would gain distinction as they helped to lift New World hospitals out of the traditional darkness. The New York Hospital Training School produced *Nora Livingstone* who, for thirty years guided nursing instruction at the Training School of Montreal General

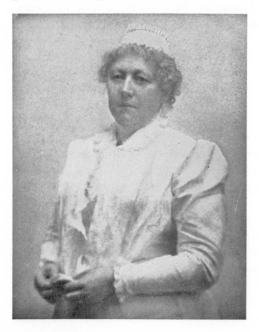

Figure 53.   Nora Livingstone. (From "Pioneers of Nursing in Canada," published by the History of Nursing Society of McGill University, Montreal, under the auspices of the Canadian Nurses' Association.)

Hospital. From the New York Hospital, too, was graduated *Clara Weeks (Shaw)*, author of what was known always as the "Clara Weeks" textbook of nursing, one of America's first and for many years a favorite.

Two other young graduates of the New York Hospital discovered a new field to pioneer. Thousands of sick people were still without benefit of the new nursing. The rich knew the luxury of the trained nurse on private duty, but the poor in their homes had little or no nursing care although it was fairly customary for hospitals to try to send nurses to them. To carry the skill of the trained nurse where it was still unknown in an American city, *Lillian D. Wald* and her friend, *Mary Brewster*, ventured into New York's slums. In 1893 these two went to live where the poor lived. Their new home on an upper floor of a tenement in Henry Street grew by a very simple process into the Henry Street Settlement, now famous as a center of public health nursing.

The poor brought all sorts of problems besides illness to their kind neighbors, and the nurses tried to solve them as best they could. What they heard and saw, while nursing the sick or sharing the family troubles, taught them the life of the poor man as a whole. They learned to recognize social causes lying behind those bacterial causes that the nursing school and the hospital had brought to their attention. They tried to prevent the things that harmed these unfortunate people, helpless because of their complete ignorance of how to protect themselves. The nurses had, indeed, stumbled upon the road to public health and, visiting nursing acquired a new outlook.

School Nursing. It was natural that school nursing should follow in the wake of visiting nursing. With knowledge of the plan in operation in England, Miss Wald visited some New York public schools, observing the pupils and conferring with the teachers. She made a report to the city health officers concerning the symptoms of communicable diseases that she discovered. A medical inspection of the schools was made soon thereafter, with recognition of the possibilities for improvement through use of the services of school nurses.

In order to demonstrate what could be done to conserve the health of school children, *Miss Lina L. Rogers*, graduate of the Toronto Hospital for Sick Children, was loaned for a month, in 1902, from Henry Street Settlement. So much was accomplished by this capable and tactful nurse that the institution of school nursing on a permanent basis followed. Later, Miss Wald and Miss Rogers were requested to visit schools of other communities to tell them of the experiment, with the result that school nursing was added to visiting nursing in a number of large cities. School nursing and visiting nursing became, very soon, a wedge for participation by the school and hospital in a social service that reaches into the homes of the school child and the discharged patient and removes deterrents in the way of their adjustment to society.

Boston Graduates. Boston as well as New York contributed its share toward supplying leaders for nursing schools. *Linda Richards, America's*

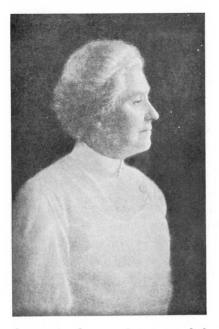

Figure 54. Anna Caroline Maxwell. (From "Early Leaders of American Nursing," published by the National League of Nursing Education.)

first trained nurse, interpreted the role of nurse missioner quite literally and went far beyond New England. She carried the Nightingale message west to Kalamazoo, Michigan, and in 1885 to Japan where she founded the first training school for nurses in that country. In all, Miss Richards took opportunity to inject reforms through the medium of nursing into at least twelve important hospitals. Some of these were specialized mental hospitals in which she followed up the work of Dorothea Lynde Dix by organizing nursing staffs and, sometimes, by initiating training schools in which students of mental nursing received a period of training in general hospitals.

From Boston City Hospital Training School in 1874 came *Anna Caroline Maxwell* who served in the position of superintendent of training schools at Montreal General, Massachusetts General, St. Luke's, and Presbyterian of New York. From the last-mentioned school she continued to radiate a helpful influence on nursing affairs for twenty-nine years.

English Graduates.   While the pioneers in America were building up schools for nurses, two other young women had taken places among leaders of nursing in England. *Mrs. Bedford Fenwick*, starting at the early age of twenty four, had organized in the ancient St. Bartholomew's Hospital of London a school which became sister in importance to the one at St. Thomas'. Mrs. Fenwick was a graduate of the Training School of the Royal Infirmary at Manchester. After six years of building, she resigned to be married. *Isla Stewart*, a Nightingale graduate of 1879, succeeded her. For the next twenty-five years, Miss Stewart gave generously of many talents, not only to the school at "Bart's" but also to the building of a new profession.

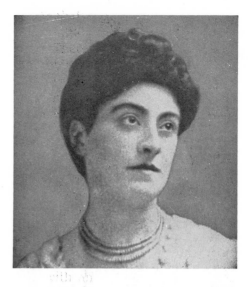

Figure 55. Mrs. Bedford Fenwick. (Courtesy of *The Trained Nurse and Hospital Review.*)

FIRST PRELIMINARY COURSES

In the early days of training schools for nurses, a common criticism on the part of their students seems to have been the dearth of instruction. Inquiring minds like those of Isabel Hampton Robb or Lavinia L. Dock were apt too often to feel a lack of mental satisfaction in the hurried nursing practice that was theirs. A course of preliminary instruction would have helped, but Kaiserswerth had not been imitated in this respect. It was in 1893 that *Mrs. Rebecca Strong*, a Nightingale nurse of Glasgow, Scotland, devised a plan of having such a preliminary course of instruction provided for her students at St. Mungo's Medical College before they entered training. Here, under the same regulations as other college students, they were taught all classroom subjects, and the training which followed was confined to the realm of nursing practice. In 1901 the first preliminary course in America was introduced by Miss Nutting at the Johns Hopkins Hospital in Baltimore. Three years later Simmons College, Boston, offered a course in sciences applicable to nursing for students preparing to enter the Massachusetts General Hospital Training School for Nurses, Boston. These appear to have been among the very earliest attempts to assure for the new schools of nursing the advantage of methods of general education.

FIRST TEXTBOOKS

Textbooks and manuals of nursing began to appear. The Connecticut Training School published, in 1878, "A Handbook of Nursing" written by a committee. Bellevue soon had its own manual. Some that had been written in England after Florence Nightingale's "Notes of Nursing" were also in use. There was a text available on midwifery, and one on the care

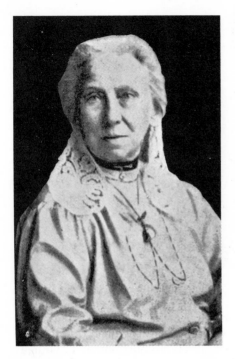

Figure 56. Mrs. Rebecca Strong, the centenarian (1843–1944). Graduated from Nightingale School in 1867. (From *American Journal of Nursing,* August, 1927. Also in *Nursing Times,* May 6, 1944.)

of the mentally ill. There were the texts on nursing, nursing ethics, and materia medica written by Clara Weeks Shaw, Isabel Hampton Robb, and Lavinia L. Dock. Huge medical books quite often were presented to the schools, especially if they were antiquated, and some ambitious nursing students personally invested in Gray's "Anatomy" and Osler's "Practice of Medicine." Classroom work, where it existed, centered around procedures, ethics, anatomy, physiology, materia medica and hygiene. Schools were extremely individual in teaching method, although in daily routine they were not.

PREVAILING METHODS

Applicants for training were required to show evidence of refinement, youth, and vigor. The preferred age was between twenty five and thirty five. Education requirements were consistent with times when private schools or convents gave finishing touches to a mother's careful rearing. Public schools, it was feared, might damage a refined personality. A great many students in the nursing schools began their careers as teachers or wished to avoid entering this traditional gateway to genteel employment. Nursing schools in distant great cities had a mysterious attraction. To thousands of girls of high intelligence the flight to them was toward freedom. It was the first time since the Middle Ages that women of the better classes had left their homes in such numbers to care for the sick.

Students were admitted to schools, not in classes or groups, but one at a time, to take the place of graduates as they left. Courses covered one year, in many instances, but gradually were lengthened to two and, finally, to three years. Some schools were administered by hospitals specializing in the care of one type of patient only and having a very limited number of beds. Some hospitals were entirely under the control of a small group of people. Accommodations, when provided in a nurses' residence, were monastic in simplicity. Emphasis was set on care of the patient and self-sacrificing service on the part of the nurse. The more worn-out her physical appearance, the better she could overlook personal discomfort or fatigue, the nearer did she approach the ideal of a good nurse.

British traditions of discipline were carried to other countries, and the life of the nurse came to be regulated by a curious mixture of military rule and custom inherited from the army and military orders combined with a good deal of that asceticism which the monastery fostered. Much deference for authority had to be learned. The student nurse must *do*. She was not asked or expected to *think*. If she could not learn to take an order, carry it out, and talk not at all when doubts or desire for knowledge overcame her, she went home. If her knowledge of house-keeping failed her, she was apt to take the same road. Punishment for lack of precision in filling medical orders was severe. In America the nurse who succeeded in graduating was free to follow her own bent, and in the private duty field, which attracted her most, expanded more quickly than trained nurses could be found to fill it. The building up of a capable supervisory group for the schools was, consequently, a slow process.

ADOPTION OF UNIFORMS

The New World nurse wore no uniform in the beginning and, strange to say, was opposed to wearing one. At Bellevue, very early in the history of the school, the authorities were in sympathy with the idea of adopting a uniform mode of dress for motives of economy and cleanliness, as well as for that psychic influence which moves a group in uniform toward improved morale and loss of self-consciousness. As early as 1875 some type of cap was worn in the hospital since the minutes of their Board Meeting of December 1st stated that, ". . . it should be impressed upon our nurses that the caps were intended to cover the hair and not to be simply coquettish ornaments, also that long dresses in the Wards are most objectionable."

Finally, in 1876, it was decided to ask one student to wear the cotton dress proposed and see what effect her appearance would have on the prejudice of the others. Happily, there was in the school an exceptionally good looking girl, *Euphemia Van Rensselaer,* member of the socially elect of New York, who agreed to go home for two days' leave during which time she would have a uniform made for herself. When Miss Van Rensselaer returned to the wards, her tall and elegant figure was arrayed in blue and white striped seersucker, with white apron, collar, cuffs and cap. Of course, all the girls wanted uniforms after that.

Other schools soon wanted uniforms, too, and cotton dresses, aprons, cuffs, fichus, caps, took on variety as they became badges of distinction between schools. Until the meaning of the word *uniform* was understood in its literal sense, distinctive individual touches were apt to be added. Prevailing fashions had their influence. A dress common to particular groups of women was often the inspiration for the uniform's design. The garb of Catholic and English Episcopal religious orders, the dress of Quakers and other Protestant sects, Deaconesses — all contributed ideas. The long full skirts were spread out by several layers of starched petticoat beneath them. Frequently they were lined as well to a depth of eighteen inches from the bottom, and for modesty's sake they escaped the floor by not more than two inches. Waists were fitted tightly to the figure, and also lined. The popular apron followed European peasant style, being similar to that worn by Sisters of Charity. It was made of several widths of sheeting gathered into a belt that was sometimes tied behind by a huge bow of ruffled strings and had a bib to cover the front of the waist.

The lineage of the cap goes back to medieval days and even to those earlier times when woman's humility and obedience were signified by her assumption of a bridal veil. The nurse's cap was the symbol of her service to humanity. It tried with varying success to fulfill, also, another purpose demanded of it by an age awakening to consciousness of germs. Caps were intended to promote hygienic care of patients by covering up heads adorned with more or less complicated arrangements of hair that might reach far below the waist when let down. In the absence of the beauty parlor as known today, hair washing was a long and tedious function, not undertaken oftener than could be helped.

School uniforms came to be worn in the home by the graduate on private duty. Patient and doctor learned the particular virtues concealed beneath each school costume. Pride in individual achievement lost itself in school pride which gradually assumed an intense form. Inevitably, the barrier raised grew higher and symbolized itself in devotion to a school uniform which assumed a fixity that made any future modification very difficult. At the same time the uniform caught the imagination of the public, for the lure of spotless simplicity and soothing uniformity enhanced the lure of the nurse's youthful charm, enthusiasm, and kindly service.

OTHER SOCIAL REFORMS

Between 1860 and 1893 the Florence Nightingale reform of nursing and attendant regeneration of hospitals had started in Canada, Australia, New Zealand, Scotland, Ireland, Sweden, Germany, India, Holland, United States, and Japan. It was one among many social reforms that were now beginning to take the place of the lost monastery. All were based on religious ideals, but were outside of church authority. In them women as well as men were taking part, the share assumed by the former being generally important. Many world-wide organizations, existing in great power today, had their origin during this time. Especially was the condition of the poor, gathered and then neglected by industry in the large cities, an incentive to these beginnings of organized social work.

SALVATION ARMY

Outstanding among the new leaders was *William Booth* who began a mission among the poor of London. In 1877 his group of associates became known as the "Salvation Army" and its organization on a military basis went on from that time. By 1893 this army of peace had invaded a large part of the world. Under its protection it gathered the poverty stricken, the discharged prisoner, the old, the young, any that were miserable, as well as those who had fallen from the grace of orthodox living. Its founder wrote a book, "In Darkest England and the Way Out," and raised a sum of money to forward the plan that he had in mind.

SETTLEMENT HOUSES

Other social organizations started and soon were flourishing, each in its chosen area of misery. Typical of these was the "settlement house" which frequently developed as an offshoot of a university in answer to the interest being taken by intellectual groups in investigating conditions and trying to find remedies for distress among the poor in old lands, or the unadjusted alien immigrant in a new land. It was a new means of reestablishing the old idea of human brotherhood. *Toynbee Hall* in London was one of these settlement houses which arose to prominence. It was founded as a memorial to a social worker among the poor and began as a residence for a few students from the neighboring university of Oxford. Under a clergyman director, these young men studied community problems and devoted some time to helping, in whatever way they could, the people who lived in its sordid neighborhood.

It was Toynbee Hall in which *Jane Addams* found answer to a long quest for means to express her own urge to know intimately, and to socially uplift, all who were held back by difficulties that might be removed. In 1889 she found a large house in Chicago which she furnished as her home, then invited all her neighbors to visit. Among these neighbors were representatives of over thirty nationalities — people who clung to their own customs and, at the same time, wanted for their children the education and the opportunity that they felt America had to offer.

Many of the mothers worked in factories. Some of them worked for meager pay in their homes. A day nursery, a kindergarten, and a library soon answered very obvious needs. In any time of distress there was some remedy to be found at Hull House, and the community learned to look to Miss Addams as its standby. Her settlement, like the one at Toynbee Hall in England, came to be typical of many others developed about this time in America.

Y.M.C.A. AND Y.W.C.A.

Even before the Civil War another social organization had spread from England across the Atlantic. The *Young Men's Christian Association* had been organized in Canada and the United States. It had also spread to Europe, for Henri Dunant was a member of it, and some of his enthusiasm for humanity is traceable to this influence. The work of the Y.M.C.A. grew in popularity and in efficiency. Character building, body building, recreation, education, relief, sick visiting, and employment gradually took their place among its growing functions. In 1894 a corresponding movement among women culminated in the world's Y.W.C.A.

MEDICAL MISSIONARIES

A unique phase of social work which had its beginnings about this time found a setting in Labrador. Here, in a region of icebergs and arctic cold, fishermen and trappers lived with their families under the most primitive conditions. They were English subjects on a far-off frontier; the barren land which they called home attracted no one else. Their lives were passed in such hazardous work, their food supply was so uncertain and so unbalanced in quality, that disease no less than accident levied heavy toll among them. They were without any medical care.

In 1892 an English physician who had chosen the missionary field as his sphere of work procured a small ship, had it fitted up as a hospital, and set out to see what need existed in Labrador for the medical service that he was prepared to give. *Dr. Wilfred T. Grenfell* found work for life-time effort — work that has been appreciated the world over. Beginning with one small hospital, "Grenfell of Labrador" undertook to develop a chain of hospital centers along the coast of Labrador and the northern part of Newfoundland as well. No person in need of care was ever refused for lack of money, and those who could, paid according to their means. Doctors and nurses, as well as college students, gave volunteer service to the Labrador mission. Land travel in winter was made possible through use of dog teams, and in summer the hospitals could be reached by boat. A complete health service to cover physical and spiritual needs was developed as the years went by.

The honor of knighthood made the missionary doctor "Sir Wilfred Grenfell." Always, to him, the need of Labrador stood as a challenge to the "chivalry of the Christ service." The way in which he and his associates met that challenge seemed to a contemporary, "one of the most simple, direct, and vital applications of the Gospel of Christ to human needs that modern times have met."[9]

Sir Wilfred Grenfell's work was a part of that great expansion in the foreign missionary field which took place during the latter part of the nineteenth century. Medical missionaries in great numbers were spreading Christian teachings into the heart of India, Africa, China, Japan, and other countries sorely in need of their influence. Hospitals, schools of nursing, and dispensaries were established as pivotal points of friendly contact where nurses and doctors, some of whom were of international reputation, devoted their lives to adding a share toward making the world a better and happier place in which to live.

Salvation Army, settlement houses, Christian associations of young people, missionaries, nursing of the poor in great public hospitals—all these and many others are examples of a tremendous social turmoil that was going on everywhere. After a Dark Period of more than three hundred years, the idea of human brotherhood was asserting itself again in new forms and to suit changed ideas. Christianity was acknowledged to be a creed that was to be lived rather than argued or fought about. Business grew apace. The west of America was being settled. The tide of immigration from Europe to the New World had few restrictions. Hospitals and nursing, of necessity, followed the people to every new frontier.

THE NEW NURSE

The nurse of this period was, typically, a bedside nurse whether in the hospital or in the home. In both fields she gave unstinted devotion to her work and radiated an unaffected enthusiasm. Hundreds of attractive young girls, immaculate and eager to please, were replacing the "Sairey Gamps" who had so long held sway. Here and there, too, were head nurses with natural aptness for teaching who delighted in their ward housekeeping, enjoyed the scope that nursing offered to their ingenuity, and delighted in developing efficient duplicates of themselves.

There were superintendents of nurses in the new schools who faced and solved problems without the aid of precedent. The names of only a few of these earnest pioneers have been carried in historical records, but institutions and local communities had honor in their hearts for many more. Among "career girls" in this transition time, the nurse stood out as particularly attractive. Here was one form of "new woman" who could

---

[9]The Challenge of Labrador, p. 15. (A pamphlet issued in 1928 by the International Grenfell Association, Boston, Massachusetts.)

be loved, who needed not to defend herself against public opinion, who had nothing masculine about her, and who was led into no strange forms of behavior. Her virtues were those admired in all women for many years, the skills she displayed attained a new efficiency under trained hands. The public lavished praise upon her.

It was an age in which the great cobweb of organization, which operates so efficiently today, was in its initial stages. The new woman was showing that she intended to do her part in the world's work and to make use of organization as another tool. It was natural that the next phase of nursing development should see its various groups drawing together in small units for friendly reasons, for consultation and ultimately, as we shall see, for protection.

MEDICINE ENTERS A REVOLUTIONARY PERIOD

In spite of the development of medical schools and the work of many individual scientists, medicine in its actual practice had so far changed little. Medical men had stumbled on ways of preventing smallpox by inoculation or vaccination, of avoiding scurvy by use of citrus fruits, or of curing malaria by use of quinine. They did not know what action took place in the body to bring about the effects observed and, aside from a few specific measures, applied medieval methods to diagnosis and treatment, too.

Sydenham, it is true, had re-directed the doctor's attention to study of symptoms and observation of differences in the pictures of disease. Experience had shown that segregation of some diseased persons permitted healthy persons to remain healthy. There was more accurate knowledge of anatomy and physiology. Many diseases had been described. Individuals here and there had ideas on how the microscope might be used to examine tissues, on the value of cleanliness in surgery and midwifery, on military and naval, as well as municipal, hygiene, and even on the prevention of illness, but few had a true scientific basis for their beliefs.

By the middle of the nineteenth century the slow-working leaven of science began to show more clearly. Its precise methods, invading the medical field, brought into common use a number of precision instruments to increase accuracy. *The stethoscope, the mercury thermometer, the microscope, and the Roentgen ray* changed the whole trend of medical examination and medical care. After 1860 great scientific minds made discoveries that set up, for all time, a dividing line between past and present in medicine and surgery.

The pathway toward understanding of causes and means of transfer of contagious diseases was disclosed by a French chemist, *Louis Pasteur*

(1822–1895). His conception of living bacteria as the source of infection contributed toward a change in medicine more rapid than any it had known hitherto. Through experiments with chicken cholera and anthrax, Pasteur also established a principle on which vaccines could be produced for use in preventing disease. His contemporary, *Robert Koch* (1834–1910), a German doctor who spent his spare time with the microscope, discovered the causes of tuberculosis and cholera, and published methods of laboratory technique that enabled others to verify his work.

Surgery was a field that offered the bacteriologist dramatic possibilities. The germs which the laboratory was discovering had easy access to the body, for there was little care in the treatment of wounds to keep them out. *Lord Joseph Lister* (1827–1912), another contemporary of Pasteur, set about finding means to destroy germs while they were still on the hands, instruments, and dressings that came in contact with broken tissues. His method was the use of antiseptics, and his choice was carbolic acid. His success marked the beginning of scientific surgical procedure and of the preventive procedure used in operating rooms today, although asepsis has almost wholly superseded antisepsis.

The treatment of disease was revolutionized speedily as men learned causes of illnesses and cooperated in devising means to rout them. After 1880 the germs of many infectious diseases were discovered according to principles laid down by Koch. About 1894 *Emil von Behring* introduced a new principle, that of using serum from immunized animals to prevent diphtheria. The year 1898 saw *Pierre Curie* and his wife, *Marie Curie*, isolating the precious radium now applied to treatment of certain types of cancer. It was the ethical spirit of true science that moved its discoverers to put radium at the service of mankind. No fault of theirs was the accident of commercial monopoly that hampered the interpretation of this spirit and set the price of radium too high for common use.

Soon after 1900 it was proved that yellow fever is transferred by a species of mosquito, and that the common housefly is a source of many dangers. It was logical to investigate the carrying facilities of other insects, so that today it is possible to control even the typhus transferred by the body louse which once, unhampered, carried a trail of epidemics through ages of European history. In 1910 came a cure for syphilis in the form of arsphenamine introduced by *Paul Ehrlich*. This is but a small part of the contribution of science to the advance of medicine. Many, many are the men who have devoted their lives to developing its resources, offensively and defensively, for the service of humankind.

It was appropriate that the people of France should subscribe to the foundation, in 1888, of an institute for research in application of preventive methods in the control of infectious diseases. Louis Pasteur became director of the *Pasteur Institute*, and thousands of cases of rabies alone have been prevented through this center from which scientific medical knowledge radiates to all the world.

In 1901 millionaire John D. Rockefeller gave to America a corresponding institution which likewise has international significance. *Simon Flexner*, eminent in the field of bacteriology and pathology, as director of this *Rockefeller Institute for Medical Research* was able to gather around him men whose names are famous in the records of medical science. Human knowledge and protection in the presence of communicable disease were further advanced. Here *Alexis Carrel*, for example, found opportunity to conduct studies of cancer and to develop histology. Other brilliant minds have helped to dispel some of the obscurity that surrounded other infectious diseases or have contributed to improvement of laboratory method.

In order to keep up with the sudden change in the tempo of medical events, both Europe and America found it necessary to increase educational facilities for students of medicine. Attempts were made to reform the schools by introducing higher requirements for education and by requiring better preparation of students who entered them. About 1870 public recognition of the problem was secured by organized medicine in America, and in the next twenty years State Boards of Medical Examiners were established. Still it was hard to make people understand what constituted a good school. Although many were eliminated by failure of their graduates to pass state examinations, and commercial schools were given up as added requirements became too expensive for profit, improvement of remaining schools was slow. What seemed to be needed was a concrete model to go by. A large endowment made it possible to establish, in 1893, the Johns Hopkins Medical School in Baltimore, Maryland, on lines worthy to be followed. Some schools reorganized according to its pattern.

By 1908 the number of medical schools in the United States and Canada had been considerably reduced, and it was decided to grade them in order to have a basis for determining the requirements of a satisfactory school of medicine, and to permit schools to see in what measure they attained these requirements. The Carnegie Foundation commissioned an educator, *Abraham Flexner*, brother of Simon, to make a study of medical schools in the United States and Canada. Mr. Flexner, in his travels, visited one hundred and fifty five schools, recording his observations. Both good and bad facts were uncovered and published in a general report, along with suggestions for improvement, in 1910. Many schools soon closed their doors, and since this time the work of improving medical schools has gone on, and a long step has been taken toward coordination of school and hospital in the teaching program.

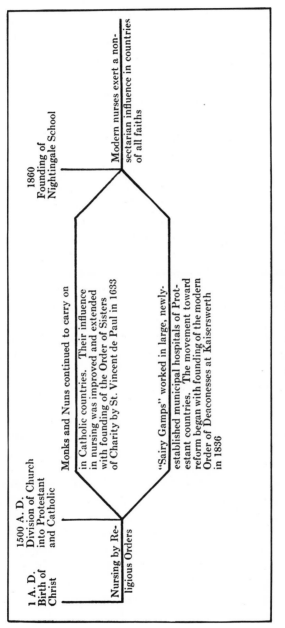

Figure 57. General World Pattern of Nursing.

Suggestions for Study

1. *(a)* Where, when, and by whom was modern nursing established? *(b)* How was the new school financed?
2. Explain the general principles on which Miss Nightingale founded this model school for nurses.
3. For what special work were the nurses of the Nightingale School prepared?
4. Name some prejudices of the time that had to be met and overcome.
5. *(a)* What Biblical character is credited with being the first district nurse? *(b)* What events led to founding of district nursing of the modern era?
6. Describe the beginning of reform in workhouse infirmaries.
7. *(a)* What experiences of Henri Dunant led him to devote much time and energy to founding of Red Cross societies? *(b)* In what way did Florence Nightingale influence him in this work?
8. Where, and in what year, did fourteen countries first sign the Treaty of Geneva?
9. *(a)* Compare date of founding the Nightingale School with that of the beginning of the American Civil War. *(b)* Was it possible for trained nurses for army service to be procured at this time?
10. *(a)* Discuss the problem of nursing care for soldiers during the Civil War. *(b)* Name several people who gave volunteer nursing service. *(c)* With what poems of Walt Whitman's are you familiar?
11. Compare activities of the Sanitary Commission of the Civil War with those of a national Red Cross society.
12. *(a)* What influences led to founding of the American National Red Cross? *(b)* Who is now its president?
13. *(a)* Why were women of America restless after the Civil War? *(b)* Name some of the public services in which they engaged.
14. Who is regarded as the first trained nurse of America and where and when did she graduate?
15. Name several women, not Nightingale nurses, but familiar with the Nightingale system, who were of value in founding early schools in America.
16. *(a)* What "trio of training schools" was founded in 1873 according to the Nightingale plan? *(b)* Name and locate several other early schools. *(c)* Collect data in regard to the founding of your school of nursing.
17. Name several outstanding problems of early schools of nursing in America.
18. Discuss the history of the following: *(a)* First preliminary courses of instruction; *(b)* First affiliations in nursing; *(c)* First textbooks.
19. Trace the transfer of the Nightingale System for training nurses from England to other countries.

20. Make an outline of a number of early nursing leaders, with their schools and outstanding achievements.

21. Where, when, and by whom was district nursing introduced into America?

22. How does district or visiting nursing differ from public health nursing?

23. *(a)* Where, and by whom, was the first nurse's uniform worn in America? *(b)* Discuss the advantages and disadvantages of wearing a uniform.

24. *(a)* What were the entrance requirements of nursing schools in the late nineteenth century? *(b)* At what times did new students enter, and how long was the course?

25. *(a)* Describe the "new nurse" of the time. *(b)* Did she agree with the popular conception of the "new woman"?

26. Name a number of social agencies other than nursing that showed rapid development between 1860 and 1893.

27. *(a)* What revolutionary changes were taking place in the practice of medicine? *(b)* Show how they inevitably affected the practice of nursing.

References

Alcott, Louisa M.: Hospital Sketches. Cambridge, Mass., University Press, 1869.

Austin, Anne L.: History of Nursing Source Book. New York, G. P. Putnam's Sons, 1957, Chaps. 7, 9, and Appendix.

Baker, Nina Brown: Cyclone in Calico. (Mother Bickerdyke). Boston, Mass., Little Brown and Co., 1952.

Baker, Rachel: The First Woman Doctor (Elizabeth Blackwell). New York, Julian Messner, Inc., 1944.

Baker, Rachel: America's First Trained Nurse, Linda Richards. New York, Julian Messner, Inc., 1959.

Boardman, Mabel T.: Under the Red Cross Flag at Home and Abroad. Philadelphia, J. B. Lippincott Co., 1915.

Breckinridge, Mary: Wide Neighborhoods: A Study of the Frontier Nursing Service. New York, Harper and Brothers, 1952.

Bullough and Bullough: The Emergence of Modern Nursing. New York, The Macmillan Co., 1964.

Cooke, Sir Edward: A Short Life of Florence Nightingale. New York, The Macmillan Co., 1925.

Cope, Sir Zachary: Florence Nightingale and the Doctors. Philadelphia, J. B. Lippincott Co., 1958.

Dock and Stewart: A Short History of Nursing, 4th edition. New York and London, G. P. Putnam's Sons, 1938.

Dolan, Josephine A.: Goodnow's History of Nursing, 11th Ed. Philadelphia, W. B. Saunders Co., 1963.

Dubos, Rene J.: Louis Pasteur: Free Lance of Science. Boston, Little Brown and Co., 1950.

Dunant, Henri: "Un Souvenir de Solferino," translated from the French by Mrs. David H. Wright, The Origin of the Red Cross. Philadelphia, The John C. Winston Co., 1911.

Epler, Percy H.: Life of Clara Barton. New York, The Macmillan Co., 1927.

Frank, Sister Charles Marie: The Development of Modern Nursing. Philadelphia, W. B. Saunders Co., 1959.

Griffin and Griffin: Jensen's History and Trends of Professional Nursing, 5th edition. St. Louis, The C. V. Mosby Co., 1965.

Gumpert, Martin: Dunant: The Story of the Red Cross. New York, Oxford University Press, 1938.

Jones, Katherine M.: Heroines of Dixie: Confederate Women Tell Their Story of the War. New York, Bobbs-Merrill Co., 1955.

Kelly, Cordelia W.: Dimensions of Professional Nursing. New York, The Macmillan Co., 1962.

Nightingale, Florence: Florence Nightingale to Her Nurses. London, The Macmillan Co., 1914.

Nightingale, Florence: Notes on Nursing. Philadelphia, J. B. Lippincott Co., 1946.

Nutting and Dock: A History of Nursing. New York and London, G. P. Putnam's Sons, 1907, Vol. IV.

Pavey, Agnes: The Story of the Growth of Nursing. Philadelphia, J. B. Lippincott Co., 1953.

Richards, Linda: Reminiscences of Linda Richards. Boston, Whitcomb & Barrows, 1924.

Sellew and Ebel: A History of Nursing, 3rd edition. St. Louis, The C. V. Mosby Co., 1955.

Seymer, Lucy Ridgely: A General History of Nursing. New York, The Macmillan Co., 1957.

Seymer, Lucy Ridgley: Florence Nightingale. New York, The Macmillan Co., 1951.

Seymer, Lucy Ridgley: Selected Writings of Florence Nightingale. New York, The Macmillan Co., 1954.

Stewart and Austin: A History of Nursing from Ancient to Modern Times. New York, G. P. Putnam's Sons, 1962.

Trattner, Ernest R.: Architects of Ideas (Louis Pasteur and Others). New York, Carrick & Evans, Inc., 1938.

Woodham-Smith, Cecil: Florence Nightingale. New York. McGraw-Hill Book Co., 1951.

Woolsey, Abby Howland: A Century of Nursing (1876 report edited by the N.L.N.E). New York, McGraw-Hill Book Co., 1951.

Chapter 11

FIRST NURSING ORGANIZATIONS AND THREE WARS

During the latter part of the nineteenth century a long evident tendency for society to draw together once more into small units showed gathering speed. An expanding and ever more crowded world made necessary the banding together of those who had interests in common. Although *clubs*, even among women, had existed for a long time, the club as a social movement began now. All kinds of organized units sprang into being – industrial, professional, social – many of them devoted to the uplift of those whom industry had trodden down.

After the Civil War, women of the United States were eager to procure for themselves greater opportunities for professional education, for positions in trade and industry, for equality with men. Even before the war they had discovered the relationship between voting power and such advancement and by 1865 women's suffrage was also a national movement. By 1889 the strength of women's clubs scattered over the nation was consolidated in a *General Federation of Women's Clubs*. Logically, the young profession of nursing would be influenced by these trends toward grouping which affected other countries as they did the United States.

NURSING ORGANIZATIONS OF GREAT BRITAIN

The need for concerted action among nurses was felt in England first. Here, as in America, the schools were growing up in isolation from one another, and no bond was felt other than the common purpose of developing Miss Nightingale's plan for providing a better type of nurse for the sick. No legal difference had been established between the new nurse and the old. It was *Mrs. Bedford Fenwick* who, in 1887, proposed an association of trained nurses. The purpose of this *Royal British Nurses' Association* was to bring together all trained nurses for protection of their interests, to promote measures for improvement of training and, ultimately, to have graduates of nursing schools registered by the government as educated, skilled workers of definite, officially accepted preparation.

In less than a decade, a group of nurses working in opposition to this *registration movement* nullified efforts to bring it about. To this group Miss Nightingale gave her support. Nursing, to her, was a calling and could not be regulated by law. In 1894 the *Matrons' Council of Great Britain and Ireland* came into being with *Isla Stewart* as first president. In 1904 the *National Council of Nurses of Great Britain* was organized to promote unity among scattered groups of graduates of schools and to prepare for affiliation with the International Council of Nurses. Mrs. Bedford Fenwick became first president and chief motive power of the new organization, which later became known as the *National Council of Nurses of Great Britain and Northern Ireland.*

NEW WORLD ORGANIZATIONS

On the other side of the Atlantic corresponding trends toward grouping of nurses were to be observed. Individual schools interpreted, in their own way, the general outline of the Nightingale plan and brought considerable variance into the constituents of a nurse's training. Isabel Hampton (Robb), endeavoring as she was to arrange a model curriculum for a model school, had been disturbed by the lack of uniformity in the conception of nursing among head nurses who came to her from different schools. To a few like her, the need for a move toward attaining similarity of training courses for nurses was apparent.

The earliest organization of New World nurses took the form of the *alumnae association*, which arose from the simple need for companionship. If she assumed charge of another training school when she left her own, the graduate, whether in Canada or the United States, was likely to move far and work alone. If she became a private duty nurse, even in the same city as her alma mater, there was no bond to hold her to old and pleasant associations. She was a free lance, and she was alone. In 1888 the Training School of the Woman's Hospital in Philadelphia formed an alumnae association, Bellevue followed with one in 1889, the Illinois Training School of Cook County Hospital in Chicago in 1891, the Johns Hopkins in 1892, the Massachusetts General Hospital in 1895, and the Boston City Hospital in 1896.

About this time, there occurred an event of international moment which ultimately was to cement trained nurses of old and new worlds in professional union. Civilization had been moving west and, to celebrate its astounding development, the city of Chicago undertook to hold a World's Fair. This was in 1893, and the Fair buildings, significantly, were to include a Woman's Building. Among exhibits in this building was to be one arranged by the nurses of Great Britain under the charge of Mrs. Bedford Fenwick. Naturally, Mrs. Fenwick was interested in meeting other nurses wherever they might be and was thoroughly aware, too, that the difficulties which had induced organization in England were likely to affect those of other lands.

Mrs. Fenwick suggested to World's Fair officials that there be a space provided in the Woman's Building for American nurses to meet. She also planned her own trip so that she might travel by way of Baltimore and make the acquaintance of Isabel Hampton at the Johns Hopkins Hospital. The upshot was that a nursing section was arranged at the fair in connection with a group meeting of people interested in hospitals and dispensaries. Eighteen superintendents of training schools gathered to discuss their problems, and Miss Hampton was made chairman of the section. The facts elicited showed a need of united effort to keep the standard of work in training schools as uniformly high as possible. A definite established course of instruction formulated by educators for all schools would be indispensable for this purpose. To this end a private meeting of superintendents was arranged at which initial steps were taken toward organization and a committee appointed to draft a constitution. *The American Society of Superintendents of Training Schools for Nurses of the United States and Canada* came into existence in 1894. In the beginning only those at the heads of schools of large, general hospitals were admitted, but later on the policy became more liberal.

In 1897 the tide of consolidating organization reached the alumnae associations, and under the guidance of Sophia Palmer and Isabel Hampton Robb they bound themselves together in the *Nurses' Associated Alumnae of the United States and Canada.* This group, too, excluded graduates of small or special hospitals, but later found that their work would be more effective if it covered a larger field. Nurses of the two countries functioned together until legal complications interfered and the Canadians withdrew to form their own association.

The year 1908 marks the formation of a *National Association of Colored Graduate Nurses,* an organization separate from the Nurses' Associated Alumnae of the United States, by request of a group of nurses who felt that by working alone they could further the nursing cause and their own special interests more readily. These various groupings of women were responsible for producing skilled nurses to protect the public from the unskilled and mark the beginning of setting standards which could be used to make a legal distinction between them.

INTERNATIONAL COUNCIL OF NURSES

Nurses of Great Britain, Canada, and the United States were by now reaching a national viewpoint on their affairs. Finland, in 1898, and Australia and Denmark achieved the same end through their new national councils. Holland and Ireland followed in 1900, Germany in 1903, and New Zealand, China, and Cuba in 1909. National associations of Sweden and India were organized in 1910, that of Norway in 1912, and South Africa in 1914. The evolution of ideals in organization going on within the woman movement helped them to attain a still broader ideal. Women in different countries already had gathered together as members of national councils of their numerous clubs and associations and had combined to form an *International Council of Women*. Its delegates carried back to their respective clubs news of woman's progress in many areas of the world.

In 1899 this International Council of Women held a meeting in London at which nurses from different countries were present. Mrs. Bedford Fenwick was one who saw the advantage to nursing of its representative organizations being grouped similarly in international federation and placed the idea at once before the Matrons' Council of Great Britain. Representatives from those countries where nurses were organized were formed into an executive committee to arrange a plan by which an *International Council of Nurses* might be formed. Before 1899 was over they had it ready, and the avowed purpose was to be that of establishing and maintaining high standards of nursing service, nursing education, and professional ethics all over the world.

Two years later, the International Council of Nurses met for the first time at the World Exposition in Buffalo, New York, where a constitution was adopted and officers were elected. *Mrs. Bedford Fenwick* of England was made first president, *Lavinia L. Dock* of the United States became first secretary, and *Mary Agnes Snively* of Canada, first treasurer. The watchword was to be "Work" until the next Congress.

Membership was not yet through national associations, but individual, and so it remained until the second ICN Congress, held in Berlin in 1904. At that time, the *National Council of Nurses of Great Britain and Ireland,* the *German Nurses' Association,* and the *Nurses' Associated Alumnae of the United States* formed an affiliation. After that, national associations of nurses constituted the membership, which in 1965 numbered fifty-nine. At the Berlin Congress "Courage" was made the new watchword.

NATIONAL ORGANIZATIONS OF CANADA

The first national nursing organization of Canada was the *Canadian Society of Superintendents of Training Schools for Nurses,* founded in

1907 by Mary Agnes Snively. Miss Snively, who by this time was a prominent figure in Canadian nursing affairs and held the office of treasurer of the International Council of Nurses, became first president. She began immediately to work toward founding of an association that would represent all Canadian nurses and be eligible for ICN affiliation.

In 1908 a meeting of representatives of the Canadian Society of Superintendents of Training Schools for Nurses, the provincial associations of Manitoba and Ontario, seven alumnae associations of Ontario, and several other local groups was held at the Lady Stanley Institute in Ottawa. The outcome was founding of a new *Canadian National Association of Trained Nurses* with which were combined the functions of the former Society of Superintendents. Miss Snively again became first president. The smaller groups continued their activities and formed provincial associations which would become constituents of the national association.

A primary objective of the Canadian National Association of Trained Nurses was brought to fruition in 1909 when twenty five Canadian nurses attended the third Congress of the ICN, held in London, and the national associations of Canada, Denmark, Finland, and Holland were admitted to membership. At this meeting, among the guests of honor on the platform, was *Edith Cavell* whose report on "Nursing in Belgium" brought forth a comment on the "quiet, calm, and serene manner in which this small retiring woman gave her paper."[1] *Sister Agnes Karll* of Germany was elected president. The watchword "Life" was given by the retiring president.

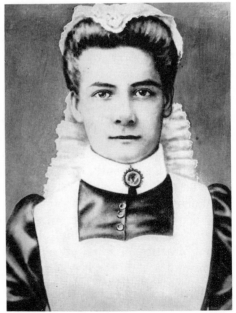

Figure 58. Edith Cavell while a probationer in London Hospital. She was then about thirty years old. (Courtesy Brown Brothers.)

[1]Quoted in "Edith Cavell" by Helen Judson. New York, The Macmillan Co., 1941, p. 142.

And so it has gone on in all countries to which the flow of nursing organization penetrated, and difficulties of one kind or another have been met. In England, especially, where doctors and hospitals were intent on maintaining their control over nurses, the opposition was particularly strong.

It is necessary to distinguish between the professional type of organization into which nurses had begun to gather, and a corresponding movement among industrial workers. Labor unions, which replaced the ancient guilds, work to procure for their members shorter hours, increased pay, and better working conditions. The professional organization, on the other hand, strives to give ever better service to the public through constant improvement in methods of education for service, together with protection of public, doctor, and nurse from invasion of the field by unqualified workers.

When the professional organization takes hold of problems of shorter hours, increased pay, and better working conditions, it sees these as contributing factors in improving its social service. This service, in the final analysis, must depend on the professional fitness of individual nurses, an ideal unattainable without health, professional growth, and that financial security which is a deep-felt human need.

First Journals and Registration.   In America there was felt a need for a journal to establish a means of communication between scattered groups of nurses and to interpret the activities of the Nurses' Associated Alumnae to the public. On October 1, 1900, the first copy of the *American Journal of Nursing* appeared, under the editorship of *Sophia Palmer,* a graduate of the Massachusetts General Hospital and, at that time, superintendent of the Rochester City Hospital. In 1920 Miss Palmer was succeeded by *Mary M. Roberts,* who maintained and then gradually raised the already high standards of the journal until 1949 when she was made Editor Emeritus. Representative of the nursing associations of Great Britain and Canada were the two official organs, the *British Journal of Nursing* established in 1888 as the first professional nursing journal in the world, and *The Canadian Nurse* established in 1905 with Dr. Helen MacMurchy, a physician, as first editor. The British Journal of Nursing has recently been discontinued.

The new magazines were begun while national associations were in the midst of a struggle to protect the public and themselves from unqualified workers. The first journals gave considerable space to a proposed program of legislation, chief objectives of which were to improve the actual practice of nursing and, by improving educational standards, to raise nursing to the level of a profession. Opposition was surprisingly strong, even though *Cape Colony (now Cape of Good Hope Province), South Africa, had succeeded in passing the first law requiring registration as early as* 1891. Throughout the United States and Canada the formation of state and provincial societies lent dignity and strength to the campaign.

The first *state* to enact a registration law was North Carolina in 1903. The first province of Canada to obtain registration was Manitoba, in 1913; but it was not until 1919, after a struggle commonly referred to as the "Thirty Years' War," that nurses of England could get a law to regulate their practice. Wherever adopted, registration has had positive results, among them the accrediting of, and a movement toward uniformity in, nursing schools.

WARS OF LATE NINETEENTH CENTURY

Two wars now intervened to add their influence to the trend of nursing development. They brought another type of organization, that of practicing nursing in groups to increase efficiency. In army nursing this system now replaced the old dependence on the work of individual nurses. Early in 1898 the United States entered upon the Spanish-American War; late in 1899 Britain began her war against the Boers of South Africa. The soldier of either nation had a better chance for good care than had been his in previous wars. National Red Cross Societies stood ready to assist both armies, although in the United States the weight of organization stood on the side of disaster relief. The United States, Britain, and Canada had schools in which nurses were being trained and through which skilled graduates could be secured. None of these countries, however, was wholly aware of its opportunity in this respect, or of the fact that nurses could be reached through their national associations. Epidemic disease, especially typhoid, turned out to be the particular scourge of the armies, and one which demanded an unusually large number of nurses to combat it.

SPANISH AMERICAN WAR

In the early days of the Spanish-American War the volunteer nursing group represented the trained, the partly trained, and the untrained, and men as well as women. System was lacking in supplying them, and a condition of emergency arose which forced itself upon the attention of both government and people. The latter were loud in their demands for better care of troops. The Nurses' Associated Alumnae of the United States was disturbed by avoidable conditions and took them under consideration at an annual meeting. The president, Mrs. Isabel Hampton Robb, suggested that the society offer itself to the government as the agent through which more and skilled nurses might be reliably secured. When, however, she and another official visited Washington for this purpose, they were disappointed to find the department of army nursing already under the direction of the Daughters of the American Revolution. This society had chosen as director of the service, *Dr. Anita Newcomb McGee,* a resident of Washington, who is described as a young and handsome woman physician. She was enrolling nurses and setting up her own standards for their selection which, fortunately, included a certificate of graduation from a training school for nurses. Nurses thus chosen were placed under direction of the Red Cross which assisted with their expenses while in service.

Several superintendents of training schools volunteered to share in the organization of army camp nursing, among them *Anna C. Maxwell,* who had leave of absence from the Presbyterian Hospital in New York. Miss Maxwell was made Chief Nurse at the camp hospital of Chickamauga Park, Georgia—one in which the nursing situation offered very difficult problems, not the least of which was the fact that fourteen of her nurses contracted typhoid fever. Her own description gives some insight into the causes of these difficulties and shows how they bore comparison with those encountered by Miss Nightingale about forty years earlier:

"Only one pound of carbolic was found, chloride of lime was secured at Chattanooga, and linen was much damaged by its use. The trenches between the tents, and the ground, saturated with typhoid bacilli, where the buckets stood, were finally disinfected, but not until the entire camp had been exposed to the infection from the millions of flies that gathered about these spots."[2]

SOUTH AFRICAN WAR

In South Africa, as in the United States, war had emphasized the need for greater preparedness for efficient army nursing through permanently organized groups of nurses, certified as to character, health, and experience, selected from the ranks of those trained in the schools. The Boer War had drawn into it contingents of Canadian soldiers and Canadian nurse volunteers who went to assist the British Army Nursing Service, which had been organized in 1881 as a result of Crimean experience, coupled with the postwar efforts of Miss Nightingale. These nurse volunteers for South African service were assembled under the direction of *Georgina F. Pope.* On their return, the Canadian Government placed them on a Reserve list in the active militia, and from this beginning, Canada built up the *Royal Canadian Army Medical Corps Nursing Service. When, in* 1904, *she gave to these first reserve nurses the relative rank of "Lieutenant," she was the first country to accord military rank to women.*

The bestowal of rank on nurses proved to be a move of high importance. Rank in armies is a system of designating the position and power to command of its holder. Without it the nurse could be classed only with the private soldier and had no authority to direct his work on the wards where he served as orderly. With it she could be assured that her

---

[2]Quoted in "A History of Nursing" by Nutting and Dock, 1907, Vol. III, pp. 207–208. G. P. Putnam's Sons, New York and London, publishers.

directions in regard to care of patients would be carried out, not only by him, but, when necessary, by those noncommissioned officers whose status was relatively below her own.

Britain also had learned that it did not do to depend on any set number of army nurses to meet the exigencies of war and reorganized her Army Nursing Service to include a Red Cross reserve that could be called upon in an emergency. The name was changed to that by which it goes today, *Queen Alexandra's Royal Army Nursing Corps.* The United States, Canada, and Britain henceforth looked to their Red Cross and their nursing schools to supply an efficient nursing service in time of war.

U. S. ARMY AND NAVY NURSE CORPS

After the Spanish-American War ended, leading nurses all over the country began to use their influence to procure legislation that would ensure an efficient army nursing service — one that would not limit itself to wartime emergency but would be effective also in times of peace. Women who had been prominent in relief work met with committees from the American Society of Superintendents of Training Schools and the Nurses' Associated Alumnae of the United States, and a joint committee was chosen to draw up a bill for establishment of an *Army Nurse Corps,* which would be presented to Congress. After many difficulties had been overcome, the bill was passed in 1901, outstanding among its sponsors being Dr. Anita Newcomb McGee, Isabel Hampton Robb, Anna C. Maxwell, and Adelaide Nutting. To the ability of the latter as chairman was due, in great part, this final success. In 1908, following the example of the army, a *Navy Nurse Corps* was established.

AMERICAN RED CROSS NURSING SERVICE

What had thus far been accomplished was provision of staffs of nurses to serve the army and navy during times of peace but this took no account of the elasticity necessary to meet the emergencies inseparable from war. By this time the new nursing organizations had had an opportunity to learn the power inherent in united effort, and they began to work toward an affiliation with the national Red Cross Society, which had demonstrated its efficiency as a medium of enrollment when additional nurses were needed.

About this time, Mrs. Robb was able to bring before the Red Cross a plan representing the ideas of the nurses' associations and herself for development of a *nursing department within the Society.* This department would enroll a nursing staff adequate to meet the demands of any emergency. The volunteer system would give way to a system providing

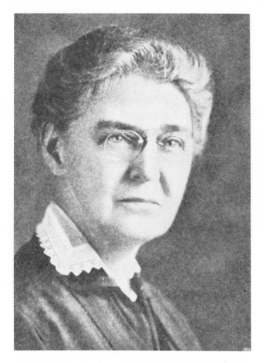

Figure 59. M. Adelaide Nutting. (Courtesy of *American Journal of Nursing.*)

salaries. Unfortunately, the plan seemed too costly to be undertaken immediately, and it was laid aside. However, *Jane A. Delano,* who was then Superintendent of the Army Nurse Corps, proved herself a valuable coordinator of Army, nursing, and Red Cross interests when, in 1909, she decided to devote herself wholly to the work of the Society.

Miss Delano served without salary until her death in France at the close of World War I. Under her capable administration the *American Red Cross Nursing Service* developed step by step and in close harmony with the ideas of Mrs. Robb and the Associated Alumnae. She made clear her aim of building up a roster of those ready to serve their country in time of war or other disaster. Qualifications would be set to determine acceptance, accepted nurses would continue with their regular work until needed, *would not be compelled to give service,* and when on duty with the Red Cross would be paid a salary.

This method of maintaining a roll adequate to meet any emergency was in force until late in World War II, when full responsibility for recruitment and maintenance of a Reserve Nurse Corps was assumed by each of the federal nursing services. The Red Cross continues to enroll nurses, but it is now for service with the Red Cross itself.

GRADUATE EDUCATION FOR NURSES

An early opportunity to demonstrate the usefulness of their organization, as well as its professional quality, came to nurses of America about the time of the Spanish-American War. There was growing dissatisfaction with the haphazard trend of nursing education. Apparently, only two attempts had been made to link the nursing school with an institution of higher learning. In Scotland Mrs. Strong's arrangement with a college, in 1893, was for a preliminary course only. About the same time the University of Texas established a university hospital with the nursing school as part of the medical department, although it was not placed on a strict university basis. These college courses were designed solely to meet the needs of student nurses.

In 1898 the American Society of Superintendents of Training Schools for Nurses decided that solution to the problem depended on graduate education for those nurses who were responsible for the education of students in hospital schools. A committee, on which Mrs. Robb served as chairman and Miss Nutting as one of the members, found that a promising arrangement for instruction of the graduate nurse might be made with the new Teachers College at Columbia University, New York City. Here, regular courses in psychology, science, and household economics would be made available to selected graduate nurses, while such special courses as dealt with nursing school and hospital work would be financed by the Society of Superintendents. The step was taken and, in 1899, a course in *hospital economics* was offered. Mrs. Robb, Miss Nutting, and a promising young graduate of the New York Hospital, *Annie W. Goodrich,* and others lectured on special subjects, often without remuneration. Two students formed the first class.

In 1907 Miss Nutting resigned from her position as superintendent of nurses at the Johns Hopkins Training School for Nurses, to give

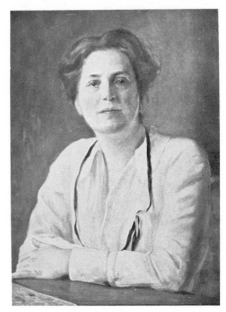

Figure 60. Lillian D. Wald.

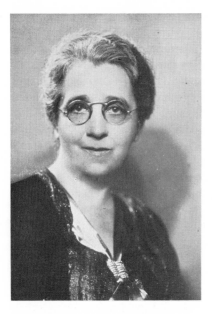

Figure 61. Isabel M. Stewart. (Photograph by G. Maillard Kesslere.)

her full time to developing this first school for graduate nurses. The College honored her with a professorship, the first to be held anywhere by a nurse. Other illustrious nurses were added to the teaching staff, including *Lillian D. Wald* of Henry Street Settlement and *Clara D. Noyes,* a graduate of Johns Hopkins. By 1909 Miss Nutting needed an assistant, and *Isabel M. Stewart,* a Canadian graduate of the Winnipeg Hospital and also a graduate of Teachers College, came to fill this position. Miss Stewart was able to arrange special courses for nurse teachers, but it was even then apparent that courses would be needed for visiting nurses, head nurses, and other specialists appearing in the nursing field. The need for financial assistance was met by Mrs. Helen Hartley Jenkins, a trustee of Teachers College, who generously endowed the department.

Time has proved the judgment of the members of the Society of Superintendents to have been wise. The vital factor in improving education has been shown to be the educator, and results of the work done at Teachers College to prepare the educator for her task are to be seen all over the world. The principle of giving the student in the nursing school an *education* designed to prepare her for giving good nursing care to the public has displaced the overemphasis once placed on practice. Her increasingly intelligent work has improved the status of nurses generally and brought them greater opportunity with greater satisfaction in their work.

The plan of raising the level of teaching in nursing schools through collective opportunity bore early fruit. Mrs. Robb had hardly dared to consider as more than a dream the possibility of some day seeing students of nursing accepted on the level of college students and taught in college classes. As early as 1909, however, a brief ten years since it had been made possible for graduate nurses to enter Teachers College, nurses in training in one school were being placed on a college level. The University of Minnesota, under the leadership of *Dr. Richard Olding Beard,* was first to institute a plan by which nurse education became a branch of college work. Thus, a new emphasis was placed on knowledge.

Nursing had thus made considerable progress in its first fifty years. It was not behind those other varied humanitarian efforts which had influenced so much the life and work of Florence Nightingale who, by this time, had seen more than ninety years of life. On August 13, 1910, she passed away, and by her own wish was laid to rest in the churchyard of St. Margaret's, East Wellow, near her old home at Embley Park, although England gladly would have placed her with those whose fame gives reason for their burial in Westminster Abbey. Monuments have been built to her memory in her own country, in Florence, Italy, where she was born, and in far distant places as well.

At the closing banquet of the first ICN Congress after Miss Nightingale's death, held in Cologne, Germany, in 1912, nurses of the world proposed as a living memorial to her some form of education work that would bring to all peoples, through their nurses, the treasure of ever better nursing. At that time it was moved by Mrs. Fenwick and seconded by Miss Nutting that such a memorial be established and that it be educational in character rather than a museum. However, wartime conditions and travel restrictions of the first World War prevented further action and years were to elapse before such a memorial became a reality.

CHANGES IN ORGANIZATION

As Miss Nightingale's life was coming to a close, a period of new developments in nursing was opening, nursing groups were forming plans to raise professional standards and improve existing methods of nursing practice and nursing education. In the United States two organizations changed their names and a new organization was founded. In 1911 the Nurses' Associated Alumnae of the United States became the *American Nurses' Association,* with a membership no longer restricted to alumnae. It persisted in its efforts to support legislation affecting the profession.

In 1912 the American Society of Superintendents of Training Schools became the *National League of Nursing Education* and continued to work for a more satisfactory type of preparation for nursing. Its curriculum for nursing schools, first published in 1917 under the leadership of Mary Adelaide Nutting, afforded a new basis for raising national standards.

A pioneer organization in the field of visiting nursing was the *National Organization for Public Health Nursing,* founded in 1912.

Its first president, Lillian D. Wald of Henry Street Settlement, was already famous for her interest in community health and social uplift. Under her direction the new association undertook, first of all, to draw into it increasing numbers of those who were filling the demand for a new type of nursing. It arranged for special courses in public health nursing, set up standards, and stimulated group interest in this rapidly expanding field.

In 1924, the name of the Canadian National Association of Trained Nurses was changed to the *Canadian Nurses' Association.* This single Canadian association, through its various national Committees, continued to carry on activities corresponding to those of three organizations in the United States.

WORLD WAR I (1914–1918)

Precipitation of World War I occurred in 1914 when Austria declared war on Serbia, Germany invaded Belgium, and France and England became involved in the conflict. Warring countries soon faced shortages of doctors and nurses, medical supplies, and other means of relief for the suffering. The Red Cross of still neutral America responded by organizing units of doctors, nurses, and other social workers to be sent out to each belligerent country. Until the imminence of America's entrance into the war caused their recall, men and women of these units did much to express the spirit of the Red Cross as they worked amid the fire and bombshells of large-scale war.

British Nursing Services. At the beginning of the war three English nursing groups were prepared to meet the emergency. *Queen Alexandra's Royal Army Nursing Corps* offered its thousands of nurses for the care of sick and wounded soldiers. *Dame Ethel Hope Beecher* served as matron-in-chief, her headquarters in close contact with the British War Office. *Queen Alexandra's Royal Naval Nursing Service,* small at the outbreak of the war, was soon enlarged. For the purpose of supplying nursing care for the newly organized Royal Air Force, the *Princess Mary's Royal Air Force Nursing Service* came into existence in 1918.

As in all warring countries, English foreign service drew so many patriotic volunteers that civilian hospitals were left in painful need. To meet the insistent demand for more assistance the British Red Cross, which had already supplied great numbers of nurses to hospitals, now became engaged in organization of a *Voluntary Aid Detachment.* Throughout the Empire laymen and laywomen took the short emergency courses offered, and many of these "V. A. D.'s" served as assistant nurses in hospitals at home and overseas. Others worked in hastily set up dispensaries and rest stations, temporary havens for tired, sick, and wounded soldiers.

Nurses of Canada, South Africa, Australia, and New Zealand expressed in many ways their desire to be of service. In Canada nurses of the Permanent Army Medical Corps Nursing Service were placed a second time under the direction of Matron Georgina F. Pope of South-African War fame. Matron Pope was stationed at Canadian army hospitals, first in England and later in France. Failing health caused her return to Canada after a little more than a year of service. The vacancy created by her withdrawal was ably filled by *Nursing Sister Margaret Macdonald.*

EDITH CAVELL.   An undoubted inspiration to many volunteers was *Edith Cavell,* whose untimely death in 1915 stirred deep feeling throughout a troubled world. Miss Cavell, an English nurse, had organized the first school for nurses in Brussels, Belgium. Here, following several battles in its vicinity, school and hospital offered care to soldiers of all

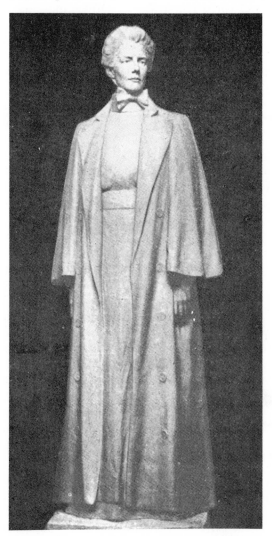

Figure 62. Edith Cavell. This figure of Edith Cavell, the martyred British nurse of World War I, is part of the Edith Cavell Memorial in Trafalgar Square, London, donated by a grateful people. The sculptor was Sir George Frampton, R.S.

armies. The Germans arrested Miss Cavell, however, and charged her with complicity in the escape to neutral territory of able bodied Allied soldiers who had been separated from their companies and were in hiding nearby. Pleading guilty, Edith Cavell was sentenced to death and executed at dawn October 12, 1915. After temporary burial in Belgium, her body was returned to England in 1919 and buried near the Cathedral at Norwich, her home town. At the same time her memory was honored by impressive ceremonies in Westminster Abbey.

American Nursing Services. America's sudden entry into the war on April 6, 1917, caught many agencies unprepared, but the American Red Cross Nursing Service, through the efforts of Jane Delano and her assistants, had enrolled great numbers of carefully selected nurses who could now be turned over for service with the expanding Army Nurse Corps and Navy Nurse Corps. Other able and experienced nurses were soon enlisted, and new recruits were actively sought and obtained.

To aid in the supply of a long-term demand for nurses, the *Army School of Nursing* was organized in 1918 with *Annie W. Goodrich* as dean. The course she organized covered three years, with a special credit of nine months to college graduates. Army hospitals and affiliating civilian hospitals offered their facilities for instruction. Applications poured in from thousands of enthusiastic women who wanted to make use of this opportunity to give service.

Another opportunity for a selected group of women was offered by the American Red Cross and Vassar College when the *Vassar Training Camp* was formed. It gave a special three months' course of preliminary instruction to four hundred eighteen college graduates, one hundred sixty nine of whom were graduated from cooperating nursing schools.

In civilian hospitals and private homes the absence of enlisted nurses created a serious problem which resulted in a new development in health education. Jane Delano's varied experience had led her to believe that women in the home could be taught to safeguard the health of their families. She advocated the establishment of classes, conducted by well-prepared nurses, in which the fundamentals of health protection and nursing care of the sick would be taught to wives and mothers.

However, this new plan for spreading health education was vigorously opposed. One objection was that such classes would draw partially trained women into the profession. Another was the old adage: "A little knowledge is a dangerous thing." Undaunted, Miss Delano, with the help of Isabel McIsaac, had already put her ideas for a course of the type suggested into a textbook now known as "American Red Cross Home Nursing Textbook." The book, the classes, and Miss Delano's planning proved so successful that providing classes in care of the sick and injured has continued as an important peacetime activity of the American Red Cross.

In spite of continuous efforts to supply nurses in civilian as well as army hospitals, the scarcity became more marked as time went on.

Enemies of public health such as pneumonia, typhus spreading over Serbia and Poland, and the great influenza pandemic of 1918 made their appearance, each claiming some doctors and nurses among its victims. Typhoid fever presented a less serious problem than during previous wars because of control by vaccination and better provision for water supply.

On November 11, 1918, the Armistice became effective and actual fighting ceased, but the ills of war continued and new problems arose. Among the ranks of the fighting men, injured and sick were still to be cared for and transported with as much comfort as possible to their homes. In addition, an underfed, discouraged civilian population of Europe offered its plea for help. War orphans, refugees, and throngs of the sick overflowed understaffed hospitals. Finally, emotional strain associated with the violent catastrophe of war left all Europe sick in mind and spirit.

It was during this period that the American Red Cross Nursing Service lost its able and energetic leader. Shortly after the Armistice, in order to study emergency problems, Jane Delano sailed for France to make a tour of inspection of nursing in military hospitals. While there she became ill and, following several emergency mastoid operations, this "Great War Nurse" died at the Base Hospital in Savenay, April 15, 1919. Burial, at first, was at Savenay in a plot of ground set apart for American soldiers; later her body was interred at the National Cemetery in Arlington, Virginia.

ROYAL COLLEGE OF NURSING

While thousands of their number were giving active service in military and civilian hospitals, English nurses became acutely aware of need for creating an organized body to work toward more uniform professional standards, as well as to deal with many other serious problems. To accomplish this end the *Royal College of Nursing* was founded in 1916. A committee was appointed to seek financial backing for the new institution, and so generous was the response of the English people that the College has been able to sponsor many progressive activities relating to nursing service and nursing education.

As a means of providing for inspection and accrediting of nursing schools, compulsory registration of nurses became of immediate concern to the Royal College of Nursing. Through its influence, in 1919, more than thirty years after founding of the Royal British Nurses' Association, the long-hoped-for legislation was procured. Other accomplishments have been establishment of special courses in hospitals and universities for sister tutors, nurse administrators, midwives, industrial nurses, and health visitors.

Student Nurses' Association. In 1925 the Student Nurses' Association of England was organized by the Royal College of Nursing and is now

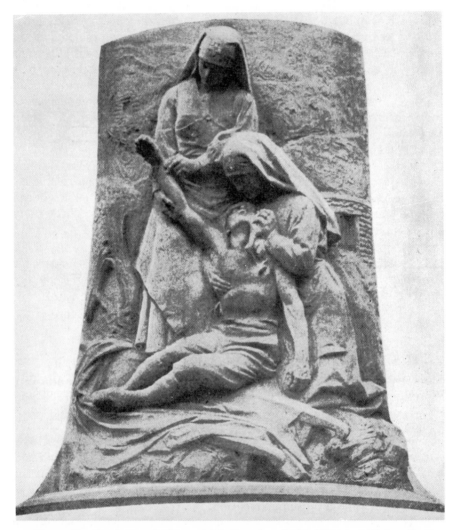

Figure 63. Panel from the Memorial to French and Allied Nurses at Reims, France. This memorial contains the Book of Gold in which are written the names of the 273 American Red Cross Nurses who died in World War I. Sculptor, Denys Puech. Architect, Charles Girault. (Courtesy *Trained Nurse and Hospital Review,* Vol. CXV, 1945.)

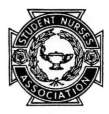

Figure 64. Symbol of Student Nurses' Association of England. (Courtesy Student Nurses' Association.)

self-governing and financially independent. Her Royal Highness, the Princess Elizabeth, graciously became first president and faithfully and conscientiously filled this office until her accession to the throne in 1952 as Queen Elizabeth II. She was succeeded in office by H. R. H. Princess Margaret, Countess of Snowden. A chairman and vice-chairman are elected.

A vacation exchange for purposes of study was arranged between the Student Nurses' Association of England and student associations of several other countries, and in 1963 sixteen students from West Germany were welcomed in London where a special program was arranged for them. Also several student nurses from Denmark, Norway, and Sweden were welcomed by the association, and two English students from Guy's Hospital in London made a study visit to the United States during their vacation of the same year.

In 1963 the Royal College of Nursing and the National Council of Nurses of Great Britain and Northern Ireland by mutual consent united into one body to be known as the *Royal College of Nursing and National Council of Nurses of the United Kingdom. Nursing Times,* a weekly journal and former official organ of the Royal College of Nursing, now represents the unified association. Her Majesty the Queen and Her Majesty Queen Elizabeth, the Queen Mother, graciously consented to be Royal Patrons.

POSTWAR RECONSTRUCTION

VOCATIONAL REHABILITATION

Great numbers of men and women, disabled by war activities, accident, or disease, were unable to earn a living. As the necessity for providing assistance became more and more apparent, vocational rehabilitation programs were initiated by a number of national governments. In the United States the first Rehabilitation Act came into force in 1920 to provide assistance for all types of handicapped persons.

A partnership between the federal government and the states was created for the purpose of developing, or restoring, the highest possible capacity of disabled persons to engage in remunerative work. The special task of returning veterans with service-connected disabilities to their rightful places in society was given over to a newly created U. S. Veterans Administration.

LEAGUE OF RED CROSS SOCIETIES

Acutely aware of need for coordinating and continuing into peacetime the work of national Red Cross societies in war-torn Europe, forty delegates of these societies met at a palatial hotel in Cannes, on the French Riviera. Among the group were several representative nurses including Lillian D. Wald of the United States. The outcome of this Cannes Conference of 1919 was founding of the *League of Red Cross Societies,* representing the greatest international agreement so far in history. From the beginning moral support poured in from all over the world.

To carry out its policies a large organized force was set up which continues to the present time to guide national Red Cross societies, assist in the medical and social fields, and provide swift emergency assistance wherever needed. A Health Section with a Nursing Division was formed almost immediately, with a nurse director of the Division and a program to furnish information about nursing, promote home nursing courses, and otherwise seek to raise the level of nursing education and service throughout the world.

POSTGRADUATE COURSES AT BEDFORD COLLEGE

Along with other pressing problems it was evident that plans must be made for instituting international postgraduate courses in public health nursing. In order to meet its overwhelming responsibility for alleviation of human misery, the League of Red Cross Societies set up temporary courses at Bedford College for Women, University of London, for nurses to be selected by their own national Red Cross Societies. In a short time courses in administration and nursing education were added to public health nursing and by 1933 more than two hundred nurses were arriving from 41 countries to take advantage of them.

Meanwhile the national Red Cross Societies of Western Europe and America made every effort to assist with civilian rehabilitation. They provided scholarships for preparation of public health nurses and helped to attract competent young people into the field of nursing. At the same time the daily newspapers depicted the civilian misery and disease which war-time activities had served to eclipse.

LEAGUE OF NATIONS

While Europe was acutely conscious of the painful effects of wholesale destruction and attempting to heal the wounds of war, plans were being directed toward securing a lasting peace. World leaders, prominent among whom was *President Woodrow Wilson* of the United States, expressed their faith in a *League of Nations* which would act as a body of arbitration between nations.

On all matters of dispute, member nations of the League were to be committed to arbitration and to postponement of hostilities until three months after a decision had been reached. Representatives of forty two countries set to work with the new objectives at the first regular meeting in Geneva, November 15, 1920. Although many citizens of the United States were strongly in favor of adding their country's influence to the League of Nations, America's traditional policy of remaining clear of foreign entanglements prevented her from ratifying its Covenant.

The new organization for world peace soon proved its value by preventing a number of conflicts. For a while it enjoyed considerable prestige and worked with increasing confidence on other problems of social significance. In time, however, lack of adequate means for enforcing decisions greatly weakened its influence.

GENERAL TRENDS IN NURSING

The general long-time trend in nursing from the beginning of its formal organization in 1893 to the end of World War I was considerably influenced by rapid expansion in the establishment of hospitals with a corresponding number of schools dependent upon them for support.

Schools increased in size as well as in number and, as a matter of economy, hospitals depended upon them to carry the chief nursing load. In line with this policy, greater and greater numbers of young women were accepted for entrance. At the same time the growing tendency toward less careful selection reached its peak during the wartime emergency. Not only was little emphasis placed on educational backgrounds but, in some cases at least, applicants with college training were suspected of being impractical and so discouraged.

Following the examples of the University of Pennsylvania and the Johns Hopkins hospitals, the length of the course in many schools had been increased to three years although the eight-hour day originally intended to be associated with it was less quickly adopted. To make up for deficiencies in education, postgraduate courses had been offered since 1890, but they were improperly financed and controlled, and offered little in the way of instruction.

Certain developments, however, were promising. The plan for a preliminary course of instruction introduced by Mrs. Rebecca Strong in Glasgow, Scotland, in 1893 and by Miss Nutting at the Johns Hopkins Hospital in 1901 was gradually put into effect in other schools. Affiliations with institutions offering experience of types lacking in the home school increased in number after Isabel Hampton arranged for her students of the Illinois Training School in Chicago to become familiar with the care of private patients at the Presbyterian Hospital of the same city. Many hospital authorities, however, were reluctant to part with their senior students at a time when they considered them of greatest value to themselves, and no law required them to do so.

By 1920 the apprenticeship system of educating nurses was coming under the fire of criticism. The efficiency of the nurse herself as a teacher of nurses was becoming apparent, and Teachers College, Columbia University, New York, offered a special course to prepare her for this work. All states except Nevada had passed laws providing for the registration of nurses. The World War, the influenza epidemic, and postwar confusion were pointing up the need for a full program of public health nursing and preparations for this program were under way.

BROADER AIMS IN MEDICINE

By the close of World War I the medical profession was coming to recognize the patient not merely as an individual who needed assistance, but rather as a member of family and community groups, all of whom could be taught the principles of healthful living. At the same time, as the services of the hospital extended into the home with development of public health nursing, more and more families were seeking advice on health subjects.

Medical Social Service. In an effort to improve and extend the services of the out-patient department of the Massachusetts General Hospital in Boston, *Dr. Richard Cabot,* working at first with *Garnet Pelton,* and later with *Ida M. Cannon,* began an investigation of home influences affecting their patients. Among other things it was disclosed that, in many instances, there were causes for emotional disturbance that contributed to illness. To ensure a knowledge of whole situations with consideration of the total patient in relationship to home, job, church, school, and community, a social worker was added to the staff of the out-patient department of the Massachusetts General Hospital. *The beginnings of Medical Social Service had been established* and today many hospitals operate a social service department.

As time went on health experts came to recognize in the patient and his family their greatest allies in the struggle against ill health and sought, by means of education, to gain their support. Public health departments accepted popular health education as a major responsibility. Hospitals, clinics, and health centers assumed a new importance as educational institutions, not only providing facilities for the education of physicians, nurses, dietitians, and others, but also guiding patients toward more satisfying ways of living.

The American Medical Association, composed of the combined membership of all county and state associations, dates back to 1847 and is the largest medical organization in the United States. Headquarters are at 535 North Dearborn Street, Chicago, and activities are made known through the *Journal of the American Medical Association,* published weekly, and national conventions. *Today's Health,* another of many publications, gives authentic information on health subjects in everyday language. Its articles are often reprinted in Braille and in foreign languages in many parts of the world. Through membership in a constituent association, a physician automatically becomes a member of the state and national associations.

Various councils, committees, bureaus, and departments carry on numerous activities of the AMA and help it to maintain a respected voice in national and international affairs pertaining to human welfare. The purpose of the *Council on Medical Education and Hospitals* is to elevate the standards of medical education and collect and disseminate information concerning medical schools. It also surveys hospitals and maintains a register of those meeting with its approval for purposes of research and for the education of interns and residents in certain specialties.

The *Council on Pharmacy and Chemistry* evaluates new drugs appearing on the market and publishes a report of their reliability, therapeutic value, and limitations in the *Journal of the American Medical Association* and also in "New and Nonofficial Drugs," a book published and revised by the Council annually. This council exerts a powerful influence toward ethical promotion of the use of therapeutic agents. A *Council on Foods and Nutrition,* a *Council on Mental Health,* a *Council on Industrial Health,* a *Council on National Defense,* and several others promote other AMA activities. A *Committee on Cosmetics* provides information relating to the usefulness, limitations, and health problems associated with the use of preparations for improving the appearance of the complexion. In 1959 a Committee on Nursing was formed, and the following year a Department of Nursing.

The American College of Surgeons and the American College of Physicians, each with strict membership requirements, came into being for the purpose of ensuring high standards of medical and surgical practice. In order to reach desired goals the American College of Surgeons, established in 1913 by practitioners of the United States and Canada, soon initiated a campaign of hospital standardization, a program for which full responsibility was carried until a Joint Commission on Accreditation of Hospitals was formed in 1952.

The American Society of Dental Surgeons and the first dental college, opened in Baltimore, had their beginnings in 1840. Each gave evidence of the fact that dentistry was attaining recognition as a science and a profession. Today it plays an essential part in the health services as an oral specialty of medical science. The subject of anesthesia has always been of considerable concern to dentists. Dr. W. T. G. Morton, of ether fame, was one of their number.

The American Hospital Association was founded in 1899 *"to promote the public welfare through the development of better hospital care for all the people."*[3] Membership consists of institutions and citizens of the

---

[3]Bylaws of the American Hospital Association, Article 1.

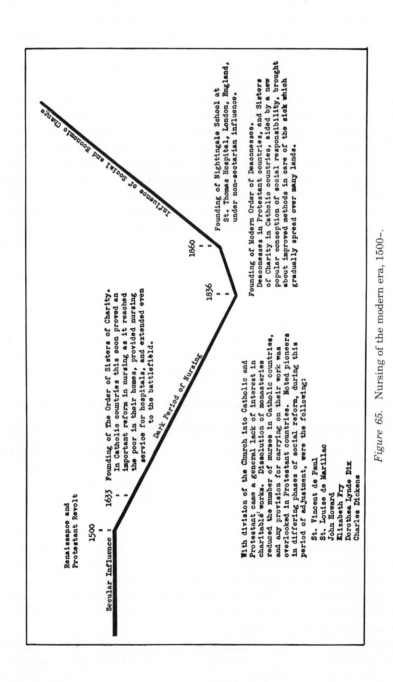

Figure 65. Nursing of the modern era, 1500–.

United States and Canada. Activities of the association are made known through *Hospitals*, an official monthly journal. Conventions, institutes, and refresher courses for administrators and department heads are held annually.

Other activities of the AHA include assistance with plans for hospital construction, equipment, administrative methods, and other factors basic to successful operation. It assists with building sound public relations programs and with the legal aspect of problems that may arise. Its influence is broadened through working in conjunction with other health organizations and groups concerned with hospital policies. Close cooperation is maintained with the American Psychiatric Association and the national nursing organizations for the purpose of providing satisfactory care for the mentally ill, who today occupy more than one-half of all hospital beds. The AHA is the national parent body of the Blue Cross, all policies of which must meet with its approval. Its headquarters are at 18 East Division Street in Chicago.

In 1964 an *AHA Council on Nursing* was established, and the incoming president of the organization referred to nurses as "this body of people who enjoy the greatest contact with our patients, represent our greatest cost of providing care, carry the heavy responsibility of dovetailing their talents with those of our men of medicine, and must be available all hours of all days for patient security."[4]

The Catholic Hospital Association of the United States and Canada, founded in 1915, and the **American Protestant Hospital Association,** founded in 1924, represent religious viewpoints and work closely with the American Hospital Association. Their energies are directed chiefly toward the special interests of institutions founded and administered by churches.

Suggestions for Study

1. Compare the first form of organization among nurses to appear in England with that in the United States and Canada.
2. Why is the World's Fair of Chicago, held in 1893, of significance in the history of New World nursing?
3. Make a list, with dates of founding, of the first nursing organizations to appear in your country.
4. When, and through whose influence, was the International Council of Nurses founded?
5. Differentiate between the objectives of a labor union and those of a professional organization.
6. Give reasons for the fact that soldiers of the Spanish-American and South African wars had better provision for nursing care than soldiers of previous wars.

---

[4]R.N. Magazine, October, 1964, p. 23.

7. Show how problems encountered by Anna C. Maxwell during the Spanish-American War resembled those of Florence Nightingale during the Crimean War.

8. What circumstances led to organizations of (a) The U. S. Army Nurse Corps? (b) The U. S. Navy Nurse Corps? (c) The American Red Cross Nursing Service?

9. (a) What country was first to grant military rank to women? (b) Does your country grant such rank?

10. At what institution in the United States was a program first developed to provide graduate study for nurses expecting to fill educational and administrative positions?

11. To what stage of development had nursing progressed when Miss Nightingale's life ended?

12. Add to your list of early nursing organizations the names they later assumed.

13. How did provision for nursing care during World War I differ from that of any previous war?

14. What nurse was executed, and for what reason, during World War I?

15. The problem of shortage of nurses for care of patients in the home was met in what ways?

16. What were the chief problems to be dealt with during the postwar period of reconstruction?

17. What two new organizations of international importance developed about this time?

18. What field of nursing was making great strides by the end of the war?

19. The emphasis in medicine was shifting in what direction?

20. What factors led to the beginning of hospital social service?

21. Make an outline of the headquarters and activities of the American Medical Association, the American College of Surgeons, the American Society of Dental Surgeons, and the American Hospital Association.

22. Who is now president of the American Red Cross?

23. Using the Official Directory of the American Journal of Nursing, make an outline of the names of nurses now at the head of each of the following federal services, with titles of their positions: (a) American Red Cross Nursing Services; (b) U. S. Army Nurse Corps; (c) U. S. Navy Nurse Corps; (d) U. S. Air Force Nurse Corps; (e) U. S. Veterans Administration Nursing Service; and (f) U. S. Public Health Service – Department of Health, Education, and Welfare.

24. Which of the above services were inaugurated during the period just studied, and which are of more recent origin?

25. Discuss the general long-time trends in nursing education from the time of beginning organization in 1893 to the period of reconstruction beginning about 1920.

References

American Hospital Association: AHA—What It Is, What It Does. American Hospital Association: AHA in Action (pamphlets). 18 East Division St., Chicago, 1955.

American Medical Association Guide to Services (pamphlet). 535 North Dearborn St., Chicago, 1955.

Breckinridge, Mary: Wide Neighborhoods: A Story of the Frontier Nursing Service. New York, Harper and Brothers, 1952.

Cabot, Richard C.: The Goal of Social Work. Boston and New York, Houghton Mifflin Co., 1927.

Cannon, Ida M.: Social Work in Hospitals. New York Survey Associates, Inc., 1913.

Clarke, Ida Clyde: American Women and the World War. New York and London, D. Appleton & Co., 1918.

Cushing, Harvey: The Life of Sir William Osler. London, Toronto, and New York, Oxford University Press, 1940.

Dulles, Foster Rhea: The American Red Cross: A History. New York, Harper and Brothers, 1950.

Gladwin, Mary E.: The Red Cross and Jane Arminda Delano. Philadelphia, W. B. Saunders Co., 1931.

Hampton, Isabel, and others (N.L.N.E., editor): Nursing of the Sick—1893. New York, McGraw-Hill Book Co., 1951.

Hoehling, A. A.: A Whisper of Eternity: The Mystery of Edith Cavell. New York, Thomas Yoseloff, Inc., 1957.

Judson, Helen: Edith Cavell. New York, The Macmillan Co., 1941.

Kernodle, Portia B.: The Red Cross Nurse in Action. New York, Harper and Brothers, 1949.

Koch, Harriet Berger: Militant Angel (Annie W. Goodrich). New York, The Macmillan Co., 1951.

Munson, Helen W.: The Story of the National League of Nursing Education. Philadelphia, W. B. Saunders Co., 1934.

Nutting and Dock: A History of Nursing. New York and London, G. P. Putnam's Sons, 1907-1912, Vol. III.

Pavey, Agnes: The Story of the Growth of Nursing. Philadelphia, J. B. Lippincott Co., 1953.

Roberts, Mary M.: American Nursing—History and Interpretation. New York, The Macmillan Co., 1954.

Sigerist, Dr. Henry E.: American Medicine. New York, W. W. Norton & Co., Inc., 1934.

Stewart, Isabel M.: The Education of Nurses. New York, The Macmillan Co., 1943.

Werminghaus, Esther A.: Annie W. Goodrich: Her Journey to Yale. New York, The Macmillan Co., 1951.

Wyche, Mary Lewis: The History of Nursing in North Carolina. Chapel Hill, University of North Carolina Press, 1938.

Yost, Edna: American Women of Nursing. Philadelphia, J. B. Lippincott Co., 1955.

Chapter 12

NATIONAL SURVEYS OF NURSING AND MEDICINE

Medicine's new aim of teaching the principles of healthful living to as many citizens as possible raised the question of supplying teachers for this purpose. Were nurses equipped with the scientific background necessary for health teaching, or should this be the province of women with more specialized education? Nursing leaders were of the opinion that the nurse should assume this new responsibility. Here again arose a problem for public health administrators. How could adequate numbers of such nurse-teachers be supplied? Now that the war was over, no exciting cause attracted young women into nursing. Should entrance requirements be lowered in order to attract greater numbers of applicants? Standards had already been appreciably declining for a number of reasons and, with them, interest in nursing was declining too. Obviously, further lowering was not the solution to the problem.

ROCKEFELLER SURVEY (1920-1923)

To make a study of ways and means of providing well qualified public health nurses, the Rockefeller Foundation called a special conference in December, 1918. Approximately fifty health leaders including doctors, nurses, and representatives of hospitals and health agencies met and, after much discussion, reached an opinion that the usual three-year course was inadequate preparation for public health work. To gain more information the delegates named a *Committee for the Study of*

274

Nursing Education, whose efforts were to be financed by the Rockefeller Foundation. *C. E. A. Winslow,* of the department of public health of Yale University, was made chairman, while actually in charge of the investigation was the secretary of the group, *Josephine Goldmark,* well known in the field of social research.

At a second meeting called by the Rockefeller Foundation about a year later the entire field of nursing was discussed, and the Committee requested to investigate all phases of nurse activity. The survey which followed covered public health groups, private duty nursing, and twenty-three representative schools connected with hospitals, large and small, public and private, over a wide territory. An educator from the field of nursing and another from the field of education, both experts, made detailed studies. The results of the survey, together with some definite conclusions, were published in 1923 in the volume, "Nursing and Nursing Education in the United States," popularly referred to as the "Winslow-Goldmark Report."

Public Health Field. Findings in the *public health field* made clear the need for teaching personal hygiene in the home. Efforts to get the cooperation of parents of school children were a new development arising from the discovery that while communicable diseases were comparatively rare, physical defects that could be either prevented or cured were legion. Children too often had organic heart disease, hearing and visual defects, infected tonsils and enlarged adenoids, defects of joints and foot arches. In other directions mental defectives and drug addicts needed psychiatric guidance. Maternal and infant mortality rates offered yet another challenge to the ability of the public health nurse. Undoubtedly it was she, health experts were coming to agree, who possessed the greatest opportunity for health teaching.

Private Duty Field. Investigation of the field of *private duty* revealed a number of interesting facts. A nurse so engaged became acquainted with and cared for only one patient, and her opportunity for teaching principles of hygiene was limited to him and his immediate family. At the same time, some physicians regarded her as too expert and too high-priced for many of their patients. Nurses themselves were failing to recognize the need for a subsidiary type of worker whose preparation could be regulated by a system of grading comparable to registration.

It was apparent also that skilled care was available only for those in comfortable circumstances and for the very poor. For the rich there were the services of the private duty nurse and the private hospital; for the poor, the visiting nurse and the free hospital. Those of moderate means were left unprovided for, although a few insurance plans for the benefit of this group were just coming into existence.

Nursing School Field. A study of *nursing schools* brought to light the fact that courses of instruction had received meager attention during the period of rapid expansion. Moreover, many nurses in responsible positions had little preparation beyond that of the basic course. Senior students were often used as head nurses, or were kept on night duty for long periods. They were sent out on private cases, and the financial return made to the hospital. Full time instructors were little known. Lecture rooms, demonstration rooms, laboratories, and libraries were generally inadequate. A great lack of uniformity in courses of instruction increased the general confusion. Such courses were often based on ward needs, and frequently modified to comply with pressure of work in the hospital. As a means of remedying deficiencies of all three phases of nursing studied, the following recommendations of the Winslow-Goldmark Report stand out as significant:

1. "That as soon as may be practicable, all agencies, public or private, employing public health nurses, should require as a prerequisite for employment the basic hospital training, followed by a postgraduate course, including both class work and field work, in public health nursing.

2. That steps should be taken through state legislation for the definition and licensure of a subsidiary grade of nursing service, the subsidiary type of worker to serve under practicing physicians in the care of mild and chronic illness, and convalescence, and possibly to assist under the direction of the trained nurse in certain phases of hospital and visiting nursing.

3. Superintendents, supervisors, instructors, and public health nurses should in all cases receive special additional training beyond the basic nursing course.

4. That the development of nursing service adequate for the care of the sick and for the conduct of the modern public health campaign demands as an absolute prerequisite the securing of funds for the endowment of nursing education of all types; and that it is of primary importance, in this connection, to provide reasonably generous endowment for university schools of nursing."[1]

As an immediate answer to the recommendation that nursing schools be independent of hospitals and on a college level, two endowed university schools of nursing were developed, one in connection with Yale University, New Haven, Connecticut, and the other with Western Reserve University, Cleveland, Ohio. The Yale School of Nursing was financed by the Rockefeller Foundation as an experiment to prove the feasibility of planning both classroom instruction and ward practice in accordance with the educational needs of students. Patients of a type and number suitable for teaching were to be selected for care during the course in each special subject, and emphasis was to be placed on the social and health aspects of nursing.

Annie W. Goodrich, leaving her position on the faculty of the Department of Nursing Education at Teachers College, Columbia University, became dean of the Yale school. After five years the experiment proved so successful that it was put on a permanent footing with a large endowment by the Foundation. The school at Western Reserve University was made independent by endowment from *Frances Payne Bolton*, and with

---

[1]Committee for the Study of Nursing Education: Nursing and Nursing Education in the United States, 1933. By permission of The Macmillan Co., publishers.

the able assistance of *Carolyn E. Gray* as dean, also proved successful. Along with the Yale School of Nursing, it demonstrated the value of university standards in the field of nursing.

GRADING OF NURSING SCHOOLS (1926–1934)

A second and far-reaching result of the Rockefeller Survey was a proposal by the National League of Nursing Education to undertake a comprehensive study of nursing education which would lead to actual grading of nursing schools. Grading, it was believed, would set up standards to which all schools would be compelled to conform. Results within the medical profession, after a similar practice had been adopted, lent probability to this belief.

The first move toward securing support for this undertaking was made when a committee of the National League of Nursing Education met with a committee of the American Medical Association for study of nursing education. The outcome was appointment of a *Committee on the Grading of Nursing Schools*, its purpose to be a cooperative study of nursing practice in all its aspects. The following organizations, all vitally interested in the project, elected representatives: National League of Nursing Education, American Nurses' Association, National Organization for Public Health Nursing, American Medical Association, American College of Surgeons, American Hospital Association, and American Public Health Association.

In addition to these groups there were representatives of university education and of the public at large. *William Darrach*, M.D., of the American Medical Association, was made chairman of the committee, and *May Ayres Burgess*, Ph.D., statistician, became director of the investigation. The services of committee members were voluntary, while the cost of extensive studies and publications was met by contributions from various sources including the AMA, the AHA, the American Public Health Association, and the three major nursing organizations. Mrs. Frances Payne Bolton and Mrs. Helen Hartley Jenkins made large contributions. Grants were received from the Rockefeller Foundation and the Commonwealth Fund and there were other special contributions.

The general purpose of the Committee on the Grading of Nursing Schools was early defined as "The study of ways and means for insuring an ample supply of nursing service, of whatever type and quality needed for adequate care of the patient, at a price within his reach."[2] In 1926 a five-year program was adopted to cover three projects judged to be worthy of study over such a period, as follows:

1. Supply and demand for nursing service.

---

[2] A Five-year Program for the Committee on the Grading of Nursing Schools (a pamphlet), p. 10.

2. Job analysis of nursing and nurse teaching.
3. Actual grading of nursing schools.

Supply and Demand for Nursing Service.   For investigation of the first problem—*supply and demand for nursing service*—the questionnaire method was used. Replies from hospitals, public health directors, registries, patients, nurses, and physicians throughout the nation formed the basis of conclusions. "Nurses, Patients, and Pocketbooks" is the title of the book published in 1928 in which opinions were expressed as to how much and what type of nursing service were necessary, as to urban and rural distribution of nurses, and as to costs associated with satisfactory care of patients.

Analysis of Nursing and Nurse Teaching.   The goal of the second project—*a job analysis of nursing and nurse teaching*—was to discover all activities that constitute nursing. Such information would be used as a scientific basis from which a satisfactory revision of the national curriculum could be constructed. Results of studies made by nurse educators were gathered together in book form by *Ethel Johns* and *Blanche Pfefferkorn* and published, in 1934, in "An Activity Analysis of Nursing."

"What is good nursing?" is the question raised in the first chapter. Opinions of patients, physicians, hospital administrators, and community laymen answered the question. Briefly, patients looked for skill combined with kindness and willingness to adjust to their particular situations. Physicians expected skill, reliability in transfer of information, and personal loyalty. The need of hospitals was for nurses who would satisfy both patients and physicians, who would assume responsibility for smooth functioning of their departments, and interpret the spirit of the hospital.

Grading of Nursing Schools.   The third project—*a comparative study of nursing schools*—encouraged each school to evaluate its own system with the help of monthly outlines provided by the Committee. All schools were identified by numbers and, as the investigation proceeded, results were returned to them in printed form. The graphs included showed the relative standing of all schools on a given subject. The position of the individual school in the general picture was checked in red.

Those concerned frequently discovered their schools to be excelling in some particulars but lagging far behind in others. All associated with a given institution, from nurses to trustees, could see how it stood in the whole scheme of American nursing education. Not only were deficiencies discernible by comparison, but new incentive was offered for removing them, and many schools took immediate steps in that direction.

Second Grading.   In 1932, to determine what had been accomplished, *a second self-study* under supervision of the Committee on the Grading of Nursing Schools was undertaken. This *Second Grading of Nursing*

Schools did not cover as wide a scope of investigation as the first, but was given more publicity. The information gathered was gratifying. Several hundred of the poorer schools had closed their doors. The others showed improvement in about three fourths of the items investigated.

The final report of the Committee on the Grading of Nursing Schools, with specific suggestions for improvement, appeared in book form in 1934. This volume "Nursing Schools Today and Tomorrow," showed the chief purpose of hospitals to be the care of patients, with their nursing schools operated as paying service departments and student nurses regarded as employees. It showed that the training offered provided efficient hospital workers, but gave little or no insight into the private duty or public health fields. It criticized the existent form of apprenticeship teaching and emphasized the need for instruction on a college level.

Certain absolute requirements for all schools of nursing were listed. They must be connected with an institution on the Hospital Register of the American Medical Association, approved by the American College of Surgeons, with a daily average of at least fifty patients. They must be accredited by the State Board of Nurse Examiners, and entering students must have no less than high school graduation as preparation. The report also stressed the necessity for a more even distribution of nursing service, for its recognition as a public responsibility with appropriation of public funds that would put nursing education on a level with other essential lines of education.

Joint Committee on the Distribution of Nursing Service. In answer to disclosures of the Rockefeller Survey and the Committee on the Grading of Nursing Schools that many areas suffered from lack of nursing care, the three national nursing organizations — American Nurses' Association, National League of Nursing Education, and National Organization for Public Health Nursing in 1928 appointed a *Joint Committee on the Distribution of Nursing Service.* This was to serve the twofold purpose

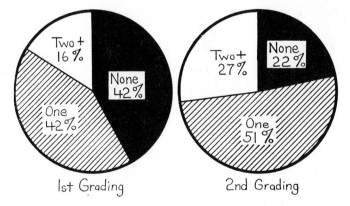

Figure 66. Grading of Nursing Schools. Per cent of schools having no instructor, one instructor, and two or more instructors, in the first and second gradings. (May Ayres Burgess in American Journal of Nursing, June, 1932.)

of making essential care available to each citizen and of ensuring needed employment among nurses during a period of great financial depression.

SURVEYS IN CANADA AND ENGLAND

While nurses of the United States were thus showing both a critical spirit and a disposition to right old wrongs, no less conscious of need for change were those of Canada and England. In 1927 three delegates from the Canadian Medical Association and three from the Canadian Nurses' Association made up a committee which proposed an investigation. Nurses on the committee were *Jean I. Gunn,* Superintendent of Nurses, Toronto General Hospital; *Kathleen Russell,* Director of the Department of Nursing, University of Toronto; and *Jean Browne,* Secretary of the Junior Red Cross Society of Canada. Chairman of the group was *Dr. G. Stewart Cameron.* All were in favor of studying educational facilities in nursing schools and were agreed further that an expert from outside the two professions would be needed to visit and investigate them. Such an expert was found in *Professor George Weir,* head of the Department of Education of the University of British Columbia.

Work on the project began in November, 1927, and drew to a close July 31, 1931. The expense had been borne by the two professions: 70 per cent by the nursing group and 30 per cent by physicians. Sufficient funds were furnished for Dr. Weir to cover every province and make

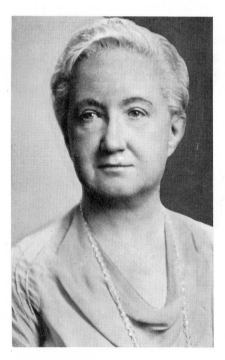

Figure 67. Jean Isabel Gunn, O.B.E., LL.D. (Courtesy of Toronto General Hospital.)

many visits to hospitals and schools. His investigations took in economic and sociological, as well as public health, implications of the nursing field, and his report was published in the volume, "Survey of Nursing Education in Canada."

In England the decline in numbers of students entering nursing schools and a corresponding decline in candidates for hospital positions led to a critical attitude toward prevailing methods. An investigation of certain phases of nursing activities was conducted in 1930 by the medical group through the *Lancet Commission*, which was made up of nurses, doctors, educators, sociologists, economists, and hospital trustees. The method followed was that of self-rating through the use of questionnaires. After studying the data returned, the Commission set down its conclusions in a published report. Disciplinary problems, poor educational opportunities, long hours of work, and salary difficulties figured prominently among deterrents to increased entrance into the profession.

REVISION OF NURSE PRACTICE ACTS

Following completion of the two national surveys of nursing education by the Rockefeller Foundation and the Committee on the Grading of Nursing Schools, interest became centered in revision of nurse practice acts. By this time it had been discovered that existing laws afforded inadequate protection for the general public, the physician, and for the nurse herself. For some time increasing numbers of "practical" nurses had been coming into employment when long-time care was needed in the home, or when housework was to be combined with nursing. At the same time no standards had been fixed for the training of a practical nurse, and she bore no guarantee of adequate preparation for the tasks which she undertook.

At the same time, even though the law set apart the Registered Nurse as one who had met certain educational requirements, anyone might call herself a nurse and accept remuneration from those who were willing to employ her. The law prohibited her from placing the letters *R.N.* after her name, but it did not prohibit her from nursing. While it had long been a requirement that all who practice medicine first meet certain fixed educational standards and become *licensed,* or legally permitted to practice, those who practiced nursing had been granted the privilege of obtaining state recognition as Registered Nurses, but were not legally required to make use of it. Laws were *permissive* rather than *mandatory.*

A pioneer in the movement to regulate all nursing practice, the State of New York enacted, in 1938, a law requiring licensing of all who nursed for hire. The law established two groups, one entitled to practice as registered professional nurses, the other as licensed practical nurses and made it unlawful for any person not so licensed to be employed in any capacity for the care of the sick in the State of New York. It was soon discovered, however, that the situation thus created was incompatible with the demands of World War II, and the law was suspended until April 1, 1949, when its mandatory provisions came into full effect. Other states followed the example of New York with the enactment of similar, but often less inclusive, legislation.

From time to time the question of a *national* licensing system which would permit the nurse to practice in any state of the union has been agitated but has met with stumbling blocks in the form of provision for "States' Rights" in the Constitution of the United States and also in differing standards for state accreditation of schools. Unfortunately, progress toward all types of revision of nurse practice acts was interrupted by participation in World War II. As a result, all thought and energy were diverted to the task of providing a hitherto unheard-of number of nurses as quickly as possible.

SURVEY OF MEDICAL PRACTICE (1927–1932)

During the period of investigation by the Committee on the Grading of Nursing Schools, an extensive survey of medical practice was also going on in the United States. Public criticism of shortcomings in provision for medical care during illness had been growing louder and louder, and the causes for complaint were many. On the one hand, scientific knowledge had increased to a phenomenal extent. Potentially it was possible to greatly reduce the incidence of illness and to prolong life. On the other hand, with improved facilities had come higher costs, and opportunity to benefit by modern methods had been carried further and further away from the average person.

In order to meet the insistent clamor for more and better medical service a *Committee on the Costs of Medical Care*, composed of physicians, economists and other specialists, was established in 1927. A research staff was engaged and a five-year plan of fact-finding formulated which developed into a nation-wide study of differences between the medical care needed and that being received by the people. The costs of such care and its distribution were also taken into consideration. At the same time, statistics relating to annual incomes of physicians, dentists, and nurses were accumulated and shown to be unsatisfactory. Because of the financial depression many professional people were suffering from lack of employment while patients were suffering from lack of care.

Conclusions reached by the Committee on the Costs of Medical Care made more apparent than ever that citizens of the country were not receiving the full benefits of what medicine and related sciences had to offer. Medical and nursing services were unevenly distributed, with some areas left entirely without them. The remedy suggested was that governmental bodies assume considerable responsibility for the health of citizens. Adequate medical services could be provided by means of group insurance, with costs distributed over great numbers of people. The question as to whether the carrying of medical insurance should be made compulsory or voluntary was regarded as controversial and has remained so in the United States up to the present time.

SOCIAL SECURITY ACT OF 1935

Satisfactory provision for care during illness was only one of many questions of a social nature as yet unanswered. Society was confronted with a complexity of problems, the solution of which involved development of methods never before employed in history. With an economic depression of global proportions, heralded by a spectacular crash of the stock market in 1929, vast throngs of people, regardless of personal abilities or years of service, were thrown out of employment with little or no hope of securing other positions. As poverty mounted, the incidence of illness increased and more and more insistent grew the demand that society as a whole assume responsibility for the welfare of its citizens.

In a number of European countries, social laws which made easier the lot of the average man were put into effect about this time. In the United States, the Social Security Act of 1935 recognized a wide range of social needs, as indicated by the following statement:

"The act was devised to alleviate phases of economic distress such as are found even in normal times among the temporarily unemployed, dependent children, the aged, and the blind, and to strengthen maternal and child welfare, public health, and vocational rehabilitation service."[3]

The U.S. Department of Health, Education, and Welfare now cooperates with state governments to administer the various projects, funds for which are provided by means of social security taxes paid by employers, employees, and the self-employed. Activities relating to hospital and public health facilities are carried on by the U.S. Public Health Service, while Maternal and Child Welfare and Crippled Children services are the immediate concern of the U.S. Children's Bureau.

U.S. National Health Surveys. In order that benefits of the Social Security Act might reach all for whom they were intended, and to secure a comprehensive picture of health conditions throughout the nation, a National Health Survey was carried on during 1935 and 1936 by the U.S. Public Health Service. There had been lesser surveys, including that of the AMA Committee on the Costs of Medical Care, but this was a greater undertaking than any that had preceded it. In the past the chief concern

---

[3]Informational Service Circular No. 1: A Brief Explanation of the Social Security Act, page 1.

of governments had been to control the transfer of communicable disease from one area to another but now statistics were required in relation to prevalent types of illness, injury, and disability.

The facts elicited revealed that an uneven distribution of medical and nursing services and inadequate facilities of hospitals and public health institutions were largely responsible for failure to meet the health needs of the people. That one-third of the population was receiving little or no medical attention, and an even larger proportion was suffering from economic burdens as the result of illness, were among the alarming conclusions.

As time went on data of this first National Health Survey became of little value while, at the same time, expanding responsibilities of health agencies of all kinds were requiring a corresponding expansion in the field of health statistics. In 1956 a National Health Survey Act was passed by Congress and signed by the President, which authorizes the Surgeon General of the U.S. Department of Health, Education, and Welfare to conduct a continuing survey of illness and disability throughout the country.

National Health Conference. Preparatory to instituting a National Health program of wide proportions, a National Health Conference was summoned to Washington in 1938. Official representatives of the American Medical Association, of hospital and social service groups, and of the three major national nursing organizations attended. Annie W. Goodrich was the only speaker representing the nurses. Discussion centered on provision for adequate and equable distribution of medical and nursing services.

As a means of accomplishing desired ends, it was recommended that each community be held responsible for coordination of effort of its own hospitals, health centers, clinics, and laboratories, and for putting them within reach of all the people. The greatest expansion of hospital and public health facilities in history followed. The best scientific knowledge and methods that modern medicine has to offer were afforded hitherto neglected areas. The services of great numbers of doctors and nurses with special preparation were secured and, through allotment of USPHS scholarships, provision was made for training others.

FLORENCE NIGHTINGALE INTERNATIONAL FOUNDATION

The proposal for a living, educational memorial to Florence Nightingale, made at the ICN Congress in Berlin in 1912, was discussed at a meeting of representatives of the British Red Cross, the League of Red Cross Societies, and the International Council of Nurses held at St. Thomas Hospital in 1932. A constitution was outlined and two years later the *Florence Nightingale International Foundation* became a reality with representatives of the LORCS and the ICN on its advisory council.

National Florence Nightingale Memorial Committees were formed in various countries to promote a Trust Fund to carry on the work of the memorial and to provide scholarships for postgraduate study. A Trust Deed, registered under English law as an Educational Trust, was obtained in order to ensure continued use of the Fund for its intended purpose. Headquarters were to be in London because, "it is there that Miss Nightingale's spirit still lives in fullest radiance, as libraries, museums, hospitals, churches, indeed the very streets, bear testimony."[4]

About this time the League of Red Cross Societies was planning to discontinue its postgraduate courses at Bedford College as responsibility for meeting the postwar emergency neared completion. Recognizing an opportunity, the FNIF took over this work on a permanent basis from the fall of 1934 to the beginning of World War II in 1939 when all new arrivals were required to return to their respective countries. During this five year period certificates were granted to 341 nurses from 47 countries who completed courses in Education, Administration, and Public Health Nursing and went out to open nursing schools in countries where none had existed and otherwise raise the level of nursing practice in many areas.

The first headquarters of the FNIF, at 15 Manchester Square in London, had previously been used by the LORCS with its scholarship program at Bedford College and was turned over to the FNIF fully furnished and equipped and with a long term lease. *Olive Baggally,* a graduate of the Nightingale School, was appointed FNIF secretary and administrator. Early in World War II the house was closed for safety reasons and its library and other valuables stored. Later it was greatly damaged by bombs.

FNIF ASSOCIATED WITH THE ICN

In 1949 the Florence Nightingale International Foundation was reorganized, and to ensure strength and protection was brought into association with the International Council of Nurses and given responsibility for its education programs. In 1957 structure changes were made in the ICN at the Congress held in Rome, Italy, when a new *Nursing Service Division* and an *Education Division* were created, the latter to be the responsibility of the FNIF and known as the *Florence Nightingale Education Division.*

The identity of the FNIF as a separate organization and its Trust Fund were retained but it was necessary to have the Trust Deed amended in order to allow the income to be used for a specific educational activity. Representatives of the Nursing Division of the League of Red Cross Societies continue to serve on its advisory council. In 1961 a new *Social*

---

[4]American Journal of Nursing, Sept., 1938, p. 795.

and Economic Welfare Division of the ICN was created at the Congress in Melbourne, Australia.

The FNIF Education Division of the ICN maintains an information center and advisory service in regard to all aspects of nursing education. The annual income of the Trust Fund is allowed to accumulate until such time as the amount is sufficient to undertake special projects, two of which have been international seminars on research methods applied to nursing problems, one held in France and the other in India, and with the help of grants from the World Health Organization, four studies of various aspects of nursing education have been undertaken.

The International Council of Nurses today is a federation of national nursing organizations, and the oldest international association of professional women in the world. The affiliated organizations, not individual nurses, constitute its membership. All nurses who belong to a national nurses' association affiliated with the ICN are entitled to its privileges and contribute to its support through their national dues.

In 1966 headquarters of the ICN and the FNIF were moved from London, England, to 35–37 rue de Vermont, 1200 Geneva, Switzerland. Here a professional and clerical staff works closely with ICN committees to carry on their various programs. Activities are directed toward promoting high standards of nursing on a worldwide basis, strengthening international good will, and protecting the interests and professional status of nurses.

A major ICN responsibility is that of maintaining relationship with other international groups interested in promoting social welfare and world health. It has special relationships with several Specialized Agencies of the United Nations concerned with international health, and sends a representative to congresses of the World Medical Association, the International Hospital Association, the International Dental Federation, and the World Federation for Mental Health. An ICN representative is present also at meetings of the Nursing Advisory Committee of the League of Red Cross Societies.

Journals and Congresses. Communication with the membership and other interested persons is maintained through bimonthly publication of the *International Nursing Review,* in which some articles appear in French, German, and Spanish. ICN Congresses are held quadrennially where nurses from many lands, representing peoples in far distant corners of the world, meet to exchange greetings and discuss mutual interests.

Suggestions for Study

1. Account for the fact that, with medicine's new aim of teaching personal hygiene to many people, the prevailing method of preparing nurses came under the fire of criticism.

2. What was the nursing situation at this time in regard to supply of workers for the public health field, and the number and type of students in the schools?

3. (*a*) What institution, closely associated with the public health movement, undertook a survey of the nursing field? (*b*) What committee was appointed, and who were its chairman and its secretary?

4. (*a*) List important findings of the Committee, and some conclusions at which it arrived. (*b*) What two endowed university schools of nursing were founded in answer to one conclusion?

5. (*a*) The appointment of what Committee was another and far-reaching result of the Rockefeller Survey? (*b*) By whom was it sponsored? (*c*) Members of what organizations served on the Committee?

6. During its five year program, what three projects were undertaken by the Committee on Grading of Nursing Schools?

7. Why was a second survey made by the Grading Committee, and what were its findings?

8. What circumstances led to appointment of a Joint Committee on the Distribution of Nursing Service?

9. What do you know of similar surveys of nursing education in other countries?

10. (*a*) In what project did organized nursing become interested after completion of the surveys by the Rockefeller Foundation and the Committee on the Grading of Nursing Schools? (*b*) What circumstances led to the new undertaking?

11. (*a*) What public criticisms led to an extensive survey of medical practice? (*b*) What Committee was appointed for this purpose? (*c*) Enumerate several conclusions reached.

12. (*a*) What changes in social outlook led to enactment of the Social Security Act of 1935? (*b*) What provisions were made for enforcement of the Act? (*c*) What field of nursing has it most vitally affected?

13. How did the U. S. National Health Survey of 1935 and 1936 differ from others that had preceded it?

14. Have any other health surveys taken place since that time?

15. Where and when was the first National Health Conference held, by whom was it attended, and what were its accomplishments?

16. (*a*) What type of memorial to Florence Nightingale was founded in 1934? (*b*) How was money raised to carry on its programs?

17. What was the first educational undertaking of the FNIF, and why was it discontinued?

18. What circumstances brought about association of the FNIF with the ICN, and what are its present title and responsibility?

19. What new Division of the ICN was created at the Congress in Melbourne, Australia, in 1961?

20. (*a*) Of what is the membership of the ICN composed? (*b*) How is communication maintained with them?
21. Where are the headquarters of the ICN and the FNIF located, and toward what general purposes are their activities directed?
22. With what other international groups has the ICN relationship?

References

Committee for the Study of Nursing Education: Nursing and Nursing Education in the United States. New York, The Macmillan Co., 1923.

Committee on the Grading of Nursing Schools: Nurses, Patients, and Pocketbooks, 1928.

Committee on the Grading of Nursing Schools: Nursing Schools Today and Tomorrow, 1934.

Committee on Costs of Medical Care: Medical Care for the American People. Chicago, University of Chicago Press, 1932.

Curriculum Committee of Canadian Nurses' Association: A Proposed Curriculum for Schools of Nursing in Canada, 1936.

Curriculum Committee of National League of Nursing Education: Curriculum Guide for Schools of Nursing, 1938.

Falk, Rorem, and Ring: The Costs of Medical Care. Chicago, University of Chicago Press, 1933.

Goodrich, Annie W.: The Social and Ethical Significance of Nursing. New York, The Macmillan Co., 1932.

Johns and Pfefferkorn: An Activity Analysis of Nursing, 1934. Published by the Committee on the Grading of Nursing Schools.

Lancet Commission on Nursing: Final Report. The Lancet, Ltd., 7 Adam Street, Adelphi, London, W.C. 2.

Roberts, Mary M.: American Nursing—History and Interpretation. New York, The Macmillan Co., 1954. Chaps. 19 and 20.

Sigerist, Dr. Henry E.: American Medicine. New York, W. W. Norton & Co., Inc., 1934.

Stewart, Isabel M.: The Education of Nurses. New York, The Macmillan Co., 1943.

Weir, G. M.: Survey of Nursing Education in Canada. Toronto, Canada, University of Toronto Press, 1932.

American Journal of Nursing
"The U. S. National Health Survey" - Lucile Petry Leone. May, 1959, p. 302.

Part Four

**ACCELERATED SCIENTIFIC
AND SOCIAL EVOLUTION**

Chapter 13

WORLD WAR II AND POSTWAR DEVELOPMENTS

Provoked by a German attack on Poland, England declared war against Germany September 1, 1939. On December 8, 1941, the United States made a similar declaration against Japan. Two days later Germany and Italy retaliated by declaring war against the United States. The world was plunged into a new and terrifying form of conflict known as "total war," involving every man, woman, and child of belligerent countries. The answer to total war was total defense, with all civilians subjected to regimentation. Every able-bodied person had his station and his duties and was trained to carry out specific tasks in the event of bombing or invasion. The aged and the children were often evacuated in great numbers out of danger zones, taking nothing with them but what they could carry. Inevitably, anxiety neuroses and emotional instability accompanied such practices.

It was inevitable, too, that rapid massing of troops in camps of the homeland would open up new channels for the spread of infection. Especially among men recruited from rural districts, the usual wartime outbreaks of children's diseases were frequent. Other varieties of disease put in their appearance with the transportation of troops to battle areas all over the globe. Lurking in the pest-ridden African desert and South Pacific jungle, along with enemy snipers, were organisms causing malaria, dysentery, typhus, and other diseases.

Advances in Medical Treatment. As in previous conflicts, advances in medical treatment were great in some directions. The prevention and treatment of shock and infection showed marked improvement. Many a war veteran owes his life today to the effectiveness of blood plasma, which could be transported to the battlefield and administered by a

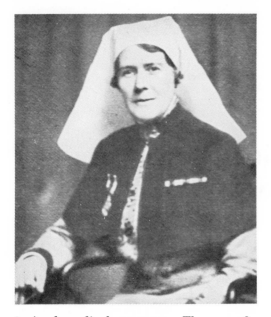

Figure 68. Dame Katherine H. Jones, D.B.E., R.R.C., S.R.N. Matron-in-Chief Q.A.I.M.N.S. during World War II. (British Journal of Nursing, July, 1942.)

trained medical corpsman. The use of penicillin and the sulfonamides in relation to infection likewise was responsible for recovery of many of the wounded. When overseas sources of quinine were cut off by enemy action, synthetic preparations were perfected, giving promise of better results than the original. The new insecticide, dichloro-diphenyl-trichloroethane, better known as "DDT," was evolved and worked miracles in the elimination of insect-borne and rodent-borne diseases, notably malaria and typhus. Also among effective prophylactic measures introduced in World War II was the administration of tetanus toxoid and yellow fever vaccine to all members of the fighting forces.

National Nursing Council for War Service. A high incidence of disease and mounting casualties of war made it necessary that ever greater numbers of doctors, nurses, and related medical personnel be forthcoming. Recognizing the need for concerted action, a *National Nursing Council for War Service* was organized in July, 1940, to represent the nurses of the United States, and plans were formulated to (a) promote a national inventory of registered nurses, (b) expand facilities of existing accredited schools of nursing and (c) supply supplementary nursing services to hospitals and public health agencies.

The National Nursing Council for War Service soon proved effective as a coordinating link between organized nursing and the federal program for supplying an adequate number of nurses to the armed forces. Launching an intensive campaign to attract candidates to nursing schools, it disseminated information that would be helpful in judging the relative merits of nursing schools, stated minimum entrance requirements, and outlined opportunities within the field of professional nursing. By magazine, poster, letter, and radio the Nursing Council spread its message of need and opportunity. In addition, it served as a consultant to the *Procurement and Assignment Service for Physicians, Dentists, Veterinarians, Sanitary Engineers, and Nurses,* a federal agency to which had been delegated responsibility for equable distribution of professional personnel in accordance with both military and civilian needs.

Red Cross Agencies. Working side by side with the National Nursing Council for War Service was the American Red Cross Nursing Service as it campaigned to enlarge the roll of reserve nurses who would be ready to augment the Army Nurse Corps and the Navy Nurse Corps as need arose. Also, a *Red Cross Student Reserve* was set up in which senior student nurses were enrolled with the pledge to become active in war service upon graduation. At the same time graduate nurses, with special preparation and holding responsible positions, were encouraged to remain at their posts. Unfortunately, however, this plea went unheeded by many.

In a determined effort to meet the desperate need of hospitals, first-aid stations, and similar organizations for trained assistants to professional nurses, the *Red Cross Volunteer Nurses' Aide Corps* was organized. Composed of women between the ages of eighteen and fifty, many of them with homes and families, the Corps was trained by qualified nurse instructors in an eighty hour course, thirty five of which were in the classroom, and forty five in hospital wards. Their instructors were pleased by the efficient manner in which this group took hold of simple nursing tasks for which housewifely experience provided a valuable background.

Additional help came from the American Red Cross in the employment of great numbers of nurse instructors to teach courses in *Care of the Sick and Injured* to housewives and mothers in order that they might take intelligent care of their families during minor illnesses or periods of convalescence. Finally, the Red Cross greatly enlarged its personnel of instructors for teaching principles of *First Aid* to all types of people.

U. S. Public Health Service. Added to the efforts of the National Nursing Council for War Service and the American Red Cross were those of the *United States Public Health Service.* By conducting the National Inventory of Registered Nurses, promoted by the National Nursing Council for War Service, it was able to determine the total number of nurses throughout the nation, their preparation, experience, and availability. With its sanction and cooperation, federal funds were granted to schools of nursing of good standing, enabling them to increase their dormitory space and teaching facilities in order to make possible an increase in student enrollment, expansion of post-graduate courses, and institution of refresher courses for those who had been inactive in nursing.

UNITED STATES CADET NURSE CORPS. So great was the need that, despite coordinated efforts, there remained an unfulfilled demand for military and civilian nurses. In one of the most effective steps taken to meet the emergency, Congress in 1943 passed the Bolton Bill, sponsored by Mrs. Frances Payne Bolton, congresswoman of Ohio, who had previously endowed the Frances Payne Bolton School of Nursing in Cleveland. Under provisions of the Bolton Act the USPHS was authorized to establish the *United States Cadet Nurse Corps* through which young women desirous of entering schools of nursing would be extended financial aid similar to a scholarship.

In a campaign to attract great numbers of recruits it was widely advertised that students entering schools of nursing would be provided with books, indoor uniforms, all entrance and tuition fees, and paid a generous monthly allowance for personal expenses. In addition, an attractive gray outdoor uniform was designed featuring crimson epaulets, insignia of the U. S. Public Health Service, and a distinctive sleeve emblem patterned after the Maltese Cross, emblem of the Knights of St. John of Jerusalem. Students, in return, pledged themselves to remain in some type of active nursing service for the duration of the war.

In order to be approved for receiving cadet students, schools of nursing were required to accelerate their curricula so that, during the last six months, senior cadets might be available for service in military or other civilian hospitals where the need was greater. In this way cadet

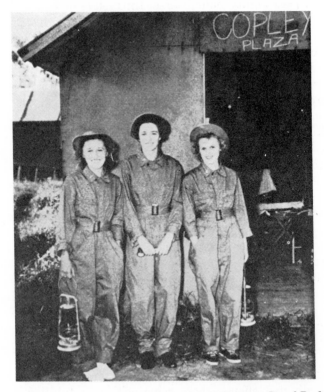

Figure 69. Trio of Army Nurses. (From Folder, "Enlist in a Proud Profession! Train as a Nurse!" Put out by the U. S. Cadet Nurse Corps during the war.)

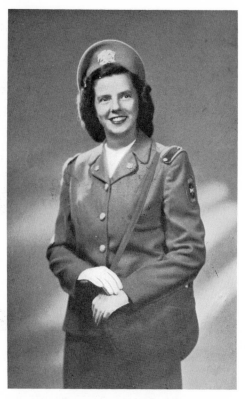

Figure 70. A member of the United States Cadet Nurse Corps during World War II.

assistance was brought quickly to many institutions, educational and dormitory facilities vacated by senior cadets were made available for new recruits, and thousands of graduate nurses were released for military service without danger of collapse of nursing service at home. At the same time nursing schools grew more and more handicapped by a shortage of qualified teachers, as doctors and nurses continued to leave for war service in great numbers.

Accepting the fact that a high percentage of their employees must be released, hospitals made heroic effort to ensure essential care for their patients. Part-time nurses and subsidiary workers were employed whenever possible. Refresher courses were instituted for retired nurses willing to return to duty, while the volunteer services of Red Cross Nurses' Aides for a few hours daily were gratefully accepted. At the same time an effort was made to discourage all types of "luxury nursing," and the employment of special nurses by patients, or office nurses by doctors, was deemed contrary to patriotic spirit.

Military Nursing. And where, one may well ask, did all those nurses leaving for active service go? The answer would cover a map of the world, for the nurse of World War II followed military operations, went with the fighting men. From Alaska to Australia, from England to Africa, from the Philippines to India, nurses of all warring countries carried on courageously, at times in face of enemy bomb, shell, and torpedo. Assist-

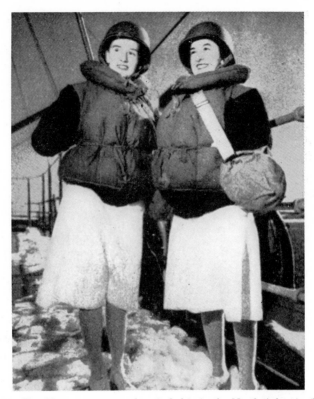

Figure 71. Two Navy nurses on a hospital ship in the North Atlantic. (From Folder, "Enlist in a Proud Profession! Train as a Nurse!" put out by the U. S. Cadet Nurse Corps during the war.)

ing in underground operating rooms, evacuating patients from bombed positions, and salvaging equipment, nurses upheld the finest traditions of their calling. Some were called upon to care for patients in the midst of tropical jungles, to part with all of their possessions as they evaded the trap of an enemy, to abandon sinking ships, to escape in submarines, to drift for days in lifeboats. Others were taken prisoner, and some were killed in line of duty.

Along with great advances in aviation prior to and during the war, it was not strange that the airplane should come to play an important role in transporting the sick and wounded, and neither was it strange that the nurse should have a place in the new method. With special training she might become a "flight nurse," caring for patients in air ambulances while in transit from battle fronts and emergency hospitals to institutions within zones of safety. A small group of selected nurses even learned parachute jumping at the Air Evacuation School set up at Bowman Field, Kentucky.

Industrial Nursing. With the production of hitherto unheard-of numbers of shells, ships, tanks, planes, and guns, *war industry* grew to vast proportions. To maintain this flood of equipment, calls for help were sent out everywhere to men, women, and children. By bus, train, and automobile they swarmed into manufacturing centers until scores of cities fairly bulged with the influx of workers. Also, in cornfields and deserts there grew like magic great industrial plants surrounded by their satellite areas of housing projects overflowing with humanity. Only in what was considered a struggle for existence could such a transformation take place so quickly.

As with the front line soldier, the health of the home front worker must be conserved if he was to remain at his post turning out the materials of war. The great expansion in industrial nursing that followed proved a further drain upon available nurse power. At the same time, with the usual wartime increase in general wage levels, more and more workers participated in prepayment and group medical plans resulting in ever greater patient loads in hospitals. With gathering speed the need for supplying doctors and nurses grew in all directions.

Like her sister in military uniform, the industrial nurse contributed her share to the war effort. Not only did she render nursing service under the direction of an industrial physician, but she also worked on safety education and accident prevention programs. Through her efforts loss of time due to occupational and nonoccupational illnesses and injuries was reduced to a minimum. In daily contact with the industrial worker and his family, she had opportunity to render assistance not only in relation to physical ills but in many psychological and emotional problems as well.

The Nurse Draft Bill. In the closing months of the war, but before it was fully realized that the end was near, the president of the United

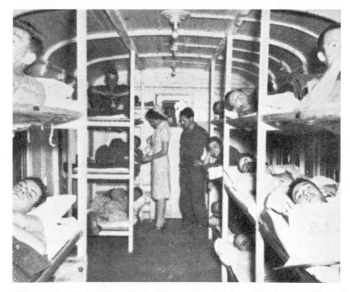

Figure 72. A hospital train. (From "Army Nursing" — a brochure published at Washington, D.C., August 7, 1947.)

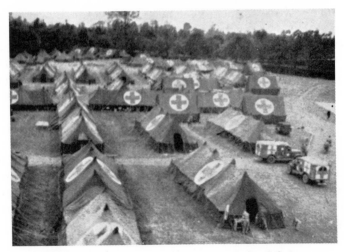

Figure 73.   An evacuation hospital near a battlefront.

States called upon Congress to prepare legislation permitting the government to draft nurses into military service. Although a large proportion of active professional nurses were in service, voluntary enlistments were not meeting requirements. The American Nurses' Association went on record as approving such a move provided that it be made a part of Selective Service legislation to include all women.

In March, 1945, the House of Representatives designed and passed a Nurse Draft Bill and sent it to the Senate, but subsequent events invalidated need for it. Realizing the urgency expressed in the president's words, additional nurses volunteered for war service, and a survey of cadet nurses showed that approximately nine tenths of them would enter the Army or Navy Nurse Corps upon graduation. Then the war in Europe came to an end on May 8, and need for a draft of nurses was over. The bill was dropped. With final termination of hostilities in the Pacific, August 14, 1945, the greatest nurse recruiting campaign in history came to a close.

POSTWAR PROBLEMS

Like other wars before it, World War II left in its wake an aftermath of hunger, fear, sorrow, and disease. This time, however, the loss of human life and human trust was greater. With these facts in view, it is understandable that sociologists of today regard the elimination of war as the most urgent of man's problems, a practice of primitive man that can be continued only at the risk of annihilating our entire civilization. As time goes on new scientific discoveries lead to more terrible agents of destruction; but new weapons alone cannot serve as a measure of the horrors of war, for old destroyers sufficient to uproot social life always

accompany it. Moral deterioration and spread of social disease are con-
comitants of war, while poverty, broken homes, and absence of parental
guidance inevitably lead to anxiety neuroses and juvenile delinquency.

With such chaotic signposts to point the way, is it little wonder that
at least a part of the world's people are striving to lead mankind out of
old primitive pathways into a constructive era of peace and good will
toward one's neighbors? The path leading to peace is a rocky one for it
necessitates changes in long standing political and economic patterns.
Nevertheless, there are reasons for encouragement.

UNRRA

The League of Red Cross Societies was active throughout the war in
relieving suffering and, late in 1943, forty-four countries banded together to bring into being the *United Nations Relief and Rehabilitation
Administration,* a temporary organization to provide immediate assistance during a critical period. With the combined efforts of contributing
nations were included the services of many doctors, nurses, dentists,
social workers, and sanitary engineers. Surely there is cause for opti-
mism concerning the future of civilization when it is realized that so
many nations, in the midst of a war whose outcome was uncertain,

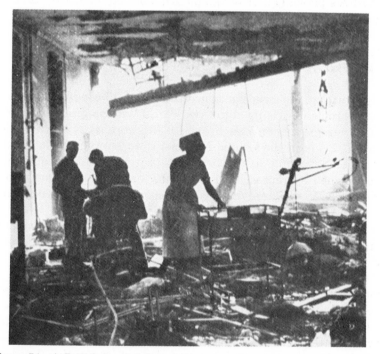

Figure 74. A British hospital after raiders passed. (American Journal of Nursing,
April, 1941.)

instituted a program to provide food, shelter, and clothing for millions of needy peoples.

Some idea of the immensity of the task confronting UNRRA can be gathered from a study of Europe in the era immediately following total war. From France to western Russia and from the Baltic to the Mediterranean, an estimated twenty million human beings suffered from exposure, malnutrition, and disease, lived a pathetic day to day existence. With a complete lack of medical supplies, or even of soap, that elementary adjunct to health, disease and moral deterioration ran rampant. Tuberculosis headed the list of causes of death while scabies, influenza, and dysentery completed the incapacitation and decimation of millions of people.

Against this holocaust UNRRA threw its might, and the vast program was carried on in the face of crippling shortages of equipment and personnel. In addition to administering to the hungry, the homeless, and the sick, it was instrumental in determining the available medical and nurse supply in a given area, establishing schools for nurses and nurses' aides, and in providing scholarships for graduate study.

Today the task of UNRRA is over. The size of that task may be measured by such statistical markers as the number of vaccines and serums administered, the tons of food dispensed, the quantity of clothing made available. Measure can never be made of the mental suffering alleviated by UNRRA's personnel, or of the message of hope that they brought to millions of hapless victims of war's ruthless desolation.

THE UNITED NATIONS

Recognizing the need for concerted action to cope with social and economic problems arising out of two World Wars, a group of representatives of nations met in San Francisco in February, 1945. Out of this gathering was born the United Nations, a world organization designed to promote peacetime teamwork and prevent future hostilities. Its charter, signed by representatives of fifty one nations, came into force October 24, 1945, the anniversary of which is observed as United Nations Day.

The structure of the United Nations consists of six principal organs: General Assembly, Security Council, Trusteeship Council, International Court of Justice, Economic and Social Council, and Secretariat.

General Assembly. At the center of the structure of the United Nations is the General Assembly, the only principal organ representing all members and having functions and powers in relation to all other UN bodies. Upon its shoulders rests responsibility for reviewing perplexing problems arising between nations and making recommendations to them and to the Security Council in the interests of international peace and security.

Procedures of the General Assembly are carried on according to parliamentary rule and recorded in English, French, and Spanish. Each member nation, whether large or small, rich or poor, has one vote, and the decisions reached exert considerable moral influence over the great family of nations.

Security Council.   The Security Council is composed of five permanent members – Great Britain, Nationalist China, France, The Soviet Union, and the United States – and ten nonpermanent members elected for two year periods by the General Assembly. It is primarily responsible for effecting peaceful settlement of disputes that might otherwise lead to war, and also for bringing about disarmament.

Any nation, whether or not a member of the United Nations, may request action if it feels that it is being imposed upon by another nation and that peace is being threatened. All sides are expected to agree to inquiry, negotiation, mediation, judicial settlement, and other peaceful means of adjustment. In all affairs of the Council world opinion exerts a powerful influence on the outcome.

Trusteeship Council.   The sacred trust of assuming supervision of Trust Territories released from control of defeated powers of World Wars I and II, as well as those voluntarily given over to it by nations responsible for them, has been assigned to the Trusteeship Council. The objective is promotion of social and economic conditions that will lead progressively to full self-administration.

International Court of Justice.   The *International Court of Justice* comprises fifteen judges from as many countries who have been elected by the General Assembly and the Security Council and provided with legal machinery to settle disputes. It is permanently in session at The Hague, Holland, and the judges, on annual salary, are permitted no other occupation. The Court of Justice makes decisions which are in agreement with the principles of international law and the general legal principles recognized by civilized peoples.

Economic and Social Council.   The Economic and Social Council of the United Nations is composed of 27 member nations, elected by the

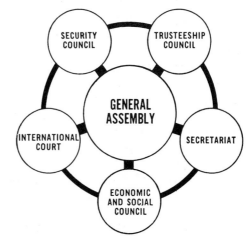

Figure 75.   The six main organs of the United Nations. (Courtesy United Nations Review.)

General Assembly for three year periods, and carries responsibility for promoting high standards of living, full employment, and educational and cultural advantages everywhere in the world. The philosophy back of all ECOSOC programs is that of assisting countries, which request their services, to reduce the incidence of poverty, disease, and illiteracy among their people. With its leadership, questions of human rights without distinction of race, sex, language, or religion, the employment status of women, and control of narcotics have made noteworthy strides forward.

Four Specialized Agencies of ECOSOC which are closely related to the field of health are the Food and Agriculture Organization (FAO), the International Labor Organization (ILO), the UN Educational, Scientific, and Cultural Organization (UNESCO), and the World Health Organization (WHO). Special responsibility for the welfare of mothers and children is assumed by the UN International Children's Fund (UNICEF), which is a Special Body that receives no financial support from the UN but with the aid of voluntary contributions works closely with the World Health Organization.

FAO. The FAO works toward provision for higher nutritional levels of peoples everywhere. So far in history more than one half of the earth's population has been constantly hungry but, with the assistance of FAO, scanty and unbalanced diets are being replaced by sufficient quantities of the right kind of food. Teams of FAO experts work with the natives to teach development of their soil and water resources, the use of modern tools and techniques for farming, fishing, and forestry, as well as improved methods of conserving and marketing foods and of carrying on campaigns against devastating diseases of livestock and poultry.

ILO. Policies of the ILO are shaped by employers and governments as well as by workers and, therefore, differ from those of an international labor union. Many of its purposes are achieved through establishment of missions in countries requesting their services. Each mission consists of a group of experts in an economic field and their families, who live among the natives and make friends with them. Missions conduct training courses for employees and teach employers and governments methods that will lead to production of more and better goods.

The ILO also aids in solution of social and economic problems associated with hours of work, wages, unemployment, and provision for injury and old age benefits. At the suggestion of the Expert Committee on Nursing of the World Health Organization, the ILO and the WHO carried on a joint investigation of causes of the world wide nursing shortage and, following its completion in 1958 the ILO published a 176 page brochure entitled, *Employment and Conditions of Work of Nurses*. In 1964 a follow up study and re-assessment of the situation was promoted by the Social and Economic Welfare Division of the ICN.

UNESCO. The preamble to the Constitution of UNESCO contains the following statement: "Since wars begin in the minds of men, it is in the minds of men that the defenses of peace must be constructed." To this end, educational facilities, scientific research, and cultural values are promoted throughout the world. Assistance is provided for building schools, libraries, and laboratories, and special studies are made of racial, religious, and social tensions that might lead to open conflict. UNESCO is now carrying on an extensive campaign to raise funds to save the archeological treasures in danger of being lost forever with the building of the high Aswan Dam on the Nubian Desert of Egypt.

WHO.   At the suggestion of China and Brazil, one of the first actions of the Economic and Social Council was that of calling a World Health Conference preliminary to drafting a Constitution for a World Health Organization, in the preamble of which is now the following:

"Health is a state of complete physical, mental, and social well-being and not merely the absence of disease or infirmity.

"The health of all peoples is fundamental to the attainment of peace and security and is dependent upon the fullest cooperation of individuals and States."

The Constitution was ratified by 26 nations April 7, 1948, the anniversary of which is celebrated as World Health Day.

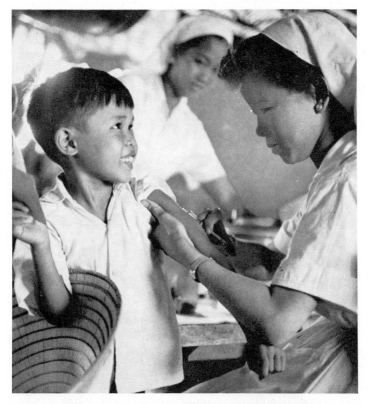

Figure 76. A BCG team, assisted by WHO and UNICEF, administers vaccine to refugees near Saigon, Viet-Nam. (Courtesy World Health Organization.)

The WHO helps nations to strengthen their own health services by sending expert consultants, teachers, and international demonstration teams, usually including nurses, to work and teach selected local personnel who are expected to carry on alone when the initial project has been completed. Fellowships are granted to native sanitary engineers, nurses, and other personnel to enable them to study outside of their own countries. Technical assistance is given to educational institutions, including medical and nursing schools, and seminars and conferences are provided. Emphasis is placed upon the necessity for educating the public to cooperate by maintaining safe water and food supplies, sewage disposal systems and effective insect and rodent control.

A chief undertaking of the WHO is a world wide intergovernmental drive to completely eradicate malaria, tuberculosis, venereal diseases, yaws, trachoma, and leprosy, all of which are now in retreat although there is some evidence of a new increase in tuberculosis infections. Great numbers of maternal and child health services have been developed, with considerable financial assistance from UNICEF. The WHO also promotes medical and occupational rehabilitation and is making a study of health problems that may arise from use of atomic energy. Through its efforts drugs have been made available in uniform strengths in many countries.

The World Health Organization has become one of the largest Specialized Agencies of the United Nations with a membership of some ninety nations. A professional staff of more than 500 is maintained including thirty public health nurses and two nurse consultants. Offices of

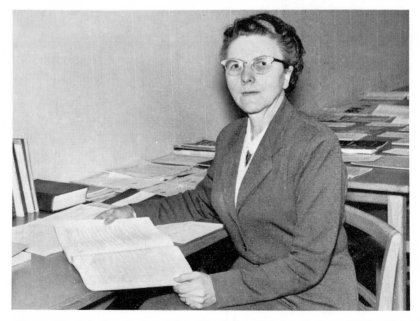

Figure 77. Lyle Creelman of Canada, Chief, Nursing Section, WHO. (Nursing Mirror Copyright.)

the latter are in the WHO headquarters building in Geneva, Switzerland. Policies are determined at World Health Conferences, held in various parts of the world and, in order to conform to health needs of specific areas, six regional offices, with a nurse in each, are maintained in the following cities: Alexandria, Egypt; Brazzaville, Congo Republic; Copenhagen, Denmark; Manila, Philippine Islands; New Delhi, India; and Washington, D.C., U.S.A.

In order to ensure a representative body of opinion, a group of non-governmental organizations (NGO's) with a basic interest in health have been granted *official relationship* with WHO. In 1947 the International Council of Nurses was admitted to this group, and nurses now serve on WHO Expert Committees on Nursing, act as advisors on subjects of nursing education and service, carry on research projects when requested, and otherwise are active in promoting nursing interests throughout the world.

The International Council of Nurses also has been placed on a *special list of NGO's maintained by the ILO* for consultative purposes, and through this relationship assisted with the ILO and WHO study of causes of the nursing shortage and employment conditions of nurses and auxiliary nursing personnel. The ICN has *consultative status with UNICEF and with the Economic and Social Council itself* by means of which it has relationship to the United Nations, and so is enabled to keep informed of all activities in the health field.

The American Nurses' Association, unlike the ICN, is concerned with programs of the United Nations as a whole and is committed to supporting it and spreading information about the United Nations System. It works through the office of public information of the United Nations as a citizen group, interested in social welfare, and sends representatives to learn about nursing activities and report them as part of the work of the United Nations.

Secretariat. Finally, the administrative body of the vast enterprise of the United Nations is the *Secretariat,* composed of a Secretary General appointed for a period of five years by the General Assembly on recommendation of the Security Council, eight Assistant Secretary Generals, and a staff of about four thousand citizens of many countries who have taken an oath of allegiance to the United Nations. Among the personnel of this permanent international civil service are many scientists, specialists in the fields of economics, social welfare and health, as well as administrators, research workers, secretaries, and others. *They are the first true international citizens,* may be of either sex, and hold permanent positions.

POSTWAR DEVELOPMENTS

Shortage of Nurses. Now that the war was over, it was at first believed that in a short time conditions along all lines would assume a normal character. Soon, however, it was apparent that a society that has been uprooted cannot return to old ground easily, if at all. Changes had taken place in homes and places of business, in those left behind as well as in those who served with the armed forces.

Hospitals and other organizations looking to the nurse returning from active military duty to relieve the emergency character of their work were soon to be disappointed. Registries reported that many war-weary nurses were taking well-earned vacations; others found means of securing advanced education, and some, indeed, were incapacitated for further professional activity. At the same time many married and retired nurses who had been giving valuable assistance suddenly left the field once more. As a final burden, termination of the benefits of the United States Cadet Nurse Corps resulted in an alarming shortage of applicants for entrance to schools of nursing.

To cope with an approaching crisis, the National League of Nursing Education and the American Hospital Association made an extensive study of the situation and soon engaged in a nation-wide recruitment program. It was not many months before interest in nursing was showing signs of reviving. Nevertheless, creation of new positions, increased hospital construction, prepayment hospital insurance, federal social legislation, together with growing public interest in health education and early treatment, were constantly increasing the demand for nurses.

Recognizing the problem to be one involving the security of every citizen, the American Nurses' Association launched a publicity campaign of considerable magnitude. The purpose was to arouse the public to an understanding of its responsibility for correcting those factors contributing to a reluctance on the part of qualified young women to enter schools of nursing.

Practical Nurses. While effort was thus being directed toward providing satisfactory nursing care for all in need of it, the necessity for supplying great numbers of well prepared practical or vocational nurses stood out clearly. To meet this demand, courses of about one year's duration began to appear in vocational and adult schools, hospitals, junior colleges, and other institutions. The *National Association for Practical Nurse Education and Service* (NAPNES), which had been organized in 1941 by leading educators in this field, gave direction to the movement and helped schools to secure improved and more uniform standards.

With headquarters at 535 Fifth Avenue, New York, New York 10017, activities of the NAPNES have expanded in many directions and now cover special educational projects including regional workshops and conferences, recruiting, and publication of a variety of materials. The *Journal of Practical Nursing* is published monthly and conventions are held annually. Membership is open to practical and professional nurses, any interested lay person, representatives of vocational education, state associations of practical nurses, and hospitals, as well as other community agencies.

The *National Federation of Licensed Practical Nurses* (NFLPN), with headquarters at 250 W. 57th Street, New York, New York 10019, is composed entirely of practical nurses. It was organized in 1949 to establish principles of ethics and promote high standards of practical nursing, obtain satisfactory licensing laws and working conditions, and otherwise look after the welfare of practical nurses. It is composed of member state associations which, in turn, are made up of local units. The *American Journal of Practical Nursing* is the official mouthpiece and conventions are held annually.

Changes in Red Cross Enrollment. In 1947 changes were made in the method of enrolling Red Cross nurses. No longer was there need for providing a reserve for the Army Nurse Corps and the Navy Nurse Corps since these services were now doing their own recruiting. Need continued, however, for the maintenance of a roster of nurses who would go into immediate action in case of an epidemic or other local disaster. An earthquake, tornado, fire, flood, explosion, or train, bus, or plane wreck, or the bombing of a city might make it necessary to give first aid to, and evacuate from their homes, great numbers of victims. Nurses would be needed to serve with the National Blood Program, to teach classes for volunteer nurses' aides, and to give instruction in Care of the Sick and Injured.

Public spirited nurses, wishing to make their knowledge and skills available in case of emergency, or to assist with another of the Red Cross Services, now enroll through their local Red Cross Chapters. A badge and membership card, designating each one as an American Red Cross Nurse, is awarded upon completion of such service. These symbols serve as identification with the humanitarian movement of the Red Cross, which knows no national boundaries.

THREE STUDIES OF NURSING

Carnegie Study and Brown Report. Progress toward the goal of ensuring to society a satisfactory type of nursing service was aided by extensive studies of educational methods in nursing schools of England, Canada, the United States, and other countries after the close of the second World War. Previous surveys had proved instrumental in bringing about better preparation of nurses.

One study in the United States was financed by the Carnegie Foundation and carried on as a final project before dissolution of the National Nursing Council. The purpose was to determine by whom professional schools of nursing should be organized, administered, and financed. *Esther Lucile Brown,* expert in the field of social research, working with both a professional and a lay advisory committee, served as director. The objective nature of the project is indicated by an early decision of the group to "view nursing service and nursing education in terms of what is best for society — not what is best for nursing as a possibly 'vested interest.' "[1]

Dr. Brown visited about fifty selected schools conducted by both voluntary and public hospitals over a cross-section of the country. Findings were evaluated as being both better and worse than had been expected. In addition, individual interviews were carried on with those responsible for nursing education and three regional conferences conducted for their special benefit. The conclusions reached, with recommendations for improvement, were published in 1948 in the volume, "Nursing for the Future," by Esther Lucile Brown.

In answer to the chief question under consideration it was recommended that "effort be directed toward building basic schools of nursing in universities and colleges . . . that are sound in organizational and financial structure, adequate in facilities and faculty, and well distributed to serve the needs of the entire country."[2] The feasibility of a combined general and professional university course, shortened to four years, was set forth, but the necessity for continuing hospital schools far into the future was acknowledged. Recommendations for providing adequate supplies of well-qualified nursing personnel included recruiting large numbers of men and minority groups into nursing schools and building integrated service teams of professional nurses, trained practical nurses and, possibly, an intermediate group of graduate bedside nurses for work in institutions.

It was pointed out that while there was a dearth of nurses with special preparation for administrative, supervisory, teaching, and public health positions, there was also a demand for specialists in certain areas of clinical nursing such as care of patients with heart disease, cancer, tuberculosis, orthopedic conditions, and mental illness. It was disclosed, too, that along with professional knowledge and skill, consumers of nursing service seek those having a calm, kindly, understanding manner and modulated voice who impart an inner sense of security and well-being.

T. C. Study and Ginzberg Report. Through the efforts of *Professor R. Louise McManus,* Head of the Division of Nursing Education, Teachers College, Columbia University, a *Committee on the Function of Nursing* was formed while the Carnegie Study was in progress. Composed of representatives of nursing and experts in the fields of medical and social science, the Committee reviewed problems centering around the current and prospective shortage of nurses. *Eli Ginzberg,* Associate Professor of Economics, Columbia University, served as chairman. *Dr. Thomas P. Murdock,* representing the American Medical Association, *Mrs. McManus,* and *Mary M. Roberts* were among committee members.

---

[1]Brown, Esther Lucile: Nursing for the Future. New York, Russell Sage Foundation, 1948, p. 11.
[2]*Ibid.,* p. 178.

Conclusions and recommendations of the T. C. study were published in 1948 in the book, "A Program for the Nursing Profession," by the Committee on the Function of Nursing. To meet the critical nursing shortage it was recommended that nursing teams be developed which would consist of four-year professional nurses, two-year registered nurses, and one-year practical nurses. The scope of nursing functions was considered difficult to define but it was stated that: "The nurse is increasingly responsible for complex technical procedures delegated to her by the doctor; she is the eyes and ears of the doctor, his interpreter, as well as an invaluable assistant in diagnosis and therapy; and she carries a large share of responsibility for health education."[3]

A.M.A. Study and Murdock Report. About this time a *Committee to Study the Nursing Problem in the United States* was appointed by the American Medical Association. Composed of five doctors, with Dr. Thomas P. Murdock as chairman, conferences were held with representatives of the American Hospital Association, the American College of Physicians, the American College of Surgeons, the American Nurses' Association and others. Conclusions and recommendations were published in the *Journal of the American Medical Association,* July 3, 1948, and the *American Journal of Nursing,* July, 1949.

Recommendations for immediate relief of the nursing shortage emphasized need for assigning auxiliary personnel to housekeeping and other non-nursing duties in institutions. To meet future needs three groups of nurses were proposed: nurse educators, clinical nurses, and trained practical nurses. Clinical nurses would have a hospital course shortened to two years.

SCHOOL DATA SURVEY OF 1949

In order to implement into action what were judged most feasible of the recommendations set forth in the Brown, Ginzberg, and Murdock Reports, the Joint Board of Directors of the national nursing organizations appointed a *National Committee for the Improvement of Nursing Services,* made up of representatives of the fields of general education, hospital administration, public health, the American Medical Association, and the nursing organizations.

The first undertaking of the newly appointed committee was a *School Data Survey.* Information gathered by means of questionnaires was used as a basis for determining the major problem areas of nursing education and nursing service and making recommendations for improvement. That the schools themselves welcomed this opportunity for evaluation of their policies is indicated by the fact that 97 per cent of the questionnaires were completed and returned.

---

[3]Committee on the Function of Nursing: A Program for the Nursing Profession. New York, The Macmillan Co., 1948, p. 101.

Interim Classification. The data received were analyzed and the schools classified in three groups according to findings. This *Interim Classification of Schools of Nursing Offering Basic Programs* was published in November, 1949, in the American Journal of Nursing and again in 1950 in the paper-bound volume, "Nursing Schools at the Mid-Century," compiled by the National Committee for the Improvement of Nursing Services. This was the first critical listing of nursing schools that had ever been published. It provided opportunity for those administering them to evaluate their practices in relation to those in vogue in all other schools of the country.

HILL-BURTON ACT

The Hospital Survey and Construction Act of 1946, popularly known as the Hill-Burton Act, provided a cooperative system of federal grants to the states for a systematic construction of greatly needed nonprofit hospitals, public health centers, and related facilities. The program is administered by the Bureau of Medical Services of the USPHS and has the benefit of advice from a nursing consultant of this Bureau. An enormous increase in ability to provide care for patients has followed its inception, but the modern hospital not only cares for those who are ill or injured but also serves as a teaching center for physicians, nurses, administrative residents, social workers, dietitians and others. In 1964 the Hill-Burton Act was extended for another five year period.

THE PRESIDENT'S COMMISSION

In a continuing effort to meet the health needs of the nation and stimulate interest in the federal government's role in maintaining a healthy citizenry, the President of the United States in December, 1951, appointed a *Commission on the Health Needs of the Nation.* For a full year thereafter representatives of medicine and allied fields, education, and consumers of health services carried on an intensive study of health conditions and requirements throughout the country. *Marion Sheehan,* NLN assistant director, represented the field of nursing.

The report of the President's Commission, submitted late in December, 1952, was embodied in five booklets titled "Building America's Health,"[4] in which information is given in regard to existing local, state, and national health facilities and recommendations are made to increase their effectiveness. Among other inadequacies, great numbers of rural areas were reported to be without provision for care during illness.

---

[4]Superintendent of Documents, U.S. Government Printing Office, Washington, D.C., 20402.

Prominent among recommendations was a proposal for creation of a Department of Health and Security within the structure of the National Government.

U. S. PUBLIC HEALTH SERVICE – DEPARTMENT OF HEALTH, EDUCATION, AND WELFARE

In 1953 the U. S. Department of Health, Education, and Welfare, with the Public Health Service as one of its members, was created within the Executive Branch of the Federal Government and dedicated to meeting today's public health needs. The chief officer of the Public Health Service is the Surgeon General, who is appointed by the president of the United States for a four year term. In 1949 *Lucile Petry Leone,* chief nurse officer, was appointed by the Surgeon General to the grade of Assistant Surgeon General, marking special recognition of the nursing profession. This position is now held by *L. Margaret McLaughlin.*

Since 1798 the *U. S. Marine Hospital Service* had cared for sick and disabled merchant seamen employed on ships carrying the nation's commerce and, in time, had been made responsible for federal quarantine activities to prevent communicable disease from being brought into the country, as well as for cooperation with local and state public health services in the enforcement of quarantine laws. As time went on responsibilities continued to broaden, and in 1912 it became the *U. S. Marine Hospital and Public Health Service,* which was abolished in 1953 with creation of the new U. S. Department of Health, Education, and Welfare, within which is the Public Health Service.

The U. S. Public Health Service is now the principal health agency of the federal government. It provides a comprehensive view of health conditions and problems and exercises leadership in public health affairs. Programs are developed in cooperation with state Departments of Public Health, universities, hospitals, and other interested groups, and the relationship is that of partnership in endeavors beneficial to all the people. An influence in international health affairs is maintained by working with the federal agencies of other countries, the World Health Organization, the Pan American Health Organization, and some other international associations.

Early in 1967, following an intensive study called for by *President Lyndon B. Johnson,* a new organizational structure for the U. S. Public Health Service was brought into effect to better enable it to exercise national leadership in meeting present and future health needs of the nation. The plan had previously been submitted by *William H. Stewart, M.D.,* Surgeon General of the USPHS and approved by *John W. Gardner,* then Secretary of Health, Education, and Welfare.

Commenting on the new structure Dr. Stewart said, "We have organized for the future. In the years ahead, the Service must provide leadership and support in the delivery of high quality health care, in the control and prevention of disease and environmental hazards, in bio-medical research, and in the development of health manpower. I believe that this plan will help us meet these goals in an orderly and efficient manner."[5]

Responsibilities of the USPHS are now shared by five *Bureaus* within each of which are several *Divisions.* Programs are coordinated and directed by the *Office of the Surgeon General,* which provides central administration and business management. It also collects, analyzes, and publishes official health statistics of the United States and prepares the nation to meet public health needs of the civilian population in the event of a national disaster. *Public Health Reports,* official journal of the Service, is edited and published.

Directly related to the Office of the Surgeon General are the *National Center for Health Statistics* and the *National Library of Medicine,* a notable contribution to the advancement of medical knowledge and prom-inent among the world's medical libraries. In 1967 the first branch of this library was opened in Boston, and about ten other regional health science libraries are being planned across the country.

The five Bureaus of the U. S. Public Health Service are as follows:

Bureau of Health Services
Bureau of Disease Prevention and Environmental Control
National Institutes of Health
National Institute of Mental Health
Bureau of Health Manpower

The *Bureau of Health Services* is the largest within the USPHS and provides national leadership for improving the quality and availability of personal health services. It supports planning and construction of health facilities and administers the *Hill-Burton Program* of cooperative grants to the states for hospital construction. Its Divisions include those for *Community Health Services, Hospital and Medical Facilities, Indian Health, Medical Care Administration,* and *Mental Retardation.* Medical programs are arranged for the *Bureau of Prisons,* the *Peace Corps, Bureau of Employees' Compensation,* and the *U. S. Coast Guard.*

The *Bureau of Disease Prevention and Environmental Control* pro-vides leadership for plans designed to prevent death and disability from infectious diseases, chronic diseases, accidental injuries, air and water pollution, and other environmental and industrial hazards to human health. It is an active partner with the states in preventing infections from crossing state boundary lines and with international organizations in activities within the field of international health.

The *National Institutes of Health* constitute the Bureau which is the main disease-oriented research center and occupies a 300 acre tract at Bethesda, Maryland, a suburb of Washington, D.C. Among its Divisions are those for *Allergy and Infectious Diseases, Arthritis and Metabolic Diseases, Child Health and Human Development, Dental Research,*

---

[5]HEW – 32, released October 11, 1966.

General Medical Sciences, the *National Cancer Institute,* the *National Heart Institute,* the *Institute of Neurological Diseases and Blindness,* and the *Environmental Health Sciences.*

The Clinical Center, where medical research is carried on, provides twice as much space for laboratories as for patients in a 14 story, 500 bed facility. Patients are referred by their own physicians and selected according to requirements of current research projects. Gigantic strides in medical science are expected, with a new and greater emphasis on health maintenance.

The *NIH Division of Computer Research and Technology* is carrying on research to develop a system of automation that will assist in prompt diagnosis and maintain continuous monitoring of symptoms of critically ill patients. The *Division of Biologic Standards* protects the public by administering federal laws to ensure the purity and potency of serums, vaccines, and other biologic products and conducts research in relation to their standardization. The *Division of Research Grants* supports training for research and stimulates expansion of research activities in medical schools, hospitals, and elsewhere.

The *National Institute of Mental Health* is the Bureau which furnishes national leadership for promoting mental health, preventing mental illness, and treating and rehabilitating the mentally ill. It conducts and supports special projects directed at problems of alcoholism, drug abuse, suicide, crime, juvenile delinquency, and community mental health.

The *Bureau of Health Manpower* has five Divisions of special interest to all health personnel, which are as follows:

Division of Allied Health Professions Manpower
Division of Dental Health
Division of Health Manpower Education Services
Division of Nursing
Division of Physician Manpower

The *Division of Nursing* of this Bureau, of which *Jessie M. Scott* is Director, carries on a continuing review of national and international nursing manpower and its utilization, and serves as a center of information and guidance in relation to all aspects of nurse education, nurse practice, and nurse manpower. It provides consultation to public and private groups who are planning for community nursing services and extending the use of community facilities.

Responsibilities of the USPHS Division of Nursing include also consultation and technical assistance to hospitals and related institutions on the administration and evaluation of institutional nursing services. It conducts research to determine the supply and distribution of nursing services and methods of improving nursing practice, and it predicts future needs and supply. Programs for public health nursing personnel are promoted, with application of the concept of continuing education for all nurses.

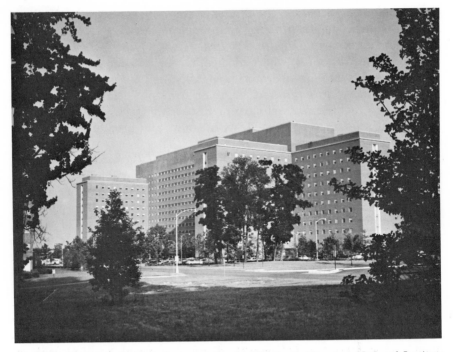

Figure 78. The Clinical Center, Bethesda, Maryland. (Courtesy National Institute of Health, Public Health Service, U.S. Department of Health, Education, and Welfare.)

Still other responsibilities of the Division of Nursing of the USPHS Bureau of Health Manpower include administration of the *Nurse Training Act of 1964* for improvement of nursing education, construction of nursing education facilities, and provision for student loans (see p. 353). It administers the *Professional Nurse Traineeship Program,* which is designed to prepare increased numbers of specialists in all fields of nursing (see p. 386). Assistance is provided for developing recruitment programs, administering a program of grants and fellowships for nursing research and research training, and promoting application of research findings.

STRUCTURE CHANGES IN ORGANIZED NURSING

Changing concepts of health care for all of the people and a wide expansion of hospital facilities were accompanied by new patterns of nursing service and assumption of wider and more varied responsibilities by nurses. In order to keep in step with the times, structure changes were made in the national nursing organizations of various countries, each of which was preceded by exhaustive studies of the existing structure and of possibilities for improvement.

In the United States a structure study was sponsored by the national nursing organizations and conducted by the Raymond Rich Associates, specialists in social studies. A report of their findings and recommendations was presented to the ANA, NLNE, and NOPHN conventions and followed by studies and discussions in district, state, and national associations over a period of about four years. A plan for one all inclusive national association and another for two associations were given serious consideration.

There were at this time the following seven national associations, each working within a field limited by the provisions of its constitution or articles of incorporation and without authority to enter another:

Major Organizations
     National League of Nursing Education (NLNE)
     American Nurses' Association (ANA)
Organizations representing special groups
     National Association of Colored Graduate Nurses
     National Organization for Public Health Nursing
     American Association of Nurse Anesthetists
     Association of Collegiate Schools of Nursing
     American Association of Industrial Nurses, Inc.

In 1950 a detailed plan for two major associations was placed before the ANA biennial convention in San Francisco and approved by the membership. Finally, in 1952 two companion organizations emerged with the common goal of providing the best possible nursing care for the American people. These are as follows:

American Nurses' Association (ANA), reconstructed in 1952
National League for Nursing (NLN), founded in 1952

The constitution and bylaws of the former American Nurses' Association became the nucleus of the reconstructed association, and the structure of the National League of Nursing Education became the nucleus for the new National League for Nursing. A Coordinating Council, composed of the boards of directors of the two organizations, provides for teamwork between them.

First of the special groups to disband was the National Association of Colored Graduate Nurses, which was absorbed by the ANA in January, 1951, leaving a notable record of forty three years of achievement. The next year the NLNE, NOPHN, and ACSN, along with several national committees, combined their programs and resources to become the new National League for Nursing. However, the *American Association of Industrial Nurses, Inc.* and the *American Association of Nurse Anesthetists* retained separate status, and in 1957 a new *Association of Operating Room Nurses* was formed, making three groups which are independent of the major associations but eligible for membership in them.

NATIONAL ACCREDITATION OF NURSING SCHOOLS

It has long been recognized that nursing, like other disciplines, should assume responsibility for its own educational programs, and among the first undertakings of the new National League for Nursing was the development of accreditation criteria for nursing education and the establishment of measurements for a system of national accreditation of nursing schools, including those offering masters degree programs.

Eligibility for NLN accreditation requires that schools conducted by hospitals have current approval of the Board of Nursing of the state in which located, while those under the aegis of junior and senior colleges or universities have current approval by the appropriate regional accrediting body as well as state approval. Two current lists of schools to which national accreditation has been granted are published annually in *Nursing Outlook*, one of those for beginning students and the other for registered nurses. However, national accreditation does not guarantee permanent accreditation. Since all forms of education are soon outmoded, each school is required to undergo periodic re-evaluations, information for which is obtained by progress reports and personal visits of an NLN representative.

As the profession evolves, higher educational standards will be developed by the membership of the NLN Division of Nursing Education while, at the same time, opportunity for flexibility and creativity will be provided so as to encourage valid experimentation and evaluation. The entire project continues to be a democratic venture, initiated and carried through by nurses, all participation in which is voluntary. This carefully worked out plan of action is preferable to any which might be imposed by an outside group.

NATIONAL ACCREDITATION OF HOSPITALS

Hospitals as well as nursing schools seek accreditation, and a *Joint Commission on Accreditation of Hospitals* was formed in 1952, made up of representatives of the American College of Physicians, the American College of Surgeons, the American Hospital Association, and the American Medical Association. Standards set by the Commission cover hospital construction and facilities for service, their administration, and the responsibilities of their medical staff and nursing department. Accreditation provides a badge of recognition that can be displayed by hospitals to show that they conform to high standards of patient care.

To be accredited by the Commission hospitals must be so constructed as to ensure the safety and welfare of patients and provide the following essential facilities for service: dietary, medical records, pharmacy, clinical laboratory and pathological services, radiology, and medical library. The governing body, whose chief representative is the administrator, is morally and legally responsible to patients, the sponsoring organization, and the community for efficient service.

The medical staff is responsible to patients and the governing body for the quality of all medical care and for the ethical and professional practices of its members. No less than twelve staff meetings must be held annually, the sole objective of which is improvement in the care and treatment of hospital patients. Professional nursing care is to be available to all patients at all times.

The Commission on Hospital Accreditation gives close attention to the ratio of graduate nurses to auxiliary workers as well as their ratio to patients. Moreover, the nursing staff is to hold monthly meetings for discussions of problems relating to nursing care of their patients and the administration of their departments. Minutes are to be kept of those meetings. Recently an *ANA Joint Subcommittee on Hospital Accreditation,* composed of nursing leaders, was formed for the purpose of examining current evaluation criteria used to survey nursing service programs in hospitals and advising in regard to improvement if necessary.

Through the untiring efforts of individual doctors and nurses, their representative organizations, the public, and contributing social factors, hospitals have become a reflection of the health consciousness of their communities with doctors and nurses as expert advisors interested in the whole life of man. As emphasis on physical, mental, and spiritual welfare continues to increase, the possibility for health education for all increases also. More and more the world of today works toward these ends, bringing the elimination of ignorance, poverty, and disease ever nearer to man's realization. Nevertheless, the strength of this movement depends upon the dedication of its membership.

Partnership for Progress. A major effort to upgrade hospital care of patients was initiated in 1964 by the American Hospital Association and several other agencies and universities when the W. K. Kellogg Foundation agreed to finance a five year program directed toward keeping hospital personnel informed of up-to-date developments in the health field. This new educational venture, *Partnership for Progress,* is to develop a continuing education program for all grades of hospital workers in an effort to improve and sharpen their skills. Projects are to be included that will increase the knowledge and ability of nurses working in hospitals and allied in-patient agencies; provide correspondence-residential or extension courses for hospital administrators; and initiate a pilot project to develop inservice education and training for all hospital personnel concerned with the care of patients.

RISE OF PSYCHIATRY

Two world wars, with emphasis on mass destruction, inevitably focused medical attention on the care of patients with nervous and mental disorders. A revolution in study of the human mind, which has followed, has restored many chronic invalids to health, and criminals and other social outcasts to their rightful places in society. Mental hygiene programs have come into being, child guidance clinics and psychiatric social work have been established in the large cities, all of which contribute to the peace and security of countless persons.

National mental health programs are in operation in many countries, and, in 1948, the *World Federation for Mental Health* came into being, the aims and purposes of which are defined as follows:

"To promote among all peoples and nations the highest possible standard of mental health, in its broadest biological, medical, educational, and social aspects.

"To work with the Economic and Social Council of the United Nations, UNESCO and the World Health Organization, with all of which the Federation has a consultant role."[6]

Membership of the World Federation for Mental Health is composed principally of societies "concerned to some degree with the establishment and maintenance of good Mental Health and better Human Relations in the home, the community, the state, and between nations."[5] Nurses can by justly proud of the fact that the ANA and ICN are two of these societies.

In the United States passage of the National Mental Health Act of 1946 was followed by wide expansion of educational facilities to equip personnel for the practice of preventive psychiatry in all its aspects.

Psychosomatic Medicine. The practice of psychosomatic medicine has followed in the wake of psychiatry. This science recognizes the body as a delicate instrument which, through the subconscious mind, responds to everything in its environment. It concerns itself with the whole pattern of everyday living of all patients and treats them as total organisms with mental and spiritual as well as physical requirements. Problems of life experiences, beginning in childhood, as well as disturbing social relationships encountered all through life, are known to be the cause of many physical as well as mental illnesses.

It has been demonstrated that many patients gain courage and substantial help through their particular interpretation of religion, and their

---

[6]Folder of the World Federation for Mental Health, 19 Manchester Street, London W. 1, England.

minister, priest, or rabbi becomes a valuable addition to the health team. In contributing to its success, the capable nurse with sympathetic understanding of the healing power of all religions cooperates with prescribed forms of treatment, whether they be medical or surgical, psychological or spiritual, in character.

EXPANSION OF REHABILITATION SERVICES

To meet the postwar needs of thousands of men and women with disabilities that prevented them from earning a living, the Federal-State Rehabilitation Program was expanded in 1943 and again in 1954. Extensive vocational guidance services were added which included placement in suitable positions and a follow-up program to ensure satisfaction of employer and employee. The employment by many large companies of thousands of persons handicapped by disease, accident, or congenital conditions has followed.

Rehabilitation centers, sponsored by public or private funds or both, have been established in every state, and Puerto Rico, all requiring the services of psychologists, speech therapists, prosthetic specialists, vocational counselors, and specially prepared doctors and nurses. Many hospitals are opening rehabilitation departments and clinics. In Canada an interesting and extensive Workmen's Compensation Board Rehabili-

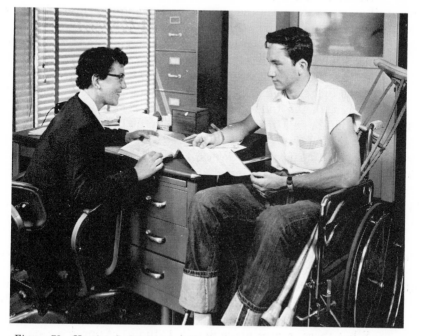

Figure 79. Harriet C. Lane, rehabilitation counselor, assisting a young man with partial paraplegia to make plans for his future. (Courtesy Liberty Mutual Rehabilitation Center.)

tation Center was opened in 1947 at Malton, Ontario. It covers twenty-seven acres of ground and has its own hospital, clinic, fire department, post office, and theater.

Rehabilitation has beome an integral part of the total care which makes up medical treatment, regarded as complete only after the individual has returned to gainful employment. In all of this work, nurses are in a particularly advantageous position for helping to solve emotional problems accompanying disabling conditions and for building that strong desire for recovery so essential to full restoration to society.

Suggestions For Study

1. How did the conduct of World War II differ from previous wars, and what was the effect on the civilian population?
2. What diseases were prevalent, and what advances made in treatment of these and other conditions?
3. In making plans to provide nurses for war service, what coordinating link was developed between organized nursing and the federal government?
4. Through what agencies and by what ways and means were ever increasing numbers of nurses made available for war service and civilian needs?
5. Tell what you know of industrial nursing and the effect of the war upon it.
6. What great relief agency was organized during the war to provide immediate assistance to destitute peoples?
7. Make an outline of the structure of the United Nations, its principal organs and specialized agencies, putting emphasis on those with which medicine and nursing are closely associated.
8. Show how the relationship of the ICN to the United Nations differs from that of the ANA.
9. Tell what you know of the World Health Organization.
10. Give reasons for a continued shortage of nurses following World War II and state the various means used to overcome it.
11. Why do the American Red Cross Nursing Services no longer provide a reserve for the U. S. Army Nurse Corps and the U. S. Navy Nurse Corps?
12. What does ownership of a membership card and the badge of the American Red Cross Nursing Services signify today?
13. Explain the differences in membership and purposes of the National Association for Practical Nurse Education and Service and the National Federation of Licensed Practical Nurses.
14. (a) What three groups made detailed studies of nursing soon after the close of World War II? (b) What three reports were submitted by them in 1948?
15. (a) What do you know of the School Data Survey of 1949? (b) What

was the Interim Classification of Schools of Nursing Offering Basic Programs? (c) What did it accomplish?

16. Explain the effect of the Hill-Burton Act upon the nursing shortage.

17. What were the findings and recommendation of the Commission on the Health Needs of the Nation appointed by President Truman?

18. (a) Discuss the founding of the U.S. Department of Health, Education, and Welfare with the Public Health Service as one of its members. (b) How does the U.S. Public Health Service differ from the health service that preceded it?

19. Name the five Bureaus of the USPHS, and tell something of the responsibilities of each.

20. Who holds the following offices at the present time? (a) Secretary of Health, Education, and Welfare; (b) Surgeon General of the USPHS; (c) Chief Nurse Officer of the USPHS; (d) Director, Division of Nursing, Bureau of Health Manpower.

21. How is it possible to determine whether or not a nursing school is at the present time accredited by the NLN?

22. What standards have been set by the Joint Commission on Accreditation of Hospitals for an institution to attain recognition as an accredited hospital?

23. What two branches of medical science have greatly expanded since World War II?

24. What do you know of the National Mental Health Act of your country and of the World Federation for Mental Health?

References

Allan, W. Scott: Rehabilitation—A Community Challenge. New York, John Wiley and Sons, Inc., 1958.

Brown, Esther Lucile: Nursing for the Future (Brown Report). New York, Russell Sage Foundation, 1948.

Bureau of Labor Statistics: *The Economic Status of Registered Professional Nurses, 1946–7.* Bulletin No. 931. Superintendent of Documents, U.S. Government Printing Office, Washington, D.C., 20402.

Canadian Nurses' Association: *C.N.A.—The First Fifty Years* (historical pamphlet). Ottawa, Canada, 1958.

Committee on Medicine and the Changing Order of the New York Academy of Medicine. Medicine in the Changing Order. New York, The Commonwealth Fund, 1947.

Committee on the Function of Nursing: A Program for the Nursing Profession. (Ginzberg Report). New York, The Macmillan Company, 1948.

Committee on the Nursing Problem: "The Murdock Report". *Journal of the AMA,* July 3, 1948, pp. 878-879.

Coyle, David C.: The United Nations and How It Works. New York, Columbia University Press, 1966.

General Assembly of the U.N.: *Universal Declaration of Human Rights.* U.N. Dept. of Public Information, Lake Success, New York.

Hume, Edward H.: Doctors Courageous. New York, Harper and Brothers, 1950.

ILO: Employment and Conditions of Work of Nurses. International Labor Organization, Geneva, Switzerland, 1960.

Joint Commission on Accreditation of Hospitals: *Standards for Hospital Accreditation* (pamphlet). Chicago, 535 North Dearborn St., 1956.

Morrissey, Alice B.: Rehabilitation Nursing. New York, G. P. Putnam's Sons, 1951.
Murdock, T. P.: "A Physician's Viewpoint." (Murdock Report). *American Journal of Nursing,* July, 1949, p. 439.
Roberts, Mary M.: "We Work for Peace through Health." *American Journal of Nursing,* Dec., 1956, p. 1539.
U.N. Dept. of Public Information: Everyman's United Nations, 1945–1955. United Nations, Dept. of Public Information, New York, 1956.
West and Hawkins: Nursing Schools at the Mid-Century, Nat. Comm. for Improvement of Nursing Service, 10 Columbus Circle, New York, N.Y. 10019, 1950.
World Health Organization: The First Ten Years of the World Health Organization. WHO, Geneva, Switzerland, 1958.

Journals

American Journal of Nursing, 10 Columbus Circle, New York, N. Y. 10019.
American Journal of Sociology, University of Chicago Press, Chicago, Ill.
Journal of the American Medical Association, 535 N. Dearborn St., Chicago, Ill.
The Canadian Nurse, 1522 Sherbrooke St., West, Montreal 25, Canada.
UN Monthly Chronicle, Columbia University Press, 2960 Broadway, New York, N.Y. 10027.
WHO Newsletter, Division of Public Information, WHO, Geneva, Switzerland.
World Health. Columbia University Press, 2960 Broadway, New York, N.Y. 10027.

Chapter 14

MODERN TRENDS IN NURSING

Today the practice of nursing, like other professions, finds it necessary to make continual adjustment to the greatest and most rapid transition phase in the evolution of society that mankind has so far experienced. A new concept of the rights of peoples of all races, religions, and levels of society to personal liberty and a fair share of the essentials to ensure health and happiness has become a principal issue. Speed in transportation, ease of communication, mixing of populations, all are contributing to an awakening to the possibilities of a peaceful world in which every citizen will benefit from the goods and services that it can be prepared to offer.

To represent nurses of the United States and guide them through a critical period, are our two national organizations, the American Nurses' Association and the National League for Nursing, the former promoting all phases of professional advancement and the social and economic welfare of registered nurses; and the latter, with the aid of community representatives, promoting high standards of all institutions offering nursing services and educational programs in either professional or practical nursing. Nurses of Canada have one all inclusive Canadian Nurses' Association to represent them and promote their interests.

STRUCTURE CHANGES OF 1966 AND 1967

Following reorganization of the American Nurses' Association in 1952 and founding of the National League for Nursing in the same year, the structures of the two organizations did not prove satisfactory in all of their relationships, and members expressed a need for assistance in meeting emerging clinical responsibilities as well as growing expec-

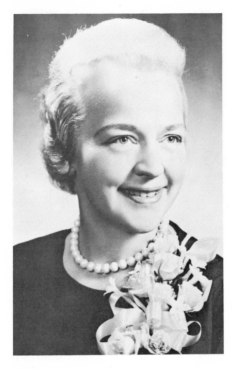

Figure 80. Jo Eleanor Elliott, ANA President, 1964–. (Courtesy of the American Nurses' Association in Convention Journal, June 19, 1964.)

tations of the public for quality patient care. In an effort to adjust to changing patterns of the health services, a *Study Committee on the Functions of the ANA* was appointed in 1959, and the following year a corresponding *NLN Task Force on Organizational Structure* was formed, each with the responsibility of reviewing the existing structure and considering all aspects of nursing responsibility for providing adequate care for all the people.

Extensive investigations and studies were carried on and many conferences held, and articles denoting progress appeared in the nursing journals. Finally, at the ANA biennial convention of 1966, held in San Francisco, nurses from all parts of the United States participated in history-making decisions to bring about a major structural rearrangement of the American Nurses' Association. The following year similar action took place at the NLN biennial convention, held in New York City, which brought about a new structure for the National League for Nursing. A Coordinating Council, composed of the Boards of Directors of the two organizations, continues to ensure teamwork between them.

AMERICAN NURSES' ASSOCIATION

Responsibility for fostering high standards of nursing practice, professional and educational advancement, and the economic and social welfare of nurses is assumed by the American Nurses' Association to the end that all the people may have better nursing care. This association is a federation of fifty four constituent state and territorial associations, including those of the fifty states, the District of Columbia, Panama Canal Zone, Puerto Rico, and the Virgin Islands. The majority of these, in turn, are made up of constituent district associations. A nurse who joins a district association automatically becomes a member of the state association and the ANA as well, and dues are apportioned among them. Nurses residing outside of the United States may join the ANA directly.

ANA membership is composed exclusively of graduates of state-accredited schools of professional nursing, who are licensed to practice as registered nurses. *Active membership* is open to all; *associate membership,* with limited privileges, is open only to those who do not expect to practice during the current calendar year. Associate members do not vote, serve as delegates, or hold office.

The ANA structure created in 1966 consists chiefly of *three Commissions, five Divisions on Practice,* and an *Academy of Nursing.* The Commissions are as follows: Commission on Nursing Education, Commission on Nursing Services, and Commission on Economic and General Welfare. Each Commission consists of nine members serving terms of four years, three of whom are elected by the House of Delegates and one is appointed by the Board of Directors biennially. Every fourth year, two members of each Commission are appointed.

The five Divisions on Practice are as follows:

Community Health Nursing
Geriatric Nursing
Maternal and Child Health Nursing
Medical-Surgical Nursing
Psychiatric and Mental Health Nursing

Each Division is responsible for establishing standards for nursing practice within its own area of responsibility and making appropriate recommendations to the Commissions. It is responsible also for stim-

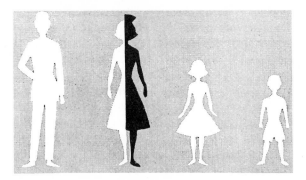

Figure 81. Part-time nurse—full-time homemaker. The "average" part-time nurse has a husband and two children, one under 10. She is between 30 and 39 years old, a graduate of a diploma program, works 20 hours a week. (American Journal of Nursing, Jan., 1964. p. 89.)

ulating studies and research and disseminating information to improve patient care.

The purpose of the Academy of Nursing is the advancement of knowledge, education, and nursing practice, and it is expected to evolve as nurses, known as *fellows,* are selected from among ANA members who have been endorsed by Division Certification Boards and are otherwise deemed qualified by the Academy.

ANA Constituent Associations. These consist of state and territorial associations whose members have joined through a district association and designated the *State Section* which represents their particular area of service. To ensure contact with the sections and provide a medium for discussion of pertinent subjects at biennial conventions, the ANA maintains the following corresponding Occupational Forums:

Educational Administrators, Consultants, and Teachers (EACT)
General Duty Nurses
Private Duty Nurses
Nursing Service Administrators
Occupational Health Nurses
Office Nurses
Public Health Nurses
School Health Nurses
Head Nurses
Operating Room Nurses

Activities of the American Nurses' Association are carried on to a considerable extent through the programs of its Commissions, Divisions on Practice, and the following Standing Committees: Bylaws; Convention Program; Ethical, Legal and Professional Standards; Finance; Legislation; Membership Promotion; Nurses' Professional Registries; Nursing in International Affairs; Professional Credentials and Personnel Service; and Research and Studies. Members of these Committees are nurses in various parts of the country who have been recommended by their state associations and appointed by the ANA Board of Directors. They work closely with the Commissions and Divisions on Practice.

National Headquarters. The national headquarters of both the ANA and the NLN, as well as those of the National Student Nurses' Association, are located at 10 Columbus Circle, New York, New York 10019. More than one hundred staff members are employed, including specialists in the areas of economics, business administration, research, and public relations, as well as nursing. The ANA keeps in close touch with the state and district associations and supplies many types of services to them. Each nurse, through membership in a district association, has opportunity to voice an opinion on all matters under consideration and to help shape future activities and policies.

The ANA acts as national spokesman for nurses and disseminates educational and other informative materials to allied professional and health groups, and to government agencies and the public. It stimulates

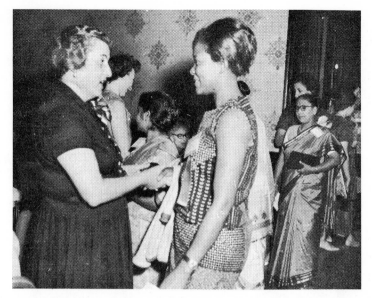

Figure 82. Welcome to international visitor is extended by Miriam Cole, director ANA International Program, to Elizabeth Gaida, Liberia, West Africa, at 1964 ANA Convention in Atlantic City. (Courtesy of the American Nurses' Association in Convention Journal, June 18, 1964.)

research relating to scientific and educational developments affecting nursing practice, carries on studies of changing health requirements, and is empowered to make grants for such studies, in all of which it encourages community participation.

Washington Office. An ANA office with a full-time staff is maintained in Washington, D.C., which keeps headquarters informed in regard to proposed legislation and supports that which seems favorable to nurses, nursing, and the health of the nation. It depends upon the state associations for their prompt support of that which is desirable and opposition to any that seems detrimental to nursing interests.

The ANA is the official United States representative of nurses in the International Council of Nurses and conducts the *ICN Exchange of Privileges for Nurses Program* in this country. It supports the United Nations and its Specialized Agencies, the Institute of International Education, the Agency for International Development (AID), as well as other groups concerned with international affairs. It conducts the *Exchange of Visitors Program of the U. S. Department of State,* as it relates to nursing.

First Position Paper. At the ANA biennial convention of 1966 the "First Position Paper on the Educational Preparation for Nurse Practitioners and Assistants to Nurses," which had previously been adopted by its Board of Directors, was presented to the membership and accepted by it. This prescribes a long-range goal of bringing all nursing education into institutions within the general system of education, and states that education for assistants in the health service occupations should be short,

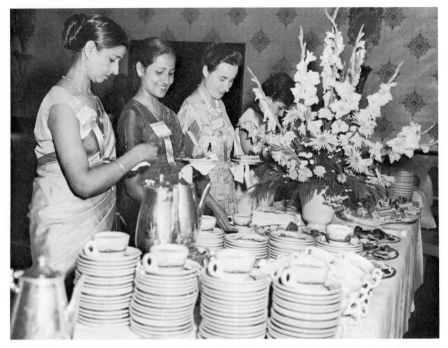

Figure 83. Teatime at the Shelburne found Anjna Malhotra, India; Arati Kerketta, India; and Doreen Hayward, England; enjoying refreshment during the ANA Convention in Atlantic City, 1964. They were among 102 nurses from 28 countries. (Courtesy of the American Nurses' Association in Convention Journal, June 18, 1964.)

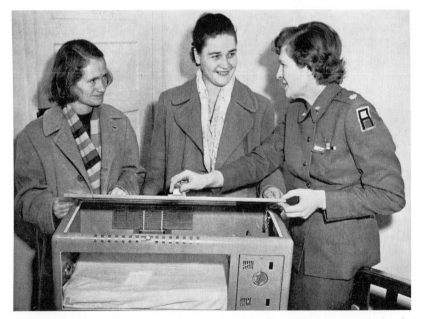

Figure 84. Two refugee nurses, being assisted by the ANA, look over an incubator with Major Lassiter. (U.S. Army Photo.)

intensive, preservice courses in vocational education institutions rather than on-the-job training in hospitals. At the same convention a *National Salary Goal* of not less than $6,500 annually for beginning practitioners was presented and adopted.

PC and PS Offices.   The *ANA Professional Credentials and Personnel Service,* formerly known as the Professional Counseling and Placement Service, cooperates with corresponding state services to provide assistance, without charge, for ANA members seeking new positions or making plans for advanced education. The ANA PC and PS compiles biographies of nurses seeking assistance, including education and experience, with letters of reference, that will be sent to prospective employers upon request.

The state PC and PS offices provide information and counseling concerning the supply and demand for nursing services over a wide area, including opportunities in foreign countries. Through these channels, the ANA is enabled to assist in establishing sound personnel practices and in solving employment problems. The aim is to ensure patient and employer satisfaction in nursing and nurse satisfaction in work.

Code of Ethics.   The American Nurses' Association and the International Council of Nurses each publish a Code of Ethics which expresses the basic concepts of ethical nursing practice and personal conduct that have been agreed upon by these organizations and can be of help to all nurses. Pocketsize copies may be purchased from headquarters.

ANA-NLN Nursing Careers Program.   This joint undertaking of the American Nurses' Association and the National League for Nursing has for its purpose the recruitment of qualified young people into accredited nursing education programs for the preparation of licensed practitioners ranging from practical nurses to those with baccalaureate and higher degrees.

ANA Journals and Conventions.   The *American Journal of Nursing,* the first issue of which appeared in October, 1900, is the official organ of the American Nurses' Association. It deals with current interests and problems of nurses and keeps them abreast of developments in the fields of nursing education and nursing practice. A Student Page is designed especially for nursing students and usually includes articles written by them. *Nursing Research,* first published in 1952, is a bi-monthly journal cosponsored with the NLN which provides comprehensive information on research projects.

Twice each year the *American Journal of Nursing* publishes an official *Directory* of international, national, and state nursing organizations, as well as governmental organizations concerned with nursing. Semi-annually also state approved nurses' *Registries* are listed. In addition to the *AJN,* the American Nurses' Association publishes and circulates to its membership a bi-monthly newsletter entitled, *ANA in ACTION,* and it publishes annually the handbook, "Facts about Nursing," a statistical summary on nurses and nursing.

The ANA holds conventions biennially in the even numbered years.

Each state nurses' association also holds annual conventions and many of them publish a magazine or bulletin. Through these media and other channels members of nursing and allied professions have opportunity for communicating with one another. They are the means whereby all concerned exchange ideas, discuss problems, learn of new developments, and share progressive thinking of the day.

ANA-NLN Film Service. This is a joint undertaking of the two major national associations which maintains a film library on nursing and health, publishes reviews of new films of interest to nurses, and assists in the production of films and filmstrips. New films are often shown at national conventions and can be purchased, or sometimes rented, from the ANA-NLN Film Library, 267 West 25th St., New York, New York 10001.

NATIONAL LEAGUE FOR NURSING

The purpose of the National League for Nursing is "to foster the development and improvement of . . . nursing education and nursing services through the coordinated action of nurses, allied professional groups, citizens, agencies, and schools to the end that the nursing needs of the people will be met."[1] In contrast to the American Nurses' Association, which is concerned with promoting high standards of nursing practice, educational advancement, and the general welfare of nurses, the National League for Nursing is concerned with promoting high standards of *organized nursing services and nursing education,* but the ultimate objective of both is to provide better nursing care for all the people.

Membership of the ANA consists entirely of registered professional nurses while that of the NLN is open to other individuals and agencies concerned with promoting the development and improvement of nursing services and nursing education. *Individual members* are professional and practical nurses, nursing aides, men and women in allied fields, as well as lay people interested in good nursing. *Agency members* consist of hospital and public health nursing services and all types of institutions offering educational programs in nursing.

The structure of the NLN that was voted by the membership at their biennial convention of 1967 consists of two main Divisions, the *Division of Individual Members* and the *Division of Agency Members,* within which are various Councils representing special interest groups, the number of which may be increased as authorized by the NLN Board of Directors. These are as follows:

I. Division of Individual Members
    Council on Community Planning for Nursing
        Committees or other groupings may be formed as follows:
            Education for Nursing Personnel
            Nursing for Health Care
            Nursing Manpower

[1] NLN Bylaws, 1967.

II. Division of Agency Members
     Council of Associate Degree Programs
     Council of Baccalaureate and Higher Degree Programs
     Council of Diploma Programs
     Council of Practical Nursing Programs
     Council of Hospital and Related Institutional Nursing Services
     Council of Public Health Nursing Services

All individuals become members of the Council on Community Planning and they may also be admitted to *one* other grouping in the Division of Individual Members or to *one* Council in the Division of Agency Members that has voted to accept some individuals. All Councils have general concern for either the continuous development of nursing education or the improvement of nursing services.

Constituent Leagues for Nursing. Constituent or regional Leagues are made up of local Leagues which may embrace a state, two or more states or parts of states, or other designated section of the country with similar interests and needs that desire to work together toward their goals. Constituent Leagues are subdivided into *Departments,* each representing the special occupational interests of its members. By joining a local League an individual automatically becomes a member of the regional and national Leagues as well, and membership dues are apportioned

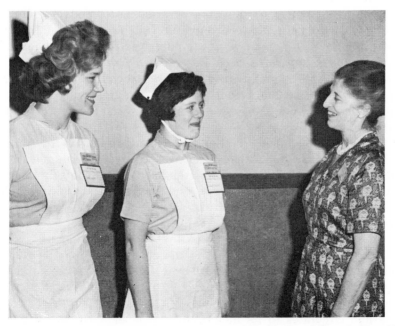

Figure 85. Jose Haigh and Elizabeth Beaton of England and Francis Tompkins, NSNA Executive Secretary, on Uniform Night, 1963 Atlantic City NLN Convention. (From American Journal of Nursing, June, 1963.)

among them. Agencies achieve membership by joining the national association directly.

Functions of the National League for Nursing include a broad program for assisting all types of educational institutions from practical nursing through professional nursing at the master's degree level. Consultation services are available to help with pressing problems, and NLN consultants travel all over the country to help schools to reach high levels of achievement.

To aid in reaching higher goals the program of *Accreditation of Nursing Schools,* both practical and professional, is carried on by the League, and special recognition granted to those meeting specified standards. While not mandatory for state approval by the appropriate legal authority, NLN accreditation is indicative of a school's concern for conducting a superior educational system. In this way it is a protection for society as well as for the institution.

A program of *Accreditation of Community Nursing Services* is now under way which is cosponsored by the National League for Nursing and the American Public Health Association. The purpose is "to improve and preserve the quality of nursing care in the home in the face of rapid expansion of home nursing services and mushrooming health care agencies."[2] Plans are being formed also for accreditation of hospital nursing services.

Committees of the NLN include the *Committee on Perspectives,* which is engaged in a continual search for the implications of broad social and professional trends on the practice of nursing and has recently centered on care of the patient. Their key consideration is "the delivery of nursing care to the patient in whatever environment he is found."[3] In 1965 a report, *Perspectives for Nursing,* was published in pamphlet form. The *Committee on Historical Source Materials in Nursing* is of particular interest to students of nursing history. It urges constituent associations to seek out, accumulate, and preserve reliable historical and contemporary nursing records which can serve as a bridge from the past to future developments in nursing.

National Headquarters.   National headquarters of both the ANA and the NLN, as well as that of the NSNA, are located at 10 Columbus Circle, New York, New York 10019. In 1961 the League opened its first regional office in San Francisco, California, and this Western Office is able to give more highly skilled and direct assistance to constituent Leagues of the west than previously was possible.

NLN Journals and Conventions.   *Nursing Outlook,* a monthly journal first published in January, 1953, is the official organ of the National League for Nursing, directed toward assisting nurses to keep abreast of trends and developments in all fields of nursing. *Nursing Research* is cosponsored with the American Nurses' Association. The NLN also publishes and circulates to its membership a paper entitled, *NLN News.*

---

[2]*Nursing Outlook,* March, 1967, p. 58.
[3]NLN Biennial Reports, 1965–1966, p. 20.

League conventions are held biennially, in the odd numbered years, in cities of the country to which they have been invited by the regional associations.

NATIONAL STUDENT NURSES' ASSOCIATION

Formal organization of a National Student Nurses' Association of the United States took place in 1953 at the NLN convention in Cleveland when a constitution and bylaws were adopted. The NSNA, which is sponsored by the Coordinating Council of the ANA and NLN, is a federation of fifty constituent student nurse organizations in forty-nine states and the District of Columbia, each of which, in turn, is made up of district associations. Membership is composed of students of state accredited professional schools of nursing. Four advisors, two of whom represent the ANA-NLN Coordinating Council, serve in an advisory capacity to the officers and members of the association. Separately incorporated since 1959, the NSNA maintains offices in Coliseum Towers, the building which also houses ANA and NLN at 10 Columbus Circle, New York City.

The purposes of the NSNA are to encourage interest and participation in nursing organization and activity; to promote closer unity among

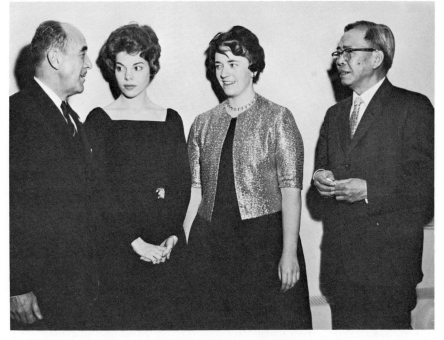

Figure 86. NSNA honored for its *Taiwan project* at the 25th anniversary of the *American Bureau for Medical Aid to China.* At the banquet, George E. Armstrong, M.D., president, ABMAC; Britt Gantt, president, NSNA; Mary Dennesaites, past president, NSNA; and His Excellency T. F. Tsiang, Ambassador from Taiwan; talk about the student association's goal of raising funds for a new dormitory for Taiwan's nursing students. (Courtesy of the American Nurses' Association in ANA in Review, Spring, 1963.)

student nurses of the country and the world; to foster good citizenship; to stimulate formation of state and district student associations; and to serve as spokesman for student nurses. It is an active, growing organization, each annual convention of which shows increasing participation and enthusiasm.

For an organization still so young, NSNA's achievements are impressive. Its National Committee on Recruitment offers suggestions to NLN and State Committees on Careers in Nursing for recruiting new nursing candidates. A model set of bylaws for use of District and State student associations and a project to stimulate improvement of student associations have been developed. The first nationwide philanthropic project undertaken by the students is that of raising funds for a new student dormitory at the National Defense Medical Center on Taiwan. The campaign began in 1961 after seeing the film strip, "Journey to Taiwan,"[4] at the 1958 and 1961 NSNA national conventions, which showed the crowded conditions under which students live at the

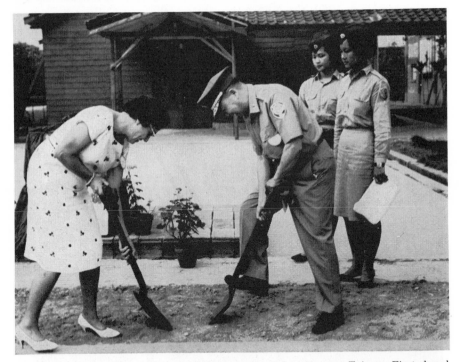

Figure 87. Ground broken for NSNA-supported dormitory on Taiwan. First shovel loads were taken up by Lulu Wolf Hassenplug and Dr. C. T. Loo on April 17, 1964, for the new *student dormitory* at the *National Defense Medical Center, Taipei, Taiwan.* Mrs. Hassenplug, dean of the school of nursing at the University of California at Los Angeles, took part in the ceremonies *as representative of the National Student Nurses' Association* of the *U. S.* Dr. Loo is *director* of the *NDMC.* (American Journal of Nursing, June, 1964.)

---

[4]Available from ANA-NLN Film Library, 267 West 25th St., New York, New York 10001.

Center. Two years later NSNA announced that the primary goal of $25,000 had been reached. Ground was broken for the new structure April 17, 1964.

In 1960 the president, first vice president, and two active members of NSNA attended the Golden Anniversary White House Conference on Children and Youth, as delegates appointed by the ANA and NLN. In 1961 the president and executive secretary of NSNA visited Taiwan and the National Defense Medical Center on their way to the Congress of the International Council of Nurses in Melbourne, Australia. Among other things, they reported that in the students' dormitory beds were in three tiers reaching to the ceiling, with no space for clothes or desks.

Journals and Conventions. Activities of the National Student Nurses' Association are made known through the Student Page of the *American Journal of Nursing* and space provided in *Nursing Outlook,* and also through its own NSNA Newsletter, published quarterly. In 1964 the *American Journal of Nursing* was adopted as the official NSNA journal.

NSNA conventions are held annually just before or after the biennial conventions of the ANA and NLN, its sponsoring organizations, and overlap them for a day or two in order that students may join the graduates at some of their meetings. The official emblem of NSNA is inscribed with the words, "Non Nobis Sed Aliis," (Not for Ourselves but for Others).

AMERICAN JOURNAL OF NURSING COMPANY

Working side by side with the nursing organizations is the American Journal of Nursing Company which came into existence two years after publication of the first issue of the American Journal of Nursing. Through the efforts of a group of able and far-sighted nursing leaders of that time, it was established on a sound business basis as a nonprofit stock company, to be owned by the American Nurses' Association. In the beginning, shares of stock were purchased by individual nurses and nursing groups, the first share going to Linda Richards, "America's first trained nurse." When funds became available these shares were taken over by the ANA, which is now the sole owner.

To keep pace with the needs of a progressive profession the services of the AJN Company have expanded and now include publication not

Figure 88. Symbol of National Student Nurses' Association of the United States. (Courtesy National Student Nurses' Association.)

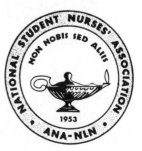

only of the *American Journal of Nursing,* official organ of the ANA, but also of *Nursing Outlook,* official organ of the NLN, and *Nursing Research,* which is sponsored by the NLN and the ANA. All three journals are owned and controlled by the nursing profession.

When sufficient funds are available, grants are made to the American Nurses' Foundation to aid in research and also to aid other projects associated with public health and welfare. In the spring of 1963 and again in 1964 the American Journal of Nursing Company and Boston University School of Nursing co-sponsored workshops of two weeks each on the basic principles of writing for various types of publications. Both terms were attended by a group of about thirty five nurses from various states, many of whom were teachers in graduate nursing programs, who completed an assigned writing project between sessions. Professional nurse traineeship grants of the USPHS were made available to them.

CANADIAN NURSES' ASSOCIATION

Following a comprehensive study, which had begun four years previously, extensive changes in structure of the Canadian Nurses' Association were made in 1954 at the 27th biennial convention, held in Banff, Alberta. A large number of nurses were present as well as

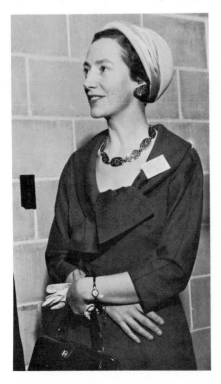

Figure 89. Isobel MacLeod, CNA President, 1964–. (Photo by Newton.)

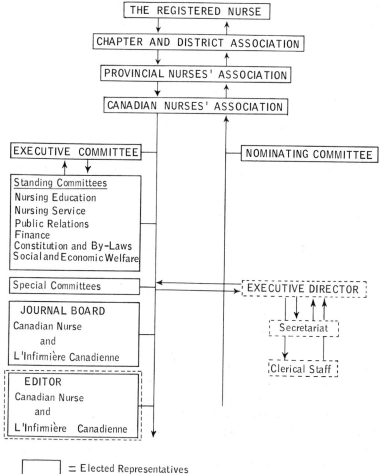

THE REGISTERED NURSE

CHAPTER AND DISTRICT ASSOCIATION

PROVINCIAL NURSES' ASSOCIATION

CANADIAN NURSES' ASSOCIATION

EXECUTIVE COMMITTEE

NOMINATING COMMITTEE

Standing Committees
Nursing Education
Nursing Service
Public Relations
Finance
Constitution and By-Laws
Social and Economic Welfare

Special Committees

EXECUTIVE DIRECTOR

JOURNAL BOARD
Canadian Nurse
and
L'Infirmière Canadienne

Secretariat

EDITOR
Canadian Nurse
and
L'Infirmière Canadienne

Clerical Staff

☐ = Elected Representatives

⌐ ¬ = Appointed, Salaried Personnel

Figure 90. CNA Organizational Chart. (Adapted from "Nursing. Its History, Trends, Philosophy, Ethics, and Ethos" by Thelma Pelley. W. B. Saunders Co., Philadelphia, Penna., 1964, p. 184.)

a group of students, many of whom had been brought by special trains across Canada from the eastern and central provinces.

The Executive Committee of the CNA now consists of the president, immediate past president, three vice presidents, presidents of the ten provincial associations, chairmen of the Standing Committees, chairman of the journal board of *The Canadian Nurse,* and four regional representatives of Nursing Sisterhoods. Because of a large proportion of French speaking nurses in the Province of Quebec, it has both an English speaking and a French speaking representative on the Executive Committee, but with only one vote.

There are six Standing Committees of the CNA, each of which, within the scope of its activities, is concerned with all fields of nursing service, and they have the common purpose of meeting the nursing needs of all the people. These are as follows:

Nursing Education
Nursing Service
Public Relations
Finance
Constitution and By-Laws
Social and Economic Welfare

There are also several Special Committees, one of which, the *Committee on Nursing Affairs,* was created by the Executive Committee in 1961 for the purpose of recommending goals to be reached within the framework and functions of the CNA in a specified period of time. During a 1963 meeting of the Executive Committee the following major goal was proposed by the Committee on Nursing Affairs and adopted by the Executive Committee:

"The Canadian Nurses' Association concentrates its efforts on nursing education in such a way that within ten years the nursing service of Canada will be provided by nurses who are graduates of university and diploma schools of nursing in the ratio of one to three."[5]

Provincial Associations. The provincial associations of Canada are autonomous, with CNA functioning largely in an advisory capacity and providing consultation services when requested. Membership in the CNA is acquired through membership in a provincial association.

National Headquarters. The Canadian Nurses' Association maintains a national headquarters in Ottawa, Canada's capital city, where several full time professional staff members and a large clerical staff assist the Executive Director to carry out activities representing nurses on a national level. The CNA is affiliated with the International Council of Nurses and also with a number of national and international health organizations. *The Canadian Nurse,* published monthly, keeps readers informed of professional activities and of current trends and developments in nursing. CNA conventions are held biennially in the even numbered years. The Patronage of Queen Elizabeth has been granted with permission for the words, "Patron—Her Majesty the Queen," to appear on all official stationery.

National Inventory. In 1963 all nurses of Canada were invited by the CNA to provide detailed information about themselves, using a specially constructed questionnaire which appeared in *The Canadian Nurse,* and now an official inventory is under way which will provide comprehensive information about nurses on a national basis that can be used to provide data on available nursing resources and also be a means toward achieving nursing goals in Canada.

---

[5]The Canadian Nurse, May 1963, p. 459

Canadian Nurses' Foundation. Establishment of the Canadian Nurses' Foundation in 1962 was a highlight of the thirty first national CNA convention, held in Vancouver, British Columbia. Made possible by the W. K. Kellogg Foundation, the purpose is to provide opportunity for nurses to prepare at the masters and doctoral levels for positions of leadership, and by the end of the following year financial assistance had been granted to nineteen nurses for postgraduate study in Canadian and American Universities. Future goals of the CNF include providing grants for research in nursing service areas.

EXPANSION OF NURSING RESEARCH PROGRAMS

Until recent years research in nursing has lagged somewhat behind that of other professions even though the national organizations for many years had been conducting it in some of their most critical areas. Studies, individual and multidisciplinary, had focused to a considerable extent on the occupation of nursing and its administrative and teaching aspects rather than on scientific inquiry into various phases of nursing practice. Changes came about with efforts to find causes and means of alleviating the nursing shortage as the possibilities to be achieved by widespread research became more and more apparent. Today research is being carried on in all areas of nursing and with increasing emphasis on clinical practice. Support is received from sociologists, psychologists, anthropologists, educators, and other groups concerned with human welfare.

Institute of Research and Service. The Department of Nursing Education of Teachers College, Columbia University, continued to carry on extensive research programs after publication of the Ginzberg Report in 1948, and in 1953 established the first permanent *Institute of Research and Service in Nursing Education,* now under the direction of *Dr. Elizabeth P. Hagen,* Executive Officer.

With a solid financial basis provided by the Rockefeller Foundation, a research center comparable to those of medicine and other established professions has been made available to nursing. Here also nurses are prepared for positions of leadership in the field of research by a staff expert in its techniques and in close contact with other fields of social service as they exist in a large university. The ultimate purpose is to raise the level of social welfare through the medium of good nursing, a contribution that will go far toward attainment of full professional status for nurses.

Chair in Nursing Research. Meanwhile the Alumni Association of the Department of Nursing Education of Teachers College in 1962 spearheaded a drive to endow the first chair in research in nursing and nursing education in honor of *Isabel Maitland Stewart* for her many contributions to nursing, including the development of organized research within the profession. Her great interest in the development of nursing was once more made evident by a bequest of about one thousand dollars to provide for "stimulation of interest in nursing history,"[6] which was received from her estate by the National League for Nursing. This amount was applied toward publication of "Three Score Years and Ten" to commemorate the 70th anniversary of founding of the American Society of Superintendents of Training Schools in 1894.

ASSOCIATE DEGREE RESEARCH PROGRAMS

Demands for increasing numbers of nurses and a high quality of nursing service made it imperative to consider all potential sources of nursing education. The Junior-Community college was judged to be one such source and a project, made possible by an anonymous donor, was initiated at Teachers College in 1952 to determine whether or not it is possible to develop an education centered program that will prepare nurses in less than the usual three years.

Mildred Montag, R.N., Ed.D., associate professor of nursing education, was made project director and the experiment was carried on in close cooperation with seven junior colleges and one hospital school in six widely separated states. All programs were developed as integral parts of the college structure, financially as well as educationally. Evaluation was based on the results of state licensing examinations, employer ratings, and opinions of the graduates themselves.

The project was completed by the Institute of Research and Service in 1957 with the decision having been reached that a carefully planned course within the organized system of education can produce well prepared nurses in two years. Furthermore such a school can give impetus to a movement of nursing education into institutions of higher learning as well as to a trend toward the use of public funds for this purpose.

An entirely new concept of nursing education, the associate degree program offers a curriculum of general education and specialized nursing education with supportive biological, physical, and behavioral sciences. Nursing subjects, including clinical experience in hospitals and other health agencies, constitute about one half the course. Inasmuch as clinical experience is rated as laboratory work, college credit is granted accordingly. Instruction in all areas of general education is provided by the college faculty while responsibility for developing and teaching the nursing course is assumed by the nursing faculty.

The majority of students are recent high school graduates but an increasing number of women are in the over thirty five age group, many married and some with families. Men, too, are admitted in somewhat larger numbers than in other types of nursing schools. Students are being attracted who wish to complete their education in a relatively short period of time, in their own communities, and in a college atmos-

---

[6]*Nursing Outlook*, April, 1964, p. 6

phere. Each must meet the requirements of a specified college for admission and graduation.

Upon completion of the course, the Associate in Arts degree is granted and graduates are eligible to take the state board examination for licensing as registered nurses. They are prepared to give quality patient care in staff nurse positions. For many, formal education stops at this point but those who are specially qualified may continue in baccalaureate programs in accordance with the policies of the particular school that they wish to attend.

Since the first associate degree nursing program came into being in 1952, there has been a steady increase in their size and number, and by the end of 1963 more than one hundred had been established in twenty nine states, some aided by grants from the W. K. Kellogg Foundation. They are no longer considered experimental and, in addition, many colleges are now offering courses for the preparation of practical nurses, also known as "vocational" nurses in some states.

ANA RESEARCH PROGRAMS

Formal programs of research in nursing are very new but those carried on within the nursing organizations and elsewhere in recent years have helped to gain national recognition of need for a critical examination of all aspects of nursing education and nursing practice. The American Nurses' Association is now continually moving forward in the field of research through the efforts of its *Research and Statistics Unit* and its *Committee on Research and Studies.* Current research activities are reported in the magazine, *Nursing Research,* and also in the *American Journal of Nursing.*

Socio-Economic Studies. A research project of considerable size was undertaken in 1946 when the National Nursing Council[7] cooperated with the Bureau of Labor Statistics of the U. S. Department of Labor in conducting a socio-economic study. The purpose was to compare the working and living conditions of nurses with those of women in other professions. The ANA, as one of the organizations represented on the National Nursing Council, took an active part in the project. The facts elicited through questionnaires sent to individual nurses and through personal interviews were published in the pamphlet, *The Economic Status of Registered Professional Nurses 1946-1947,* prepared by the Bureau of Labor Statistics. The figures therein indicate that, while the salaries of teachers in city schools were higher at that time, the average salary of urban and rural teachers combined about equaled that of nurses.

In 1956 another survey was conducted by the Bureau of Labor Statistics, this time to secure up-to-date, authoritative information on earnings and employment conditions of all hospital employees, in-

---

[7]Successor to the National Nursing Council for War Service.

cluding nurses, in approximately twenty urban hospitals. For some time such a survey had been advocated by the ANA and state nursing associations in order that the facts so obtained could be used in setting up minimum employment standards, in furthering the goals of economic security for nurses, and in providing accurate figures for Congress, state legislatures and the public.

In 1960 a third socio-economic survey was undertaken by the U. S. Bureau of Labor Statistics, this time a study in fifteen major metropolitan areas to obtain information concerning hospital employment conditions. This survey of practices involved 350,000 employees and covered various levels of nursing positions, including those of practical nurses and nursing aides, and examined health and welfare benefits as well as salaries. Although their economic status had improved since the initial study in 1946, the 1960 survey indicated that nurses had not reached a "level of compensation in keeping with their educational requirements and professional responsibilities."[8]

National Inventories. Another ANA research project, carried on through its Research and Statistics Unit, is that of making periodic national inventories of all registered nurses. Such surveys were made in 1948, 1951, and again in 1957-1958. In this way the number of active nurses, their location, age, marital status, field of nursing and type of position were determined. Information in regard to registered nurses not actively employed would prove of value in the event of a national emergency.

In 1962 the ANA, under a contract from the U. S. Public Health Service, introduced a new standard form to be filled in by nurses when applying for, or renewing, their state licenses. Recently completed, this study will provide a rich source of accurate information on the nursing resources of the nation as well as an assessment of nursing needs on both a state and national level.

Studies of Nursing F. S. & Q. The ANA took its first stride forward in research in 1950 when, at the request of the state associations and other groups, it initiated a five-year nation-wide program for *Studies of Nursing Functions, Standards, and Qualifications for Practice.* Although a number of such studies were under way in the district and state associations, it was agreed that a national program to coordinate and interpret these efforts was necessary. It was agreed also that full responsibility for determining the functions of nurses in each occupational group, their qualifications for various positions, and desirable standards of nursing practice lay within the profession itself.

Individual nurses were encouraged to participate in discussions of the subject in their district, state, and ANA sections. Statements representing a national viewpoint of all nurses were urgently needed at this time for many reasons. Advances in medical science were creating new responsibilities for nurses. A health conscious public was making de-

---

[8]American Journal of Nursing, May, 1961, p. 92

mands for more and better health services. Growing emphasis on prevention and rehabilitation as integral parts of all medical and nursing care was making it more necessary than ever before for nurses to be prepared to teach patients, their families, and community groups. In the work of rehabilitation particularly, nursing functions had been found to overlap at times with those of members of associate medical groups such as physical therapists, medical social workers, occupational therapists, and vocational counselors.

Reports of all studies were reviewed and analyzed by the ANA Research and Statistics Unit. Significant and rather consistent findings revealed wide variations in nursing practice. Many nurses were assuming responsibility for certain technical functions formerly performed by physicians, while auxiliary nursing team members were providing more direct patient care.

Final F. S. & Q. Statements were made available to nurses and the public through the medium of the July, August, and September, 1954, issues of the *American Journal of Nursing,* as well as through *Nursing Research* and other channels. A comprehensive report followed in book form, "Twenty Thousand Nurses Tell Their Story," by Hughes, Hughes, and Deutscher, sociologists who directed the study.

Implementing the Statements. The statements of nursing functions, standards, and qualifications for practice represent goals toward which the profession is moving. They provide a criterion for critical evaluation of present practices, for preparation of specifications for employment for various positions, and for all kinds of educational programs for nurses. They have relationship to development of minimum employment standards and salary figures by state associations. They are essential in case of a lawsuit for malpractice.

Using the statements of functions as a chief authority, the ANA Committee on Legislation, with the help of state attorneys, formulated legal definitions of both professional and practical nursing. These were approved by the ANA Board of Directors and recommended for inclusion in state nursing practice acts. They are as follows:

"The practice of professional nursing means the performance for compensation of any act in the observation, care, and counsel of the ill, injured, or infirm, or in the maintenance of health or prevention of illness of others, or in the supervision and teaching of other personnel, or the administration of medications and treatments as prescribed by a licensed physician or dentist; requiring substantial specialized judgment and skill and based on knowledge and application of the principles of biological, physical, and social sciences. The foregoing shall not be deemed to include acts of diagnosis or prescription of therapeutic or corrective measures."

"The practice of practical nursing means the performance for compensation of selected acts in the care of the ill, injured, or infirm under the direction of a registered professional nurse or a licensed physician or licensed dentist; and not requiring the substantial specialized skill, judgment, and knowledge required in professional nursing."[9]

[9]American Journal of Nursing, July, 1962, p. 72

Even though considerable progress had been made in defining and implementing standards of nursing practice, disparities in nursing service continued to increase as more and more nurses were carrying out functions traditionally entrusted to physicians. Mounting problems faced by nurses in practice, professionally and legally, prompted the ANA to propose the formation of committees on professional practice within the state nursing associations. With acceptance of the proposal by the ANA House of Delegates in 1962, the names of all Committees on Functions, Standards, and Qualifications for Practice were changed to *Committees on Practice.*

The new Committees on Practice assumed responsibility for continuing to study, interpret, and promote implementation of the functions, standards, and qualifications for nursing practice and for maintaining legal, professional, and ethical standards. At the same time, an ANA Intersectional Committee on Nursing Practice was formed to assist the state committees with their work.

Blueprint for Nursing Research. In an effort to move forward more rapidly in the field of nursing research, the functions of the ANA Committee on Research and Studies were broadened in 1960 to include studying the association's programs on research, identifying needs for research, and finding ways to stimulate future research. A *Blueprint for Nursing Research,* published by the Committee in 1962, outlines subject areas where research is needed now and will be needed in the future. It emphasizes a critical need for more nurse investigators, wide dissemination of research findings, and the application of new knowledge to patient care.

To the original list of subjects requiring research, the necessity for historical research has been more recently added, and the statement made that "Those individuals who cannot remember the past will be condemned to repeat it . . . we have been oblivious to the great importance which other professions, such as medicine, law, and education, have placed upon history, and the way in which knowledge of the past has guided and inspired their forward movement."[10]

AMERICAN NURSES' FOUNDATION FOR RESEARCH

Another stride forward in the field of research came in 1955 with establishment of the American Nurses' Foundation, Inc. By that time it had become evident that concern for improving nursing practice extended beyond the profession itself and that research in regard to it would continue far into the future. The Foundation is an independent corporation created by, and composed of, the ANA Board of Directors. The Foundation's Board is elected from this group and also includes several socially-minded, non-nurse members. Specialists in social science, research techniques, and statistics are employed on the staff at headquarters.

---

[10]"The Case for Historical Research"—Newton. *Nursing Research,* Winter, 1965, p. 20

The Foundation supports research in nursing and sponsors special projects. Completing the program of Studies of Nursing F. S. & Q. became one of its immediate responsibilities. The ANF is empowered also to make grants to hospitals and other educational institutions for research purposes. The ANA Research and Statistics Unit continues to carry on in areas of more immediate concern to nurses themselves, such as determination of the correct teaching load for instructors and the proper source of payment for transportation costs of public health nurses. The ANF provides a financially sound means of carrying on programs which have implications for the entire health field. Before its establishment funds for research came entirely from nurses, but the permanent and tax-free status of a Foundation is expected to attract the support of outside groups since all proposed activities will be in the public interest as well as within the purposes of the ANA itself.

The first contribution to the Foundation came from the National Institutes of Health of the USPHS in the form of a generous grant for a three-year study of nurse-patient relationships and other factors relating to public health nursing in the New York-New Jersey metropolitan area. Another grant came from the Rockefeller Foundation for an International Nursing Project involving foreign nurses in this country on the Exchange Visitor Program of the U. S. Department of State. Interviews in regard to their experiences in American hospitals are providing information which serves as a basis for improvement of the program.

In 1960 a nationwide movement was launched, with the aid of state and district associations, to seek additional funds for research purposes from corporations, organizations, and foundations, as well as from nurses and friends of nursing. The response to this appeal is making it possible for the Foundation to provide accurate knowledge of nursing requirements vital to the health needs of a growing population.

In 1962 the ANF was able to award a special grant to the Cornell University – New York Hospital School of Nursing for a study that would seek out and encourage talented students with potential for leadership in research and teaching positions. A year later a three-year project of continuing education for graduate nurses in Upper New England was supported by a generous grant from the Irene Heinz Given and John La Porte Given Foundation. This is designed to assist staff nurses from hospitals, nursing homes, and public health agencies, as well as private duty nurses, in the application of research findings to nursing care of their patients.

A further effort to stimulate nursing research in the area of patient care came about in 1963 when the ANF initiated a *Small Grants Program,* whereby awards of moderate size may be made to competent researchers to carry out specific activities, perhaps to test a research tool or to conduct a pilot study needed for development of a special research project.

Another objective was realized when the American Nurses' Foundation was able to provide, on a permanent basis, an *Abstracting Service* for the journal, *Nursing Research.* In each issue now appears a section titled, "Abstracts," which gives abbreviated accounts of pertinent research studies that have previously been published elsewhere. In addition, there are now available two retrospective sets, "Abstracts of Studies in Public Health Nursing, 1924–1957" and "Abstracts of Studies in Nursing, 1955–1958."

NLN RESEARCH PROGRAMS

The National League for Nursing takes part in research directed toward providing an adequate amount of high quality nursing services through progressive adjustments of nursing education to meet the needs of our rapidly changing social structure. It provides statistical and other information and promotes studies for the purpose of reaching desired goals.

One important study, carried out by NLN's Committee on the Future, was to estimate the future needs for nursing service in order to provide a reliable basis for development of educational programs. A report of this study, published in the booklet, *Nurses for a Growing Nation,* gives an estimate of the number of nurses that will be needed by 1970. This proved to be an increase of 42 to 92 more than the national ratio of 258 nurses for every 100,000 of the population that were available at the time of the study.

Predictions were based on past trends and took into account the demands of a growing population rate and an increasing emphasis on all aspects of health care. Need for expansion of existing school facilities and re-evaluation of educational programs was pointed out with a reminder to nursing educators that quality, as well as quantity, must be the goal.

NLN Research and Studies Service. Research activities of the League were strengthened in 1959 with establishment of a *Research and Studies Service,* set up to provide assistance to its various departments and services, to continue the annual and periodical statistical surveys of nursing practice and nursing education, and to conduct other special studies. Of great practical significance is the *Study on the Cost of Nursing Education,* supported by a grant from the U. S. Public Health Service. This project was to determine the cost of educating a student nurse in each of three types of preservice programs, diploma, associate in arts, and baccalaureate degree. The information thus far brought forth indicates that the administrative costs of diploma schools are greatest, and study of the other programs continues.

A recently completed study of widespread interest is the *Test of a Nursing Performance Evaluation Instrument,* which it is hoped will prove effective in evaluation of clinical performance. At the same time,

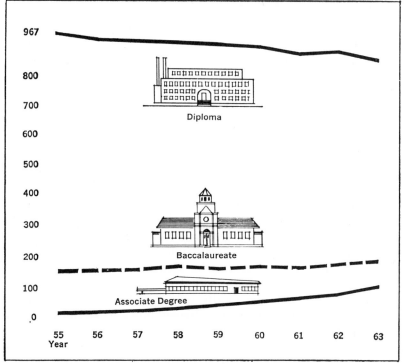

Based on data from: American Nurses' Association, Facts About Nursing, 1956-1963 eds.; National League for Nursing.

Figure 91. Number of basic nursing programs. (American Journal of Nursing, May, 1964.)

a rating device for evaluating the performance of a hospital staff nurse has been developed by the NLN Department of Hospital Nursing with the assistance of the Research and Studies Service.

Recognition of an urgent need to plan health services for patients, following their discharge from hospitals, brought about a three-year study, *Factors Influencing Continuity of Nursing Care,* sponsored by the NLN and supported by a USPHS grant, which investigated current plans for referral of patients to public health nursing services after they leave the hospital. The staff of the Institute of Research and Service in Nursing Education conducted the study and gathered information from approximately 800 patients and the same number of health personnel in six hospitals, three in metropolitan and three in non-metropolitan districts. Conclusions reached brought about strong evidence of need for continuity of nursing services following hospital discharge.

An *NLN Council on Research in Nursing,* formed in 1961 upon request of the membership, reflects the high interest of nurses and their associates in the subject of research. An Interdivisional Council, CORN provides opportunity for members to meet with fellow researchers for the purpose of sharing concepts and exchanging ideas as well as promoting research in various areas of nursing.

In the Foreword of the report are the following statements: "In the opinion of the Group, the Nation faces a critical problem in ensuring adequate nursing services in the years ahead. . . . But it will not be enough simply to increase our supply of nurses. Quality must be the constant goal of education, service, and research if nursing is to meet its share of responsibility for the health of the nation. . . . In the judgment of the Consultant Group, if the nursing problem is to be solved, there is no alternative to Federal Aid."

At the time of the report there were an estimated 550,000 graduate nurses, 225,000 practical nurses, and 400,000 nursing aides, orderlies, and attendants in the United States. During the preceding year there had been some 1,800 foreign nurses licensed to practice in this country. Three out of five graduate nurses and more than one-half of all practical nurses were serving on hospital staffs, and the total of all persons employed by hospitals comprised the fifth largest group of workers in any industry.

The Consultant Group outlined a feasible goal to be that of increasing the annual number of graduates of diploma, associate degree, and baccalaureate degree programs from the existing 30,000 to that of 51,000 by 1969, bringing the national number of graduates to 680,000 by 1970. The report emphasized also an urgent need for the number of nurses with academic degrees to be increased from the existing 55,000 to 120,000 during the same period.

Study of Nursing Education.   The initial recommendation for improving the situation was that "a study should be made of the present system of nursing education in relation to the responsibilities and skill levels required for high quality patient care."[16] In line with this statement a fifteen member autonomous *National Commission for the Study of Nursing Education, Inc.* was formed in 1967 by the ANA and NLN with the support of grants from the Avalon and W. K. Kellogg Foundations and a gift from an anonymous donor. At the head of the Commission is *W. Allen Wallis,* president of the University of Rochester, Rochester, New York. Other members include prominent persons in fields of the health disciplines, higher education, social and physical sciences, and business administration. A final report, with recommendations, is expected within two or three years.

Other recommendations of the Consultant Group were for granting federal funds for stimulation of recruitment to nursing schools and for assistance to hospitals, colleges, and universities for expanding and improving the quality of their nursing education programs. Another recommendation was for providing federal funds as project grants to nursing schools for experimentation with new and improved methods for inservice programs for graduate nurses, and on-the-job training for nursing aides in hospitals and nursing homes, as well as for continuing education programs for graduate nurses.

---

[16]Quoted in *ANA in ACTION,* Sept./Oct., 1967, p. 5

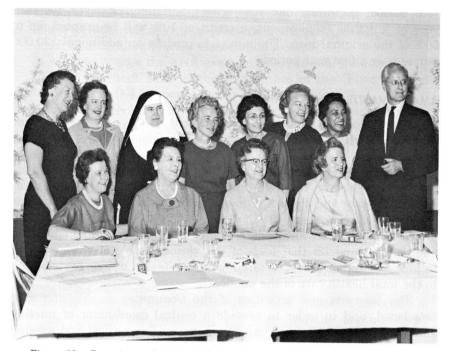

Figure 93. Committee of ANA-NLN Coordinating Council to formulate plans for a Comprehensive Study of Nursing Education recommended in "Toward Quality in Nursing." Left to right are, seated: Mrs. Judith G. Whitaker, Inez Haynes, Lois M. Austin, and Mrs. Margaret B. Dolan. Standing are Rena E. Boyle, Mrs. Margaret F. Carroll, Sister Maureen, Mrs. Lucile Petry Leone, Mrs. Minnie H. Walton, Jo Eleanor Elliott, Willetta Simonton (ANA associate executive director for sections, not a member of committee) and Robert K. Merton. Absent was William J. McGlothlin. (Courtesy of the American Nurses' Association in ANA in Review, Fall, 1963. Photograph by Jules Geller.)

To help meet a critical need for nursing leaders, it was recommended that the current federal programs of Professional Nurse Traineeships be increased and extended, with greater emphasis placed on aid for doctoral candidates, new funds for the preparation of clinicians and for baccalaureate preparation for registered nurses. Throughout the Surgeon General's Report, the need for nursing research programs is strongly indicated.

Nurse Training Act of 1964. As a direct outcome of recommendations made in the report of the Surgeon General's Consultant Group on Nursing, entitled "Toward Quality in Nursing," The Nurse Training Act of 1964 was passed by the House of Representatives and the Senate and became law in 1964. The Act is designed to offset a persistent and critical shortage of nurses by providing funds for constructing new nursing schools and modernizing existing ones; expanding and improving teaching programs; extending the traineeship program for nurses; and establishing grants for recruitment projects and student loans.

Student loans are to be limited to $1,000 a year and preference is to be given to first year students. They are to be repaid within a ten

25. What major recommendations are set forth in the report of the Consultant Group, entitled "Toward Quality in Nursing – Needs and Goals," published by the USPHS in 1963?

26. What is the Nurse Training Act of 1964? What are its major provisions?

27. Tell what you know about the AMA Committee on Nursing. In what way do you think this may affect patient care?

References

American Nurses' Association: Facts About Nursing. Revised annually by the ANA Research and Statistics Unit.

Dolan, Josephine A.: Goodnow's History of Nursing. Philadelphia, W. B. Saunders Co., 1963.

Frank, Sister Charles Marie: The Historical Development of Nursing. Philadelphia, W. B. Saunders Co., 1959.

Hughes, Hughes, and Deutscher: Twenty Thousand Nurses Tell Their Story. Philadelphia and Montreal, J. B. Lippincott Co., 1958.

Kelly, Cordelia M.: Dimensions of Professional Nursing. New York, The Macmillan Co., 1962.

McKenna, Frances M.: Thresholds to Professional Nursing Practice. Philadelphia, W. B. Saunders Co., 1960.

Meyer and Heidgerkin: Introduction to Research in Nursing. Philadelphia and Montreal, J. B. Lippincott Co., 1962.

Montag, Mildred L.: Community College Education in Nursing. New York, McGraw-Hill Book Co., 1959.

Morison, Luella J.: Steppingstones to Professional Nursing. St. Louis, C. V. Mosby Co., 1965.

Rogers, Martha E.: Educational Revolution in Nursing. New York, The Macmillan Co., 1961.

Sanner, Margaret C.: Trends and Professional Adjustments in Nursing. Philadelphia, W. B. Saunders Co., 1962.

Shryock, Richard H.: The History of Nursing. Philadelphia, W. B. Saunders Co., 1959.

Spalding and Notter: Professional Nursing: Foundations, Perspectives, and Relationships. Philadelphia and Montreal, J. B. Lippincott Co., 1965.

U. S. Department of Health, Education, and Welfare. Washington, D.C. Toward Quality in Nursing – Needs and Goals. Public Health Service Publication No. 992, 1962.

Vaillot, Sister Madeleine Clemence: Commitment to Nursing. Philadelphia and Montreal, J. B. Lippincott Co., 1962.

AMERICAN JOURNAL OF NURSING

"The Functions of the Professional Association" – Merton. Jan., 1958, p. 50.

"The Professional Status of Nursing" – Bixler and Bixler. August, 1959, p. 1142.

"Nursing Research – Its Evolution" – McManus. April, 1961, p. 76.

"Today and Tomorrow in Nursing Research" – McManus. May, 1961, p. 68.

"Current Actions Indicate Changes Ahead," September, 1961, p. 73.

"Putting Our Own House in Order" – Dolan. December, 1962, p. 76.

"Technical Education in Nursing" – Montag. May, 1963, p. 100.

"Changing ANA to Meet Changing Needs. Parts I, II, III." – Powell. March, April, May, 1964, pp. 111, 113, 117.

"Standards for Organized Nursing Services," March, 1965, p. 76.

NURSING OUTLOOK

"Nationwide Hunt for Nursing's Historical Treasures"—Goostray. January, 1965, p. 26.
"NLN at Ten"—Haynes. June, 1962, p. 372.

NURSING RESEARCH

"What is Research"—Bixler. June, 1952, p. 7.

Chapter 15

GRADUATE NURSING CAREERS

Today's graduate meets with a rapidly evolving society in which continual adjustment to changing circumstances and changing attitudes has become a necessity. Unprecedented advances in the medical and social sciences, growth of technology, explosion of knowledge, population changes, and a health conscious public making increasing demands for health services of all kinds, have greatly broadened the responsibilities of doctors and nurses. Nursing now encompasses prevention of disease and disability, health promotion, rehabilitation, along with care of the sick, and involves teaching, counseling, spiritual and emotional support, as well as the physical aspects of nursing care.

At the same time an expansion of health services outside the hospital continues, with provision for home care for the chronically ill and the acutely ill short-term patient. Meanwhile the emergence of the clinical nursing specialist as an expert practitioner, with advanced knowledge in a given field, represents a major influence in the improvement of nursing practice as well as the return of skilled nursing to the bedside.

CAREER OPPORTUNITIES

Broadly speaking, all nursing opportunities come within two fields: *Nursing Service* and *Nursing Education*. The field of nursing service covers not only the care of patients in hospitals, nursing homes, clinics, and public health agencies but also that provided by industrial organizations, doctors' offices, and elsewhere. The field of nursing education includes various teaching positions with practical and basic professional programs of nursing schools, inservice programs, and those offered

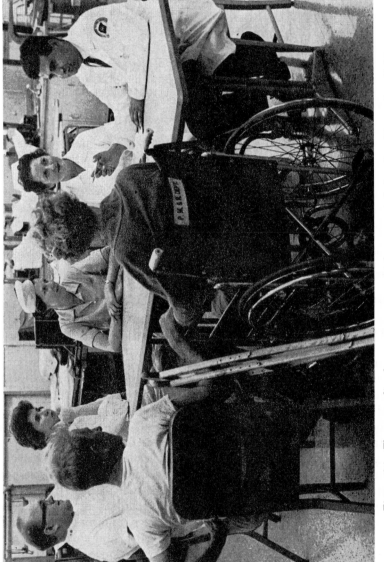

Figure 94. The expanding home care program takes concerted planning. Here a hospital team of physical therapist, occupational therapist, visiting nurse, hospital nurse, and physiatrist counsels a stroke patient and her husband in preparation for her continuing care at home. (American Journal of Nursing, May, 1964.)

As a family health teacher, the public health nurse spends considerable time in health counseling and supervision. Sometimes he or she gives bedside care in the home, and may serve also as a team leader to assist families in guiding and coordinating the work of less prepared personnel. Whether in the home, hospital, school, or elsewhere, the public health nurse works alone a large part of the time and is challenged to meet many different situations.

As an essential member of the health team, the public health nurse takes a place alongside community leaders, physicians, health educators, parents, and others to promote community health. Teaching classes for antepartum patients, speaking at citizens' group meetings, participating in disease detection and immunization programs, all are within the scope of public health nursing.

Many, but not all, public health agencies require their staff nurses to have a baccalaureate degree, with preparation at the master's level for supervisory, administrative, consultant, and teaching positions. For the well prepared public health nurse, opportunities abound for interesting and challenging work either at home or in foreign lands.

Occupational Health Nursing. A rapidly growing field, occupational health has become an important part of industry, and nurses are employed by factories, banks, hotels, department stores, large offices, and other places where they are demonstrating their value by helping to maintain a high health level among employees and their families and, at the same time, fostering a fine spirit of cooperation among all associates. While some nurses are supervisors of occupational health nursing services, the greater number work alone and are solely responsible for the services of an employee health department.

In an effort to keep employees well and on the job, emphasis is placed on preventive health measures. In general, the occupational health, or industrial, nurse offers health counseling and teaching, assists with health examination programs, provides emergency care for employees who become ill or injured while at work, and arranges for medical care when necessary. Frequently the nurse also serves on a plant Health and Safety Committee and helps to develop and implement the safety program.

While qualifications are variable, rarely is the new graduate employed in a one nurse industrial health program. Public health preparation is an excellent background for the nurse in industry and, in addition, a knowledge of personnel work, safety practices, and health education methods proves a useful asset. A nurse director is generally expected to have advanced preparation in nursing.

To meet the need in other fields, various programs in clinical specialties are available in hospitals and colleges. Since rehabilitation has become an integral part of medical care, more and more teaching centers are offering short-term courses to enable nurses to carry out rehabilitation techniques in hospitals and other health agencies.

Nursing Research. In this growing field, nurses are finding opportunities for work of absorbing interest, preparation for which requires education beyond the baccalaureate program as well as progressive experience in this field. Nurses are employed, too, in a variety of other satisfying positions including those of staff workers on the local, state, and national nursing organizations, editors of nursing journals and textbooks, and as consultants for U. S. Government agencies, Foundations, the national and international Red Cross Societies, and the World Health Organization.

Nursing Education. In this field, the need for qualified nurse educators is a major problem facing the profession. While the majority of positions are on faculties of diploma schools of nursing, an ever-increasing number of faculty members are needed for baccalaureate and associate degree programs. Furthermore, programs for practical nurses are growing steadily and offer additional teaching opportunities. Although numerous positions are open to nurses with baccalaureate degrees, increasingly nurse educators in professional schools are required to have a master's degree with the trend toward preparation at the doctoral level for positions in colleges and universities. Today many nurses are continuing their studies for higher degrees while holding teaching positions.

There is also considerable demand for qualified administrators and instructors of inservice programs in hospitals and other health agencies. Many nurses are employed to prepare the various levels of non-nurse personnel for work in health service agencies; others to conduct refresher courses for inactive nurses. The development of university extension courses for nurses marks a new area for nurse educators. Moreover, there are openings in the community to teach classes in Red Cross Home Nursing as well as in Civilian Defense and First Aid.

Men Nurses. Since the early days of Christianity, when deacons went into the homes to care for sick male members of the Church, men have assumed a share of nursing responsibilities. Throughout the Middle Ages, great numbers of men, belonging to religious and military orders, administered to the sick. Their Military Nursing Orders built and managed great fortress-like hospitals to care for sick and wounded Crusaders along routes of travel. Ultimately these supplemented the work of established monasteries all over the west and in Palestine.

Nursing Brotherhoods have had a far-reaching effect on nursing. Among the most widely spread and active were the Brothers of Mercy, the Franciscans, the Alexians, and the Brothers of St. John of God, some of whom continue in nursing today.

In the early history of the United States some hospitals accepted men as well as women students, and some established schools exclusively for men, three of which are still in existence. *The Mills School of Male Nurses* was founded at Bellevue Hospital in 1888, and along with the Bellevue School of Nursing has since become associated with the Division

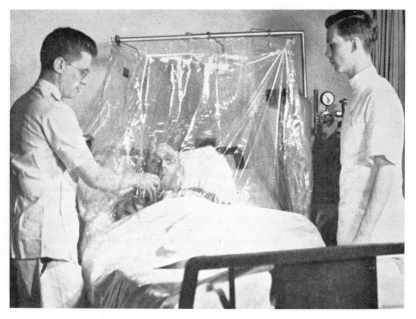

Figure 96. Oxygen tent patient receives attention from men student nurses at Alexian Brothers Hospital School of Nursing, Chicago.

of Nursing, College of Medicine, of New York University. *The Alexian Brothers Hospital School of Nursing for Men* was established in Chicago in 1894, and in 1914 the *School of Nursing for Men of the Pennsylvania Hospital* was founded in Philadelphia.

Opportunities for men nurses have expanded tremendously in recent years. Avenues which once were closed have opened wide. More than ever before they are in demand for care of men patients with fractures, heart conditions, genitourinary problems, venereal diseases, as well as for those who are alcoholics. Personnel in psychiatric wards wonder how they ever got along without them. They are found in increasing numbers in public health work, private practice, rehabilitation, and in international health work. Opportunities in the fields of anesthesia and occupational health, areas apparently of particular interest for men, are available also. Men nurses are especially well equipped for positions in mines, construction jobs, heavy industry, and prison work.

The U. S. Public Health Service and the Veterans Administration, as well as the Army Nurse Corps and the Air Force Nurse Corps, have openings for men in positions almost as varied as those for women. A few government posts, such as the USPHS Quarantine Station at the Mexican Border are open only to men.

Within recent years, men nurses have been assuming leadership roles in the national nursing organizations. They have served on the ANA Board of Directors, the NLN Staff, and have filled offices of both associations. In 1960 *Philip E. Day,* director of nursing service, Mary

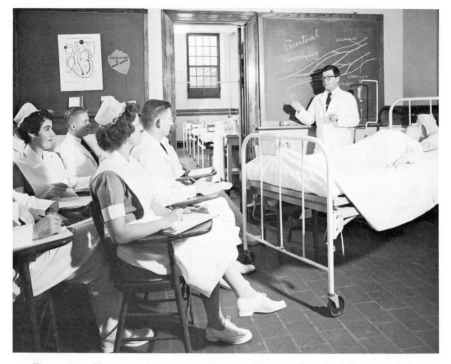

Figure 97. Classroom instruction, McLean Hospital School of Nursing, Belmont, Massachusetts. (Courtesy Hutchins Photography, Inc.)

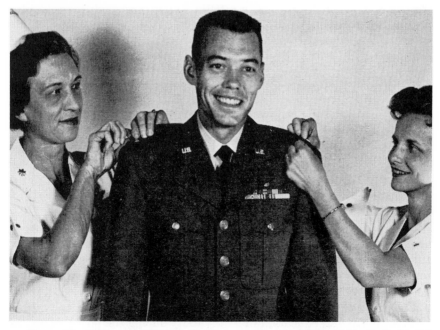

Figure 98. Gold bars of the U.S. Air Force are pinned on Richard Martin by Lt. Col. Hilda Echols and his wife, Donna, as he becomes a member of the Air Force Nurse Corps. (American Journal of Nursing, Nov., 1962.)

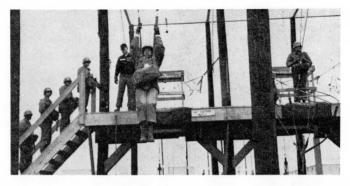

Figure 99. Men nurses practicing parachute jumping at Fort Campbell, Kentucky, in preparation for work with teams to provide immediate care for casualties. (American Journal of Nursing, Nov., 1958.)

Fletcher Hospital, Burlington, Vermont, was elected president of the Vermont State Nurses' Association and so became the first man to fill this office in any state. In succeeding years, men nurses were chosen as presidents of the Michigan Nurses' Association, the Pennsylvania Nurses' Association, and the Oregon Nurses' Association.

In 1964 Mr. Day was made executive director of the American Journal of Nursing Company. A veteran of World War II, he is a graduate of the Pennsylvania Hospital School of Nursing and the University of Pennsylvania, and holds an M.A. degree in Administration of Hospital Nursing Service from Teachers College, Columbia University. It may well be that the employment of greater numbers of men nurses will go far toward solving the "nursing shortage" problem and this term will eventually disappear from nursing literature.

GOVERNMENT SERVICES

Opportunities for nurses in the federal services began to unfold with organization of the U. S. Army Nurse Corps in 1901, and this field has gained increasing recognition with each World War and the Korean Police Action of the United Nations. Today there are six major federal agencies with responsibility for health care: the Army, the Navy, the Air Force, the Veterans Administration, the Public Health Service, and the Agency for International Development (AID).

In each service challenging opportunities are offered to nurses for contributing their share toward defending their country and guarding the people's health. At the same time personnel policies are generous and, in many instances, include opportunities for active inservice education, professional advancement, retirement benefits, medical care and, sometimes, travel in a foreign country. It may be possible, too, to acquire additional education in a university during the period of service.

Military Nursing. Necessary qualifications for appointment to the

Reserve of the U. S. Army Nurse Corps, the U. S. Navy Nurse Corps, and the *U. S. Air Force Nurse Corps* are similar and can be met by the average young graduate of an accredited nursing school. Appointments to the regular services are made from members of the Reserve. Accepted candidates are granted immediately the rank of full commissioned officers, the grade determined by age, professional preparation, and experience. Initial appointments are usually to the rank of second or first lieutenant for the ANC and AFNC and to ensign for the Navy Nurse Corps. They may be higher for those with special qualifications.

Nurses of all three Corps may be assigned to hospitals at home or abroad, caring for men of the Armed Forces and their families. Nurses of the Air Force Nurse Corps may serve also as flight nurses; while those of the Navy Nurse Corps may be aboard the Military Sea Transportation Service. Nursing functions, in addition to care of patients, may include supervision, teaching, administration, or research.

A major stride forward came with establishment of a Department of Nursing at the Walter Reed Army Research Institute, which enables nurses to collaborate in, and conduct, research in patient care on a full time basis. At the same time a nucleus of nurses is provided who are schooled in nursing, in science, and in research methodology and are available to the Army Medical Service when needed.

A course in Nuclear Nursing, which is shared by civilian nurses, is conducted by the Navy at the Naval Medical School of Bethesda, Maryland. All Air Force nurses, as key members of the Aerospace Team, have opportunity to keep abreast of new developments in Aerospace Medicine, while those who are qualified for flight nursing attend a special program at the School of Aviation Medicine at San Antonio, Texas. New arrivals are prepared for responsibilities of a "Missile Age" by the School of Aviation Medicine at Brooks Air Force Base in Texas. Further information concerning these services can be secured from the nearest recruiting office of the U. S. Army, U. S. Air Force, and the U. S. Navy.

Opportunities for Senior Students. The *Army Student Nurse Program* and the *Navy Nurse Corps Candidate Program* offer opportunities to senior, and some junior, men and women student nurses of schools approved for completion of their education under the aegis of the Reserve of the U. S. Army or the U. S. Navy. Applicants are expected to show evidence of personal ability and meet certain other basic requirements. Successful candidates of either program complete their studies in the home school while receiving financial assistance with their school expenses and a generous monthly allowance. When they have been graduated and become registered nurses, they are commissioned as officers in the Reserve of the U. S. Army Nurse Corps or the U. S. Navy Nurse Corps and are expected to give active service for a specified period of time. Information can be secured from the nearest recruiting office of the U. S. Army or U. S. Navy.

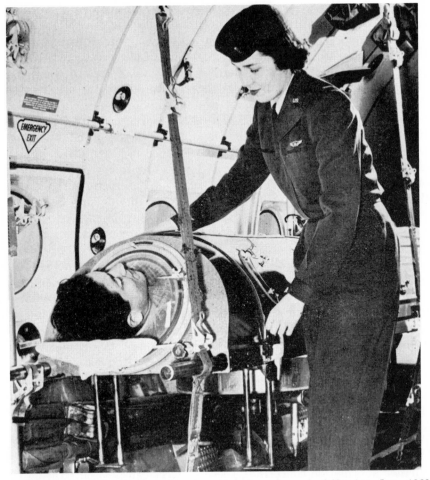

Figure 100. U.S. Air Force Nursing. (American Journal of Nursing, Jan., 1963. Official Air Force photo.)

Nursing in the *U. S. Veterans Administration Service,* largest of the federal services, involves the care of honorably discharged veterans of all wars who have service-connected disabilities. Veterans Administration hospitals are equipped with a full range of clinical services and research facilities, and many serve as teaching institutions for medical and nursing students. Home care programs have been set up for veterans who are under the care of a physician but not restricted to a hospital. Community Nursing Agencies assume responsibility for their care.

Positions are available in hospitals, out patient clinics, regional offices, and the central office in Washington. The salaries of staff nurses often compare favorably with those of nurses in advanced grades since it is believed that qualified practitioners who give skilled bedside care are deserving of the same recognition as those in teaching, supervisory, or administrative positions. Additional education or experience is necessary for promotion to each upper grade. Nurses just graduating from schools may receive temporary appointment pending state registration, providing they show evidence of having taken the state examination or having made application for so doing.

Openings in the *Public Health Service, U. S. Department of Health, Education, and Welfare* are available for men and women nurses in government hospitals and public health agencies where many patients are federal beneficiaries. Fifteen such Public Health Service hospitals throughout the United States include general hospitals, a tuberculosis hospital, two hospitals for narcotic addicts and neuropsychiatric patients, and the National Leprosarium at Carville, Louisiana. The Clinical Center at Bethesda, Maryland, is part of the National Institutes of Health, a research Bureau where the study of health problems is carried on. At this 500-bed service the nurse functions as an important member of the research team.

Other assignments of nurses to the U. S. Public Health Service may be to stations in Washington, D. C.; to regional offices in large cities; to hospitals, health centers, and public health stations for natives in Alaska; to the Division of Indian Health for work on Indian reservations; or to foreign fields for public health nursing and educational assignments. Special preparation is required for public health positions and for work in clinics, but not for clinical nursing in hospitals.

All positions with the U. S. Public Health Service are secured through Civil Service examination and appointment or by special appointment as a commissioned officer. A baccalaureate or higher degree is required for the Commissioned Corps. The greater number of nurses enter as Civil Service appointees and remain in one location, but may be rotated in accordance with their interests and the need for nurses. A commissioned officer is often rotated from one assignment to the care of Indians on a reservation, to the care of natives in Alaska, and back to another assignment. Nursing students within six months of graduation are permitted to make application for appointment and will be given provisional ratings.

Commissioned Officer Student Training and Extern Program. In an effort to attract promising students to a career in one of its services, the USPHS now offers vacation time experience to graduate nurse students in baccalaureate programs. During a three month summer period, students enrolled in the *Commissioned Officer Student Training and Extern Program* have opportunity to travel while receiving a salary and gaining experience in clinical nursing, public health nursing, or nursing research. Recently COSTEP was opened to undergraduate students enrolled in baccalaureate programs as well as to graduate nurses.

The Nursing Section of the Children's Bureau, *U. S. Department of Health, Education, and Welfare* employs a chief nurse and several regional consultants whose function is to assist state agencies with nursing matters relating to the Crippled Children's Services and Maternal and Child Health. Also nurses may be employed to work abroad as consultants and teachers. Specialized education in child and maternal health, in addition to public health nursing, is required for these positions.

The Agency for International Development (AID), administered by the U. S. State Department, is providing technical and economic assistance to more than seventy newly developing nations, during what has been called "the revolution in rising expectations."[1] Conservation of health is an important part of the program and nurse consultants are employed to assist with nursing projects. Since each activity is carried on as a cooperative venture, AID nurses work with their host country counterparts wherever possible. They may function as teachers or supervisors in hospitals while preparing those who will follow them after AID nurses are withdrawn. In 1964 *Margaret G. Arnstein,* former Chief of the Division of Nursing, U. S. Public Health Service, accepted an assignment with AID to direct a special study on international nursing problems.

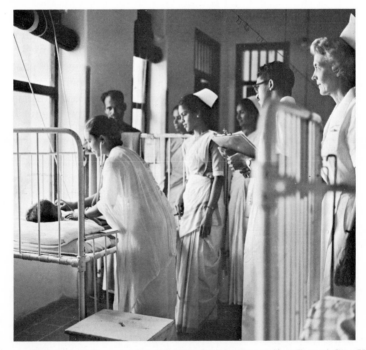

Figure 101. An A.I.D. nurse helps to organize a pilot ward at Bogotá City Hospital, Colombia. (From A.I.D. folder, "The Overseas Nurse in A.I.D." Department of State, Washington, D.C. 20402.)

---

[1]AID folder, "The Overseas Nurse in AID." Agency for International Development, Department of State, Washington, D.C. 20402.

Foreign Service Nurses are also employed by the U. S. State Department to assist with health programs at foreign posts, principally embassies, where U. S. Government agency employees and their families reside. Preference for appointment as a Foreign Service Nurse is given to applicants with a bachelor of science degree in nursing and experience of a year or more in public health or industrial nursing.

The Peace Corps. To Tanganyika on the Indian Ocean, to the Dominican Republic between the Atlantic Ocean and the Caribbean Sea, to Nepal in the Himalayas, as well as to many other areas throughout the world, Americans of the Peace Corps, representing all races, social strata, and educational levels, are sharing in an effort to promote better understanding of their country and to bring back to America a better understanding of other peoples.

Dealing first hand with health and clinical conditions seldom

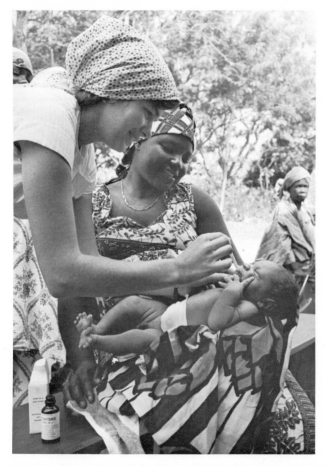

Figure 102. Ann Moore, Peace Corps Nurse of Ohio giving vitamins to a baby at an outdoor clinic in Togo, West Africa. (Miss Moore is wearing a scarf presented to her by Togolese women patients.) (Photograph by Rowland Scherman in "Registered Nurses in the Peace Corps." Peace Corps, Room 600, Washington, D.C. 20402.)

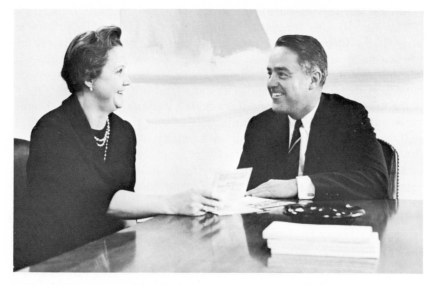

Figure 103. Nurse advisor in the Peace Corps Dorothy Sutherland shares the enthusiasm of Peace Corps Director R. Sargent Shriver for the contributions nurses make in the host-countries where they are serving. Shriver notes that native doctors are "overwhelming in their praise of American nurses." (Courtesy of the American Nurses' Association in ANA in Review, Spring, 1963.)

encountered in the United States, nurses work side by side with host country nurses. Many are assigned to senior staff nurse positions in hospitals, rural clinics, and health centers, while others assist with the clinical teaching of nursing students or auxiliary personnel. A few participate in formal classroom instruction in schools of nursing, and some are members of health teams for the control of yaws or tuberculosis. Further information can be obtained by writing to the Director, Professional and Technical Division, Peace Corps, Washington, D. C. 20402.

S. S. Hope. Since S. S. Hope first sailed for Southeast Asia in 1960, armed with people and equipment prepared to provide expert health services, it has carried medical missions to many parts of the world. Patterned after a modern hospital, this "great white ship" is set up primarily for the purpose of educating local medical and paramedical personnel in new concepts and techniques of health care and teaching preventive health practices to the people. A corps of medical, dental, and nurse practitioners is assisted by host counterparts to make sure that the work of S. S. Hope, whose name stands for "Health Opportunity for People Everywhere," is continued by native personnel after its departure.

Wherever possible S. S. Hope's health services are extended into the communities with the staff working in port hospitals and as inland teams. Staff nurses, along with their native colleagues, have set up a variety of programs pertaining to nursing and health care which have

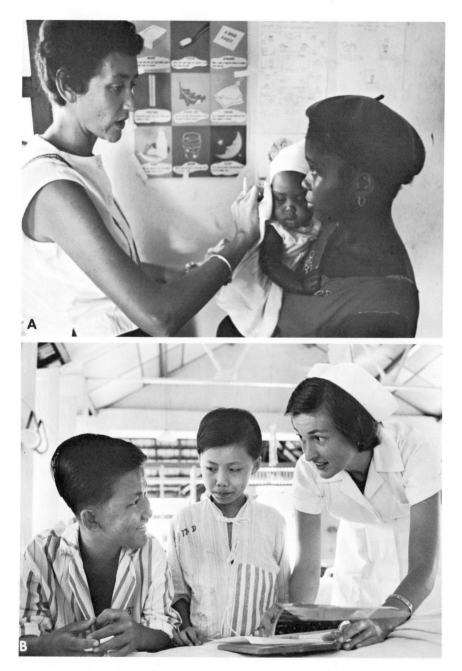

Figure 104. A, Peace Corps Nurse checks patient at well-baby clinic in St. Lucia, British West Indies. B, Peace Corps Nurse at Leprosarium in Malaya. (Courtesy of Paul Conklin, Peace Corps.)

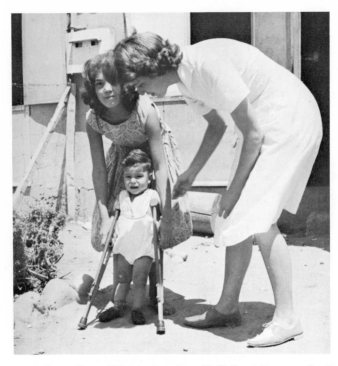

Figure 105.   Peace Corps Volunteer works with Polio victim near Santiago, Chile. (Photo: UNESCO-Gillette in The Americas, October, 1963.)

been well received. Comprehensive immunization projects have been initiated on board and carried on shore.

The People-to-People Health Foundation, 1016–20th St., N.W., Washington, D.C. 20036, which sponsors Project Hope, is providing an emissary of goodwill and peace to peoples of less privileged lands from the people of the United States. American nurses have been eager to join and about thirty serve yearly at a minimum salary.

The U. S. Civil Service Commission, whose staff is responsible for providing candidates for all types of federal civil service positions, evaluates credentials and conducts competitive examinations. Notices of the time and location of such examinations are posted in the larger local post offices, while those for nurses are published also in nursing journals. Information in regard to them can be obtained directly from the headquarters in Washington. Some examinations consist of filling out a detailed application for federal employment which is rated according to preparation and experience.

A nursing consultant on the staff of the Civil Service Commission carries on activities related to procuring nurses for the Nursing Section of the Children's Bureau, the U. S. Public Health Service, government hospitals in Alaska and two federal hospitals for civilians in Washington, D. C. These are St. Elizabeth's Hospital, a psychiatric institution, and Freedman's Hospital. The military establishments also employ a few Civil Service appointees to augment their nursing personnel.

CANADIAN GOVERNMENT SERVICES

All Canadian Federal Nursing Services are placed within three large departments of the government, the *Department of National Defense,* the *Department of Veterans Affairs,* and the *Department of National Health and Welfare.* In each department nurses find opportunities not only for interesting and rewarding experience but also for contributing to the general welfare and security of their country. Personnel policies include generous vactions and sick leaves, provision for medical and hospital benefits, and plans for retirement.

DEPARTMENT OF NATIONAL DEFENSE

Included within the Department of National Defense are the *Royal Canadian Navy,* the *Royal Canadian Army,* and the *Royal Canadian Air Force,* appointments to the nursing services of which are available to registered nurses who are Canadian citizens or British subjects residing in Canada. Other qualifications vary somewhat with the service although one or two years of nursing experience beyond completion of the basic nursing course is strongly recommended by all.

With granting of relative military rank in 1904, Canada became the first country of the world to give such recognition to its nurses. Commissions range from Second Lieutenant to Major. While serving the interests of their country Army nurses with special qualifications have opportunity for taking postgraduate courses in operating room technique, public health nursing, supervision, teaching, and administration.

DEPARTMENT OF VETERANS AFFAIRS

The Department of Veterans Affairs has a Canada-wide medical service for care of veterans who are eligible under the Veterans Treatment Regulations. In addition, the Department provides services to others at the request and expense of other federal departments, other governments, and certain corporate bodies such as workmen's compensation boards.

Registered nurses are employed under the Civil Service Commission and subject to its regulations. Following qualification, appointments are made by promotion or open competitition to a D.V.A hospital of one's choice, whenever feasible. Various levels of positions are available, including those of director, assistant director, supervisor, head nurse, and staff nurse.

Each year a specified number of registered nurses are granted the privilege of taking leaves of absence on half-pay in order to attend university courses in teaching and supervision or nursing administration.

DEPARTMENT OF NATIONAL HEALTH AND WELFARE

Indian and Northern Health Services. The Indian and Northern Health Services, largest of the Department's operating services, provides care for Indians and Eskimos and offers a rich and varied career to its nurses. In eighteen hospitals, located throughout the country from James Bay to the Pacific Ocean, nurses care for patients of Indian and Eskimo origin, many of whom are victims of tuberculosis in spite of an intensive tuberculosis control program which has been carried on for some time. Also, in numerous public health agencies stretching across Canada from the east to the west and spreading into the northern reaches of the Yukon and Northwest Territories, nurses engage in work that is primarily public health nursing. Such assignments may be to an *Out-Post Nursing Station,* a *Health Center,* a *Public Health Field Post,* a *Clinic,* or to a part-time position as *Nurse-Dispenser.*

Nursing Consultant Services. Nursing Consultants are employed by the Health Branch of the Department of National Health and Welfare in the divisions of Occupational Health, Child and Maternal Health, Mental Health, Emergency Health, and Health Insurance. They have special preparation for their work and promote education through institutes and the preparation of health education material.

Quarantine, Immigration Medical, and Sick Mariners Services. These services provide medical and nursing care primarily for immigrants and mariners. Nurses are stationed at certain sea and air ports of entry into Canada where they assist in the screening of persons entering the country. Those employed in hospitals help with medical inspection of immigrants and give first aid and nursing care to passengers and detained persons in need of them.

The Quarantine Service is responsible also for care of patients with leprosy, for whom there are two hospitals in Canada, one located at Tracadie, New Brunswick, in a wing of the Hôtel-Dieu de St. Joseph Hospital, the other at Bentinck Island, British Columbia, where patients live in separate cottages under the supervision of a graduate nurse.

Civil Service Health Division. This Division functions as an industrial or occupational health service for civil servants in the Ottawa area and employs nurses with preparation and experience in public health nursing. Activities are carried on at a *medical center* and various *health units* located throughout the city. A continuing staff education program has been developed which includes orientation for new employees and inservice training for nursing counselors. Also, facilities for field work experience are offered to students of public health nursing and of medicine in several universities.

VICTORIAN ORDER OF NURSES FOR CANADA

In 1897 Queen Victoria (1819–1901) appropriated a considerable sum of money for the establishment of a Foundation to provide nursing services for the sick and needy throughout the British Empire. This was to be in commemoration of her Diamond Jubilee celebrating the sixtieth year of her reign (1837–1901). In the same year the Victorian Order of Nurses for Canada was founded and given a Royal Charter, with a national headquarters in Ottawa and provincial and local branches scattered throughout the nation. Each branch plans its own program but is under supervision of the national office which sets up standards and policies. The primary purpose is to provide visiting nursing services for patients in their own homes, and no one is to be refused because of inability to pay.

In addition to giving home nursing care, nurses in many of the branches teach classes for expectant parents, conduct school health programs, assist with child health conferences and immunization clinics, and provide part-time health services for small industries. Increasing emphasis is being placed upon care of patients with chronic illnesses. All VON applicants are required to be registered graduate nurses and, in most cases, to have additional preparation in public health nursing. Appointments are approved by the national office. Opportunity for professional growth is provided through staff education programs

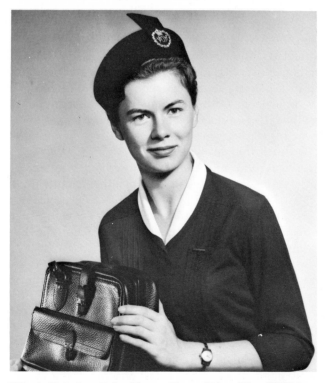

Figure 106. A Victorian Order Nurse. (From folder, "Can YOU have a Victorian Order Nurse?" Victorian Order of Nurses for Canada, 5 Blackburn Avenue, Ottawa 2, Ontario, Canada.)

and a generous policy of awarding scholarships for advanced study. In 1957 the Victorian Order of Nurses for Canada celebrated its own Diamond Jubilee.

U. S. EXCHANGE VISITOR PROGRAM

Through the International Educational Exchange Service, administered by the U. S. Department of State, a plan was initiated in 1948 to provide for an exchange of nationals between the United States and other countries for purposes of study, teaching, lecturing, or research. The purpose is to develop a mutual person-to-person understanding of the way of life, culture, and aspirations of all peoples, which can be the only true basis for harmonious living and world peace.

The American Nurses' Association has been made a sponsor of the Exchange Visitor Program and so is able to arrange for the exchange of nurses between the United States and other countries. Positions available are primarily in hospital staff nursing although some openings in public health nursing may be found. Arrangements can be made also for periods of study or observation in hospitals and health agencies.

The ANA International Unit, in cooperation with the International Council of Nurses, will provide full information in regard to employment possibilities in foreign countries. An official ICN application form, procured through the ANA Professional Counseling and Placement Service, is to be completed, following which the ANA carries on whatever correspondence is necessary. Exchange nurses are required to have current membership in a national nursing organization affiliated with the ICN, to have some knowledge of the language of the foreign country involved and to have had two or more years of nursing experience. They are responsible for all of their own expenses but receive an allowance from the agency in which they are placed.

Many colleges and universities throughout the world now have enrolled large numbers of students from other countries. During the winter of 1963–1964 nearly 75,000 students, representing more than 150 countries, attended institutions of higher learning in the United States. While the majority of students came from the Far East, an ever increasing number come from Africa.

As the world in which we live continues to shrink to ever smaller and smaller proportions bringing peoples of all ethnic cultures, religions, and degrees of social progress into close contact for the first time in history, there comes a vital necessity for willingness to discard outworn habits of thought and action. During this critical period of social adjustment, nurses everywhere with their humanitarian attitudes and social and psychological insight are in a position to be of inestimable value in the struggle to guide the trend of human affairs toward an era of peaceful co-existence.

MORAL AND LEGAL RESPONSIBILITIES OF NURSES

In the writings of Sir William Osler (1849–1919), distinguished physician of the modern era, is to be found the statement that "turning over to a stranger the care of a life precious beyond all computation may be one of the greatest earthly trials." Dr. Osler, the son of a minister and himself deeply religious, taught medical science in several of the great universities of England, Canada, and the United States, but he is best remembered by medical students for his emphasis on the necessity for thoughtful observation at the bedside and for the ethical precepts with which he filled their minds.

Today, no less than when Dr. Osler was teaching medical ethics, it is essential for a person to have full confidence in the doctor and hospital staff when entrusting himself or a loved one to their care. The nurse, as representative of both, is in a position to create a sense of security through the degree of judgment and kindly interest displayed at the bedside. It has been fully demonstrated, too, that desirable nurse-patient relationships contribute markedly to the patient's recovery.

To aid in protecting the patient, laws have been enacted to which he may resort in an emergency, laws with which the capable, ethical nurse may never become involved but with which every nurse should be thoroughly familiar. The ever mounting number of litigations involving the practice of medicine and nursing attest to their significance. It is not uncommon for hospitals, doctors, and nurses to be made defendants in lawsuits arising from alleged negligence in the care of patients. Uncertainty as to what constitutes nursing practice has complicated cases and made it difficult for courts to reach decisions.

The ANA, through its sections, has done a great deal to clarify the meaning of nursing practice by determining the functions of the various occupational groups and drafting legal definitions of professional and practical nursing which it recommends for inclusion in state nursing practice acts as they are amended.

Professional Liability Insurance.   Recognizing the need for protection against lawsuits, the ANA sponsors a Professional Liability Insurance Plan for its members, and similar plans are sponsored by some of the constituent associations. Further study is being made of areas in which protection is needed, one of which is the vulnerability of nurses when carrying out unwritten orders of physicians. A law requiring all orders to be written might be the eventual solution to this problem. Another area upon which much attention has been focused is whether nurses have the legal right to administer intravenous therapy. In some states laws relating to nursing have been extended to cover this and other new responsibilities which nurses are assuming.

The American Nurses' Association emphasizes the fact that all nurses need enlightenment on the legal aspects of their work and helps to meet this need by publishing in its journal reports of recent legal developments involving the field of nursing. Nursing schools are placing increasing emphasis on instruction in this subject and some universities are including law courses in their curricula for graduate nurses. For their own protection all senior students should review their textbooks on laws affecting nursing practice, only a few of which can be briefly touched upon here.

LAWS REGULATING NURSING PRACTICE

Of immediate concern to all who are about to graduate are state laws governing the practice of nursing. If the law of a state is *mandatory,* it will be illegal to practice for compensation within the state without first passing a state board examination and being licensed to practice. If the state law is *permissive,* it will be legal for the graduate to practice but not to affix the letters "R.N." to his or her signature or to claim in any way to be a registered, professional, or licensed nurse. In recent years the state nurses' associations and the ANA have been active in promoting mandatory legislation for professional nurses with corresponding mandatory or permissive legislation for practical nurses. In all states the annual or biennial renewal of licenses is required.

As a safeguard to society, and to nurses themselves, laws prescribing minimum standards for the accreditation of nursing schools whose graduates will be eligible to take state board examinations have long been in force in all states having such schools. However, requirements vary in regard to personal and educational qualifications and the length and content of the course. For state-accredited practical nursing schools, approved programs of one year in length are recommended by the National Association for Practical Nurse Education and Service (NAPNES). Upon graduation and passing a state board examination for practical nurses, the candidate becomes legally entitled to affix to a business signature the letters "L.P.N." or "L.V.N.," depending upon whether the term "licensed practical" or "licensed vocational" nurse is used in that state. For breach of ethical conduct, all types of licenses are revoked at times and this fact published in the nursing journals.

Interstate Licensure. The nurse who wishes to practice in a state other than the one in which a license was originally obtained will meet with the problem of *interstate licensure.* However, the development of national minimum standards for the accreditation of nursing schools, along with the use of a national licensing examination throughout the country, has simplified matters considerably.

Moreover, these same measures are steps in the direction of the long-hoped-for goal of national recognition. The State Board Test Pool for licensing examinations is now used by all of the states, although they continue to differ in regard to passing scores. At the same time, accreditation of nursing schools on a national basis by the NLN is well established. If, in time, other stumbling blocks in state requirements are overcome, a nurse who is licensed in one state will be eligible for licensing in any other state.

Before moving to another state to practice, either the professional or the practical nurse should obtain a license by writing to the Examining Board of that state, the address of which can be found in the Official Directory in January and August issues of the American Journal of Nursing. Such a license can usually be obtained without difficulty. On the other hand, it may be necessary to complete additional classwork or clinical experience and to take another state board examination. In some cases an application may be rejected entirely.

CONTRACTS OF EMPLOYMENT

Any type of contract can be a source of legal entanglement. All employed persons have contracts for their services and should know their nature and significance. A *contract of employment* is an agreement between two parties which outlines conditions of work and describes the relationships and responsibilities of employer and employee. Such agreements can be either *express* or *implied,* but only one kind can exist in any given situation. Terms of an express contract are clearly defined either orally or in writing. Nurses employed in doctors' offices and by hospitals and other agencies usually have this kind. Though the written contract is seldom required by law, it is safer, nevertheless, and may be an imposing document or merely written memoranda such as contained in letters.

In an implied contract the terms are inferred from certain known facts about a particular line of work. Nurses in private practice usually have this kind. Both express and implied contracts are morally and legally binding, and failure of either party to meet his or her obligations can result in a *breach of contract.* However, agreements with no definite time limit can be terminated without threat of liability.

In the past most contracts for nurses have been on an individual basis but there is now an increasing trend toward collective agreements which are drawn up by state nurses' associations with hospitals and other agencies employing nurses. In these instances, the state associations act as representatives for the nurses.

LEGAL STATUS OF EMPLOYED PERSONS

Every employed person has a *legal status* derived from his own contract of employment which is either that of *employee* or *independent contractor.* Differentiation between the two is important because status may become an issue in legal proceedings. The distinction, however, is not always clear, but of several factors used as criteria the most decisive relates to retention of control over the manner in which services are to be rendered. The one who performs services under the control of another has the status of an employee. Most nurses have this status. An exception is the nurse in private practice who usually is an independent contractor since his or her activities are not under the control of another person. Whether the status is that of employee or independent contractor, nurses are legally, as well as morally, responsible for the safety of their patients.

In certain cases, where the legal status is that of employee, the employer can be held liable as well as the employee. This is application of the doctrine of *respondeat superior* or "Let the master answer." However, in some states, which operate under the doctrine of *charitable immunity,* this ruling does not apply if the employer is a charitable institution but there is now a definite trend toward imposing either full or partial liability on them. In all instances, however, the employee also is held responsible, for every person is liable for the wrong he commits and there is no escaping this rule of law. In legal nomenclature, any individual can be held responsible for a *tort* or a *crime,* either of which constitutes a legal wrong.

TORTS VERSUS CRIMES

Torts. A civil wrong, or breach of a legal duty involving injury to an individual or his property, is known as a *tort.* Such conduct, whether intentional or unintentional, constitutes a wrong according to either statutory or common law. Legal action can be instituted by the injured party and is called a "civil proceeding." The defendent may be commanded to pay damages or, in some cases, the penalty may be imprisonment. The tort which is most likely to have bearing on nursing practice is negligence.

According to law, negligence is the unintentional commission or omission of an act which results in injury to a person or his property. *It is failure to exercise due care in pursuing a line of duty.* Negligence in professional performance, or failure to use the necessary knowledge, skills, and judgment in a particular situation, is called "malpractice." It is the most frequent cause of lawsuits against nurses and other professional persons. Supervisors, teachers, and administrators, as well as bedside nurses, can be held liable for negligence in the performance of their duties, and as more and more auxiliary personnel are employed, their legal implications are increased.

Other torts which may involve nurses but are less common causes of legal action are *assault, battery, slander, libel,* and *false imprisonment.* These differ from negligence in that, for conviction, proof must be given that the act was intentional. False imprisonment, when applied to the care of patients, might include unauthorized use of restraint, detention of a patient in a hospital for nonpayment of a bill or other reason, or otherwise interfering with his freedom.

Crimes. A criminal wrong or one committed against the safety, security, health, or other type of welfare of the public is known as a *crime*. It is a violation of a statutory law. Legal action is initiated by the state and called a "criminal proceeding." The defendant may be fined, imprisoned, or both, and all fines paid by him belong to the state. A wrong can be both a tort and a crime, in which case both civil and criminal action may be taken.

Crimes which come within the scope of nursing practice include violation of federal narcotic laws, state narcotic laws, laws dealing with abortion, and medical and nursing practice acts. Presenting the greatest problem at this time is violation of medical practice acts. Points at issue center primarily around the nurse's proper role in the performance of certain techniques that once came within the province of the physician. However, there is growing recognition of the fact that nursing practice now includes many such responsibilities. Evidence of this is to be found in recent medical and nursing practice acts and in judicial decisions.

A trend has developed, too, for state medical, nursing, and hospital associations to issue joint statements concerning certain controversial nursing functions in order to establish standards of nursing practice. While such policy statements are not legally binding, they carry weight in court. In all cases of legal action involving alleged negligence in the care of patients, the ANA Statements of Nursing Functions, Standards, and Qualifications for Practice can be expected to play an important part. Medical records always provide significant evidence in court, and a complete and accurately kept patient's chart, with no erasures, can become an important part of legal proceedings.

ECONOMIC SECURITY FOR NURSES

ANA Economic Security Program. Significant factors leading to the development of an Economic Security Unit of the ANA in 1946 were a rapidly rising cost of living, a critical shortage of nurses, and a need for higher salaries and improved working conditions if adequate standards of nursing service were to be maintained. On the basis of data provided by the Socio-Economic Study of 1946, and with the help of experts, an ANA Economic Security Program was set up to provide a plan for improvement that could be adopted and carried out by the state associations.

Since that time nurses have become more articulate in formulating principles and practices for the Economic Security Program which, in turn, has been strengthened and expanded. In addition, a *Technical Advisory Group,* composed of experts in the fields of economics, law, industrial relations, and education, provides assistance to an ANA Committee on Economic and General Welfare.

State Economic Security Programs.   One by one the state nurses associations were stimulated into action as various occupational groups developed their own programs under the guidance of a National Committee and a staff of consultants. Minimum employment standards were set up by the state sections for the specialty groups covering salaries, hours of work, paid vacations and holidays, sick leave and health programs, social and health insurance, retirement plans, nondiscrimination against minority groups, and other pressing subjects. Contracts then were drawn up between state nurses associations and employers, which brought about improved personnel policies with a corresponding improvement in nursing service and greater stability in nursing staffs.

The use of collective bargaining for securing desired goals, long a controversial issue, even though it received an approval vote by the membership at an ANA Convention, is gaining momentum as nurses employ it more readily to promote their economic welfare. However, major responsibility for operation of an economic security program rests with the state nurses associations, 49 of which have adopted such a measure.

Group Health Insurance Plans.   The introduction of group health insurance plans has been an important phase of economic progress for nurses. Sometimes these are offered through employers and included in collective bargaining agreements; more frequently they are available through the state or, occasionally, the district association. The type of coverage varies but, in general, includes medical and hospital benefits for accident or sickness, hospitalization, and medical and surgical payments, as well as life insurance, disability income, and retirement plans.

Professional Liability Insurance.   Group insurance plans for professional liability, endorsed by the American Nurses' Association, and similar insurance endorsed by the state associations are designed to cover the cost of legal counsel as well as any claims for damage that may arise from a lawsuit. Information is available to ANA members through the ANA Economic Security Unit, 10 Columbus Circle, New York, N. Y. 10019.

Social Security Protection.   The ANA has further helped to promote the economic welfare of nurses by supporting labor legislation and amendments to the Federal Social Security Act which are favorable to nurses. Nurses in private practice and those employed by nonprofit hospitals were not included in the provisions of this Act until 1950. Covered also for the first time were local and state government employees. In 1954 the Act was extended to include citizens employed outside the United States. The 1961 amendment extended the disability insurance and provided, on an optional basis, a retirement age of sixty-two for men as well as for women.

Life Insurance and Retirement Income.   Insurance policies offered by reputable life insurance companies are considered to be an excellent form of economic security. Various policy forms are suited to particular needs, two of which are straight life insurance and retirement income. *Straight life insurance* is the least expensive form of life insurance and is taken out to protect a beneficiary. However, it usually acquires a cash surrender value after a specified number of years. *Retirement income insurance* involves larger payments but has a greater cash value at maturity. This may be accepted as a single sum or in the form of an annuity to provide a monthly income for life.

U. S. Savings Bonds. Several types of U. S. Savings Bonds are available, some of which pay interest semiannually while others accumulate interest to be paid at maturity. They provide a sound form of systematic savings for economic security for the holder. They also provide necessary funds for the national government.

EDUCATIONAL FUNDS FOR NURSES

The qualified registered nurse of today who is seeking advanced preparation will find available an increasing number of sources of financial assistance. Competition for them is keen and the demand still exceeds the supply but each year finds new sources added to the list. Nursing organizations, government agencies, various foundations, colleges and universities, business organizations, civic groups, and many individuals are aware of the need and gradually assuming a share of responsibility for raising the level of human welfare through the medium of good nursing.

Discrimination is used in selection of candidates for awards of educational funds, with preference given to those who can be expected to make lasting contributions to nursing and society. A baccalaureate degree is required of those who wish to undertake what is designated by universities as "graduate study." Those who wish to make application for a fund for either undergraduate or graduate study are advised to consult the latest June issue of *Nursing Outlook* for selection of a college or university that has been approved for this purpose by the National League for Nursing. The Dean of the Department of Nursing of the institution of one's choice should then be contacted directly for information as to the courses offered, entrance requirements, and educational funds that may be available for nurses.

The NLN Committee on Careers in Nursing publishes a leaflet, entitled *Scholarships, Fellowships, Educational Grants, and Loans for Registered Nurses*, which contains information concerning a variety of sources of aid offered on a regional and national basis. The national nursing journals also publish articles and news items on educational funds available to men and women nurses. Some of the chief sources of such funds are described here, but there are others and new ones are being added from time to time, the majority of which are free from income tax obligations. Further information can be obtained from the nearest ANA Professional Counseling and Placement Service or the NLN Committee on Careers in Nursing.

NURSES' EDUCATIONAL FUNDS, INC.

Nurses' Educational Funds, Inc. was established as an independent corporation to gather together and administer a number of scholarships, fellowships, and loan funds for men and women nurses that had come into existence over a period of years. These include the *Isabel Hampton Robb Memorial Fund,* established in 1915; the *Isabel McIsaac Loan Fund;* the *Nurses' Scholarship and Fellowship Fund* initiated in 1952 by the alumni association of Teachers College, Columbia University; the *Shirley C. Titus Fellowship Fund* honoring the retiring executive secretary of the California Nurses' Association; the *Dr. Clara D. Hardin Scholarships* founded in 1964 by the American Journal of Nursing Company as a tribute to the late executive director of the American Nurses' Association.

The *Laura D. Smith Fund* was added to the list of available educational funds for nurses in 1962 by the National Student Nurses' Association as a memorial to the late senior editor of the American Journal of Nursing, who gave considerable encouragement and support to their organization. Preference in this instance is given to previously active NSNA members.

New funds are being added from time to time and include bequests, memorials, and gifts from individuals and professional and business organizations. Full information and application forms in regard to any of the funds may be obtained by writing to Nurses' Educational Funds, Inc., 10 Columbus Circle, New York, New York 10019.

USPHS TRAINEESHIP AWARDS

To ensure an adequate and continuous supply of specialists in all fields of nursing, the U. S. Public Health Service has initiated a *Professional Nurse Traineeship Program,* whereby teaching grants are made to approved educational institutions which, in turn, make traineeship awards to qualified candidates. To be eligible for such an award, a registered nurse must be a citizen of the United States, or have made declaration of intent to become one, and be able to meet the entrance requirements of the institution chosen for study.

Two types of awards are available: (a) Traineeships for Full Time Academic Study and (b) Traineeships for Study in Short Term Intensive Training Courses, and from their beginning in 1956 until the end of 1964 more than 24,000 nurses had taken advantage of the opportunities offered, with 10,000 pursuing full time academic study and about 14,000 taking short term intensive training courses in administration, supervision, and teaching.[2] The purpose is to *improve the quality of patient*

---

[2]California Nurses Association Bulletin, Sept. 1964, p. 4.

care by increasing the number of graduate nurses with special preparation for positions in public health nursing, psychiatric-mental health nursing, nursing research, and rehabilitation. In 1964 a five year extension of the Professional Nurse Traineeship Program was made, with an expansion to include preparation of nursing specialists in the clinical fields.

PUBLIC HEALTH NURSING TRAINEESHIPS are available for registered men and women nurses who wish to prepare for beginning positions in public health nursing through full-time enrollment in public health and related courses. Applicants who wish to prepare for a public health nursing career are directed to write to an institution having a traineeship grant in regard to entrance requirements and availability of traineeships.

PSYCHIATRIC-MENTAL HEALTH TRAINEESHIPS are awarded to undergraduate and graduate students of collegiate nursing programs who wish to prepare for responsible positions in the field of psychiatric-mental health nursing in nationally accredited nursing programs. Similar awards are made to physicians for study of psychiatry and to social workers for psychiatric social work. Upon completion of their course, nurses are prepared for leadership positions in a wide variety of positions in the psychiatric-mental health field. Information in regard to these traineeships and a list of institutions offering approved courses may be obtained from the Training Branch, National Institute of Mental Health, Bethesda, Maryland 21214.

NURSING RESEARCH TRAINEESHIP AWARDS. Predoctoral and postdoctoral fellowships are offered to nurses who wish to prepare for research in nursing or a related health field. It may be education in a university or special training in the skills and techniques of research in a research center. Qualified nurse researchers are in demand for independent research, for collaboration in multidisciplinary research, and to guide and teach research in nursing or in the biological and social sciences contributing to the health fields. Interested nurses, with a bachelor's degree, are advised to write to the Chief, Research Grants and Fellowships Branch, Division of Nursing, U. S. Public Health Service, Washington, D. C. 20201, for full information.

REHABILITATION TRAINEESHIP AWARDS. In an effort to overcome an acute shortage of qualified personnel in the rehabilitation field, traineeships are provided for the education of occupational therapists, speech and hearing specialists, vocational counselors, social workers, physicians, nurses, and others interested in activities requiring special knowledge of rehabilitation techniques. Traineeships available to nurses are for study at the master's or post-master's level in preparation for rehabilitation nursing, the clinical specialties, teaching, administration, or consultation. Awards are made also for short-term courses in special aspects of rehabilitation.

The long range objective is to prepare sufficient numbers of persons with understanding and skill to make it possible for rehabilitation to become an integral part of all health care. A list of participating

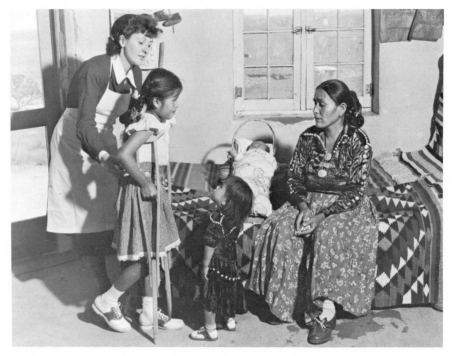

Figure 107. Rehabilitation on an Indian Reservation. (U.S. Public Health Service Photo.)

schools may be obtained from the Office of Vocational Rehabilitation, Department of Health, Education, and Welfare, Washington, D. C. 20201.

U. S. CHILDREN'S BUREAU AWARDS

Traineeships to aid in preparation of nurses for consultation and teaching in maternal and child health positions are provided by the U. S. Children's Bureau, Department of Health, Education, and Welfare. At the present time they are available through courses provided by Boston University; Teachers College, Columbia University; and the University of California School of Nursing, San Francisco Medical Center. Also several schools of public health across the country prepare qualified nurses for the care of mothers and children in public health programs.

Children's Bureau awards are available also for short programs in the care of premature infants at the Institute in Premature Care, New York Hospital, 525 East 68th Street, New York, New York 10019, and at the School of Nursing, University of Colorado, Boulder, Colorado.

OTHER FUNDS FOR NURSES

National Fund for Graduate Nursing Education. The National Fund for Graduate Nursing Education is a nonprofit organization originally financed by the Rockefeller Brothers Fund but since its establishment in 1960 the list of contributors has grown and now includes many leading industrial concerns of the country. In 1964 a generous grant was received from the American Journal of Nursing Company. The purpose is to assure optimum patient care in our hospitals through improvement of facilities and faculties of graduate nursing schools. The address from which further information can be obtained is 90 Park Ave., New York, New York 10016.

Mary M. Roberts Fellowship in Journalism. The Mary M. Roberts Fellowship in Journalism was established in 1950 by the American Journal of Nursing Company to enable promising candidates to acquire preparation in the field of writing. Nurses with such preparation are needed as editors of nursing journals and authors of all kinds of nursing literature. A generous grant is made annually for a year of study in an approved school of journalism. Each applicant is required to submit an original unpublished manuscript, in any literary form except a play or television script, which has been prepared especially to accompany an application.

Bixler Scholarship. The Bixler Scholarship was initiated in 1963 as a memorial to the late *Dr. Genevieve K. Bixler,* staff member-consultant of the *Southern Regional Education Board* (SREB) and a director of the *Southern Regional Project in Graduate Education and Research in Nursing.* This project brought about establishment of the first six graduate schools of nursing in the south, namely those of the University of Alabama, Emory University, University of Maryland, University of North Carolina, University of Texas, and Vanderbilt University.

Eligibility for the Bixler Scholarship is limited to outstanding graduates and faculty members of these schools. It is awarded annually by each school, in rotation, to help finance study at the post master's level. The purpose is to promote "her great efforts in the cause of improved collegiate and graduate education for nurses in the South and the development of research in nursing."[3]

WHO FELLOWSHIPS FOR FOREIGN STUDY

Each World Health Assembly has emphasized the necessity for international exchange of health knowledge and collaboration in training health personnel. WHO fellowships are provided for this purpose and are to be awarded to individuals who can be expected to contribute to the objectives of their own governments and the World Health Organization.

WHO fellowships are usually awarded to persons with two or more years' experience in the field selected and who can speak, read, and write the language of the foreign country chosen for study. During the course close contact is maintained between the fellow and the nearest WHO Regional Office, and immediately after its completion all par-

---

[3]SREB folder, "The Bixler Scholarship in Nursing."

ticipating persons are required to put their services at the disposal of their own national governments for a stipulated period of time.

In the United States, WHO travel fellowships are awarded for periods of two to four months to persons who are engaged in full time public health or educational work. Consideration is given not only to the ability of the applicant but also to the precise benefits which another country can be expected to derive from his or her association with their health services.

Participants with broadened viewpoints are in a position to spread awareness of the fact that each country is part of a total system of world relationships, the welfare of the whole depending upon the understanding and cooperation of each individual comprising it. For full information write to Secretary, WHO Fellowship Selection Committee, Department of Health, Education, and Welfare, U. S. Public Health Service, Washington, D. C. 20201.

FULBRIGHT SCHOLARSHIPS

Several Acts of Congress have made funds available for the Educational Exchange Program with other countries, one of which, the Fulbright-Hays Act, includes nurses among its beneficiaries. Under this Act, scholarships are granted to United States citizens with college degrees who, on the basis of their background and experience, are judged most competent to make substantial contributions to their special fields.

Since the major purpose is to increase mutual understanding between people of the United States and those of other nations, selected scholars are expected to be good representatives of their country and its form of higher education. Further information and application forms can be obtained from the Fulbright Program Advisor on the campus of a university. Scholarships are awarded through the Institute of International Education, 809 United Nations Plaza, New York, New York 10017.

Suggestions for Study

1. Name several major changes in the practice of medicine and nursing that have taken place in recent years. Cite problems in nursing practice that are due to a scarcity of graduate nurses.
2. Which of the two broad fields of nursing are you preparing to enter? What type of nursing within this field is most interesting to you? Will it require special preparation?
3. What do you consider to be the advantages and disadvantages of work with the military services? What nonmilitary federal services employ nurses?
4. It is suggested that a student write to the nearest recruiting office

of the Army Nurse Corps, listed in the AJN Directory, for information concerning the *Army Student Nurse Program;* that another write to a corresponding address for similar information relating to the *Navy Nurse Corps Candidate Program;* and a third write to the U. S. Public Health Service for information about the *Commissioned Officer Student Training and Extern Program* (COSTEP). How many seniors in your school are taking advantage of these opportunities?

5. It is suggested that a member of the class write to the ANA for personal copies of the ANA Code for Professional Nurses, available at nominal cost, and that another student write to the ICN for copies of the International Code of Nursing Ethics. Do you think that any section of either Code should be revised or deleted, or that another section should be added?

6. Enumerate reasons for seniors to review their text and reference material on the subject of legal and moral responsibilities of nurses. What questions of your own have grown out of your readings on this subject? What is the overall purpose of all laws with which the nurse may come in contact?

7. Explain the difference between mandatory and permissive licensure for nursing practice. What progress is being made toward securing mandatory licensure for professional nursing practice? Practical nursing?

8. Why is the subject of interstate licensure of considerable importance to many nurses? What are the specific responsibilities of the Board of Nursing in your state? What are the principle reasons for suspending or revoking a nurse's license?

9. In what ways can you assist practical nurses to broaden their understanding of ethical practices in nursing?

10. After making a study of the Nurse Practice Act of your state, give its definition of the practice of nursing.

11. From reference reading determine the meaning of the following terms: tort. crime. rule of respondeat superior. charitable immunity. principle of stare decisis. doctrine of res ipsa loquitur.

12. Describe specific nursing situations, either real or imaginary, to illustrate the following: negligence, libel, slander, assault and battery.

13. In what ways do the ANA and the State Nurses' Associations promote economic security for nurses? How can each nurse assist the associations in these and all other activities?

14. List four or more policy benefits provided by the ANA Registered Nurses' Professional Liability Insurance Policy.

15. It is recommended that a representative from a large life insurance company explain the various forms of life insurance policies, and that a member of the class obtain information from a bank about U. S. Savings Bonds.

16. Compare the various provisions for economic security for nurses which exist in the health agencies of your community or in the community in which you expect to reside after graduation.

17. It is suggested that students explore various sources of educational funds available for nurses, and then state which ones seem most attractive for their particular purpose.

18. Name a number of outstanding contributions of men nurses from the early Christian era, through the Middle Ages and the Renaissance, to modern times. From the current issue of *Facts About Nursing* determine the percent of professional men nurses employed in the various fields of nursing today.

19. Make a list of the types of positions in which men nurses are employed in your home community or the community in which your school is located.

20. It is suggested that a group of students set up a box of up-to-date folders and pamphlets on nursing subjects of interest to all seniors, which can be kept up-to-date by future classes.

References

Brown, Esther Lucile: Newer Dimensions of Patient Care. Part 3. Patients Are People. New York, Russell Sage Foundation, 1964.

Bullough and Bullough: The Emergence of Modern Nursing. New York, The Macmillan Co., 1964.

Creighton, Helen: Law Every Nurse Should Know. Philadelphia, W. B. Saunders Co., 1957.

Dietz, Lena Dixon: History and Modern Nursing. Philadelphia, F. A. Davis Co., 1963.

Griffin and Griffin: Jensen's History and Trends of Professional Nursing. St. Louis, The C. V. Mosby Co., 1965.

Hayes and Gazaway: Human Relations in Nursing. Philadelphia, W. B. Saunders Co., 1964.

Lambertsen, Eleanor C.: Education for Nursing Leadership. Philadelphia, J. B. Lippincott Co., 1958.

Lesnik and Anderson: Nursing Practice and the Law. Philadelphia, J. B. Lippincott Co., 1962.

Pelley, Thelma: Nursing–Its History, Trends, Philosophy, Ethics and Ethos. Philadelphia, W. B. Saunders Co., 1964.

Roberts, Mary M.: American Nursing: History and Interpretation. New York, The Macmillan Co., 1954.

Rogers, Martha E.: Reveille in Nursing. Philadelphia, F. A. Davis Co., 1964.

Simmons and Henderson: Nursing Research–A Survey and Assessment. New York, The Macmillan Co., 1964.

U. S. Dept. of Health, Education, and Welfare. Washington, D. C. Nurses for Leadership. (The Professional Nurse Traineeship Program. Report of the 1963 Evaluation Conference.) Public Health Service Publication No. 1098, 1963.

AMERICAN JOURNAL OF NURSING

"The ANA Economic Security Program – What It Is and Why" – Schutt. April, 1958, p. 520

"The Changing Role of the Professional Nurse in the Hospital" – Whitaker. Feb., 1962, p. 65

"The Law and the Nurse" – Hershey. A series beginning Feb., 1962, p. 75

"The Nature of Nursing" – Henderson. Aug., 1964, p. 62

NURSING OUTLOOK

"The Head Nurse's Changing Role" — Barrett. Nov., 1963, p. 800

"Federal Legislation: Its Impact on NLN's Accrediting Program" — Boyle. March, 1965, p. 34

NURSING RESEARCH

"Nursing Research Programs of the Public Health Service" — Vreeland. Spring, 1964, p. 148

Chapter 16

NURSING IN MANY LANDS

Nurses who gain personal knowledge of the history and geography of the countries of those with whom they come in contact will be enabled to make a substantial contribution toward improved human relationships. In the daily performance of their duties, whether at home or abroad, all nurses are in a position to exert a tremendous influence toward breaking down barriers of suspicion and ill will, barriers that have long obstructed human progress and world peace. They rank in the vanguard of those social forces struggling for international understanding and an international conscience as well. It is not chance that has placed both medicine and nursing in this role but rather the very core of their philosophy, deeply rooted as it is in principles of brotherly love, service, and implementation of the Golden Rule.

LATIN AMERICA

Latin America comprises Mexico, Central America, South America, Cuba, the Dominican Republic, and other parts of the West Indies. Puerto Rico, a territory of the United States, is also inhabited by races of Latin origin. Explorers from Spain and Portugal traveling in a southerly direction over routes and trails blazed by Christopher Columbus and Hernando Cortez were the original European settlers. Many descendants of these early conquistadors intermarried with Indian aborigines to produce a mixture of cultures, while other lines have remained of direct Spanish, Portuguese, or Indian descent. The Spanish language and Spanish customs and the Catholic faith predominate over this area, but Portuguese is the language of Brazil.

Lying largely in the Torrid Zone, the coastal regions and lowlands of the interior of many Latin American countries are areas of tropical heat while more temperate climates are found on elevated plateaus. In the extreme south, as in South Africa and Australia, the summer season falls in the months of November, December, and January. Tropical vegetation abounds, many products of which, especially coffee and bananas, are exported in great quantities and find their way to our tables.

Educational institutions, including modern universities, are provided for the cities but a high percentage of illiteracy, and the usual poverty and illness associated with it, is common in rural districts. The average citizen had little awareness of possibilities for disease prevention through application of modern principles of sanitation. As might be expected, illness is a major problem while medicine and nursing are relatively new professions which have not penetrated the masses.

Pan American Union. As early as 1890 the Republics of Central and South America and the United States united their interests in the *Pan American Union,* now the oldest international organization in the world, the original purposes of which were mutual protection from foreign invasion and fostering trade relationships. Pan American Conferences were held at intervals and, in time, new responsibilities assumed, one of which was establishment of the *Pan American Health Organization* (PAHO) in 1902 as the first health organization on an international basis. Headquarters of the Pan American Union are in a beautiful marble, Spanish style building in Washington, D. C., situated in the midst of landscaped gardens with plants and decorative details typical of Latin America.

Organization of American States. At the Pan American Conference held in Bogotá, Colombia, in 1948, the inter-American System was reorganized and a charter for an *Organization of American States* (OAS), which would function as a regional agency of the United Nations, was signed by twenty Latin American nations and the United States. The Pan American Union was made the secretariat or governing body to carry out OAS policies which include a system for pacific settlement of international disputes, research programs covering agriculture and other fields of economic activity, technical assistance services, and promotion of social and cultural relationships among all nations of the Americas. In cooperating with the United Nations, the OAS seeks to avoid any overlapping of functions.

When plans were made in 1949 to open a WHO Regional Office for the Americas, the functions of such an office were combined with those of the Pan American Health Organization since that agency was already experienced in the field of international health. Through PAHO headquarters, known as the *Pan American Sanitary Bureau* (PASB), the World Health Organization provides assistance to Latin American countries in developing their own local and national health services and carrying on campaigns against infectious disease. Inter-American seminars and workshops are conducted and WHO fellowships are awarded to native candidates who can be expected to contribute to social welfare through the promotion of health and the eradication of disease.

MEXICO

Colorful Mexico, adjoining the southern border of the United States, is possessed of such lavish stores of gold, silver, and petroleum, and such magnificent scenery as to be known as one of the richest and most beautiful of all nations. In the vicinity of Mexico City, ancient capital of the Aztec Empire and modern capital of Mexico, are the Pyramid of the Sun and the Pyramid of the Moon, ingeniously constructed centuries ago by Aztec Indians in the location where occurred, according to legend, the creation of these luminous bodies so universally worshiped by primitive peoples. Immediately surrounding Mexico City is the Federal District, just as the District of Columbia surrounds Washington, capital city of the United States. The nation is a republic composed of twenty-nine states and two territories in addition to the Federal District. A president is elected every six years and is permitted to serve but one term.

The story of the defeat of Montezuma, last of the Aztec rulers, by Hernando Cortez, invader and conqueror from Spain, is well known. Mexican tribes had attained so high a degree of civilization before arrival of the Spanish as to make them the most cultured of American races. This circumstance inevitably led to perpetuation of their culture which was modified but not eradicated by that of Spain. Then, too, the Indians survived as a race to form about one third of the present-day population of Mexico.

Notwithstanding the early attainment of a high degree of civilization, Aztecs, Toltecs, Mayas, and Incas of Mexico were guilty of a common barbaric practice in offering human sacrifices to their seemingly blood-thirsty gods. Archeologists are discovering and unearthing, one by one, beautiful temples and pyramids of an antiquity that may antedate the better known ones of Egypt, and that were once the scenes of human sacrifice. Sacrificial stones are being brought to light over which many a prisoner-of-war was stretched, as a priest held high a formidable knife before burying it deep into the chest of his victim. Removing the still quivering heart, he would display it to great throngs of worshipers who bowed down to the earth in awe and reverence.

While governor of Mexico, Cortez exerted a constructive influence in a number of directions. He was the founder of the Hospital of Jesus of Nazareth in 1524, first on the American continent, and today one of Mexico's most beautiful and modern. Built in a fashion resembling the homes of Mexican and Spanish people of means, it has rooms and porticos encircling two patios or open gardens, one of which contains a fountain. Like many homes, too, it is enclosed by a high wall.

Nursing in Mexico. For centuries nursing was carried on by Sisterhoods and Brotherhoods of the Catholic Church. However, after a political revolution, occurring about the middle of the last century, the number of churches and church officials decreased appreciably and, as might be expected, the practice of nursing soon became neglected as it had been in Europe during the Renaissance. Lay people of the "Sairey Gamp" type again flourished.

In 1911 guidance of nursing practice was taken over by the University of Mexico, and nursing education and midwifery were placed under the faculty of Medicine. Today classes are provided for student nurses who affiliate with two nearby general hospitals. Graduate courses in public health nursing, school nursing, and social work are also available.

Not only does the University of Mexico maintain high standards of

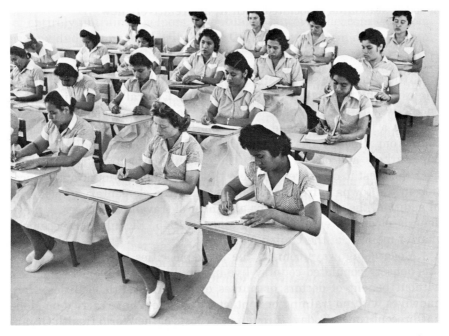

Figure 108. Auxiliary nurses trained in Mexico. Crisply uniformed student auxiliary nurses take lecture notes at Huamantla Training School in Tlaxcala, Mexico. During the course they have opportunity to practice what they learn.

Prevention of illness among mothers and children, improvement of community sanitation, and nutrition projects are among the main goals of a comprehensive training program set up by the Mexican government. Doctors, sanitary engineers, and nurses implement the well-planned public health campaigns mapped by health districts in every area of the country. The auxiliary nurses are, perhaps, the most important personnel in the rural health scene. The program is aided by the United Nations Children's Fund (UNICEF), which supplies training and medical equipment, and by the World Health Organization (WHO), which gives technical guidance. (UNICEF photo by Bernard Cole.)

the *Universidad Nacional del Litoral,* Rosario, Argentina, in 1940. Here entrance requirements are on a level with those for students of medicine, pharmacy, and dentistry, and the sciences are taught in the university.

World War II brought about closer contacts of peoples in many parts of the world than in previous history, with public recognition of need for assumption of responsibility for the general welfare. In the Western Hemisphere, the World Health Organization working with the Pan American Health Organization and other agencies, became active in a movement toward improvement of standards of living. Establishment of new hospitals, nursing schools, and health centers in Central and South America followed. Additional assistance in the form of nursing consultants and international nursing teams has been provided when requested.

Possibilities for improving the social welfare through the medium of modern health practices are beginning to be appreciated in many parts of Latin America but public awareness of the part played by sanitary measures in eradication of disease is still nonexistent in some areas. A WHO nursing consultant for the Lima Zone, covering Ecuador, Colombia, and Venezuela as well as Peru, reported in 1951 that uncovered water supplies used for drinking purposes also provided swimming facilities for pigs, ducks, and children. Pasteurization of milk was

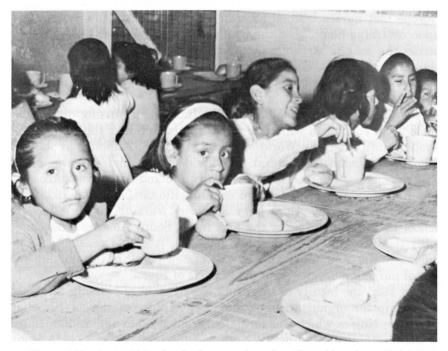

Figure 109. A nourishing lunch of cornmeal mush, milk and bread provided daily to 75,000 children in Lima, Peru. The Peruvian government constructed special dining halls. A central kitchen prepares the meals for this A.I.D. Project. (From A.I.D. pamphlet, "Food for Peace," p. 13. A.I.D., Dept. of State, Washington, D.C. 20402.)

unknown. Refuse tossed into streets made it necessary for pedestrians to use caution in crossing.

Combined national and international effort is helping to remedy the situation, and modern nursing schools are developing and extending their influence over wide areas. Although they have not arrived at uniformly high standards, South American nursing leaders are using their influence to bring about more effective laws for their control. Schools of Chile have progressed to such an extent that many fellowship students from other Latin American countries are arriving for advanced study where the language difficulty can be avoided that would be encountered in the United States or Canada. Countries with no national nursing organizations are making efforts to initiate them and to improve their nursing so as to meet requirements for affiliation with the International Council of Nurses.

FRANCE

Throughout the early history of France, religious orders of the Catholic Church carried the chief burden of nursing but, in time, city hospitals were built and wholly untrained people cared for their patients. An event of great significance in French nursing reform was organization of the Sisters of Charity by *St. Vincent de Paul* and *St. Louise de Marillac* in 1633, which proved to be the beginning of a reform movement that was to grow to international proportions. Other important changes in nursing method came about in the nineteenth century as a result of discoveries by the Frenchman, Louis Pasteur, who began a series of experiments in 1865 that would revolutionize the practice of medicine and surgery. Necessary nursing adjustments, however, did not come as quickly as might be expected.

Some improvement in nursing practice came to France and other European countries with establishment of Red Cross hospitals where nurses were trained for work in the home and for service during wartime. In the beginning little was accomplished because the courses covered a period of not more than six months and offered little in the way of instruction.

A young woman physician introduced into France reforms based on Nightingale principles. Possessed of high ethical principles, *Dr. Anna Hamilton,* as a medical student, had observed a crudeness and inefficiency in the care of hospital patients that was shocking to her. Upon graduation in 1900 her thesis, "Considérations sur des Infirmières Hôpitaux," not only exposed poor nursing methods but suggested reforms similar to those effected at the Nightingale School in London. Among her suggestions chief emphasis was placed upon having a trained nurse, rather than a physician or a layman, in charge of each nursing school. The following year when Dr. Hamilton became head of the Protestant Hospital at Bordeaux, she was able to put her ideas into practice. It was here that she founded the Ecole Florence Nightingale and placed responsibility for conducting it in the hands of a young graduate of the London Hospital.

Progress continued to be won by slow moves in France until sudden changes were precipitated by outbreak of the first World War. Working together in a common cause, nurses of Great Britain, America, and France exchanged ideas and stimulated interest in improvement. Mlle Chaptal, a graduate of the nursing school of La Pitié Hospital of Paris and particularly interested in social work, became a leader in the revitalized movement to raise the level of nursing practice, and it was through her influence that state registration of nurses became effective in 1922. In 1923 the National Association of Graduate Nurses of France was organized with Mlle Chaptal as first president. Until her death in 1937 Mlle Chaptal continued to be a prominent figure in French nursing history and, indeed, international history, for she was elected president of the International Council of Nurses at the Congress held in Montreal in 1929.

American Nurses' Memorial. The Ecole Florence Nightingale of Bordeaux has come to hold a unique interest for American nurses, for it is here that their individual contributions were used to erect the stately structure that provides classrooms and residence for student nurses. As a tribute to the two hundred and ninety six American nurses who died in service during World War I, about one hundred of whom are buried in

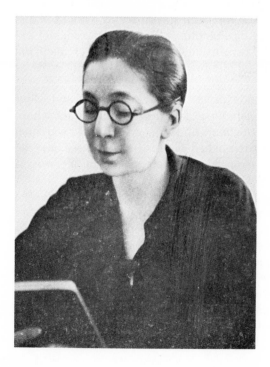

Figure 110. Mademoiselle Chaptal. (From "Mademoiselle Chaptal," by Marguerite Peltier, Editions Spes, Paris, France.)

France, it bears, engraved in stone over the main entrance, the inscription: "American Nurses' Memorial." Within, on one side of the fireplace in French and on the other in English, is the following dedication:

"To the Florence Nightingale School in memory of our comrades who died in service in the Great War, we, the nurses of America, dedicate this memorial to the higher education of nurses."

Today France is a highly socialized state with a complex health and social service program entirely under governmental control. The responsibilities of a public health nurse and a social worker are often combined in what is known as an *assistante sociale* who has completed two years of study in a nursing school and another year and one half in a school for social workers and holds diplomas in both nursing and social work. There are others who have completed a two and one-half year course in social work, the first year combined with that of students of nursing, but who have no diploma in nursing.

Assistantes sociales are prepared to look after both the health and social service needs of entire families. They teach and follow up the progress of their patients, either walking or riding a bicycle from one house to another, but they do not provide home nursing. As social workers they are prepared to accept requests for sickness and unemployment insurance and to inquire about any absence of children from school, attendance at which is compulsory. They also see that necessary immunizations are given, and they make plans for children to attend summer camps.

At combined public health and social service centers assistantes sociales weigh babies and keep records of their diets and any necessary treatments. They advise mothers in regard to preparation for deliveries, many of which take place in the home with a midwife or a doctor in attendance. A genuine interest in the welfare of whole families, and tact in limiting counseling to that which is regarded as acceptable are considered essential to success.

In recent years nursing schools have been established in various parts of France, many of which were developed and are maintained by the French Red Cross. Some are independent of hospitals but provide clinical experience in several and in outpatient clinics as well. Students often live apart from hospital or school but arrive daily for classes and ward practice. Doctors provide most of the instruction and conduct all of the state board examinations.

GERMANY

A foundation for nursing in Protestant Germany was laid during the early Christian period by the ancient Order of Deaconesses. During the hardships and perils of the Middle Ages, however, these kindly ministers of Christian service almost entirely disappeared, and it was not until 1836 that efforts to revive their Order proved successful. In that year Theodor Fliedner, pastor of a Protestant church at Kaiserswerth-on-the-Rhine, introduced into Germany a model school to prepare deaconesses for the work of teaching or nursing. Thereafter, Protestant deaconesses carried the chief burden of nursing in Germany and were transplanted far afield, even across the seas to America. At the same time, Catholic Nursing Orders also were active in some parts of Germany.

After 1863, when national Red Cross societies were being formed, about forty Red Cross hospitals were opened in Germany and soon graduated more than three thousand from their short courses in nursing. The Nightingale System finally made its appearance but not before revolt and leadership had led the way.

The motherhouse system, patterned after the custom of monasteries, had been spread throughout Germany by both deaconess and Red Cross hospitals. Under this arrangement nurses, upon graduation from schools, remained associated with them and governed by them for the remainder of their lives. While permitted no voice in matters pertaining to conditions under which they lived and worked, more and more came to be demanded of them and less and less was given in return. A working day of from fourteen to seventeen hours with responsibility for the care of as many as twenty patients, and meager remuneration, inevitably led to mental depression, invalidism, and poverty.

First to display open dissatisfaction and daring by breaking away from traditional patterns was a group of nurses who came to be known as the "Free Sisters" or "Wild Sisters" of Germany. In the attempt to earn their living these free lancers suffered many hardships. Their only hope for success lay in banding together, and in *Sister Agnes Karll* they found an able leader. Through the cooperative effort of this group the German Nurses' Association was organized in 1903 with Sister Agnes Karll as first president.

In 1904 the Congress of the International Council of Nurses was held in Berlin where a gracious welcome by Sister Agnes Karll was the beginning of a friendship among nurses of the world that was able to withstand the stress and strain of the war years ahead. In 1909, at the ICN Congress held in London, England, Sister Agnes Karll was elected president.

Since the close of World War II many new nursing schools have opened in Germany to operate according to principles in vogue in the British, American, or Russian zones of occupation. In both eastern and western zones Catholic and deaconess organizations conduct their own schools and employ their own graduates. In the eastern zone, greatly needed courses in advanced nursing education were established at the Johannes Institute, a school of social work for women. In the western zone the Red Cross Werner Schule for postgraduate work operates in association with a university.

The first basic nursing course within the organization of a university was opened at Heidelberg University in 1953, with a broad curriculum including participation in the cultural life of the university. First director of the school was *Olga von Lersner,* former matron of the Red Cross School of Nursing of the same city. In preparation for this work Miss von Lersner spent nine months at the University of Toronto taking work in administration and clinical supervision. She also visited the Yale University School of Nursing, the Skidmore School of Nursing, and schools in Sweden and Switzerland as well. The Swedish Nurses' Association offered encouragement by granting a two and one-half year scholarship to one of her instructors.

BELGIUM

Sandwiched in between France and Germany, and sensitive to happenings in both, is the little country of *Belgium,* the most densely populated of Europe. Its people are adherents of the Catholic religion and have for their official languages both French and Flemish. As in France nursing has been carried on chiefly by nuns with the assistance of untrained helpers.

An interesting medical practice began in Gheel, near Antwerp, about the 14th century, when mentally ill patients gathered around their church and were taken into the homes of the townspeople to live and work as members of their families. So rapid was their improvement that the practice has grown to care of about 250 patients and is now conducted by the state.

A hospital was built and staffed by nuns, to which each newcomer goes for diagnosis and assignment to a carefully selected home. The community is divided into districts in each of which men nurses are employed, who wear no uniforms and maintain friendly relations with all patients. Tasks are assigned to as many patients as possible for which they are paid a small sum by both the family and the state, and families also are paid for room and board by the state. The undertaking is regarded as highly successful with few disturbed episodes and rapid improvement in those who are living a nearly normal life.

The first school for lay nurses to be established in Belgium along modern lines was opened in 1907 in the city of Brussels by *Edith Cavell,* martyred English nurse of World War I. Known as the "School of the Rue de la Culture," its development was promoted by Miss Cavell in the capacity of matron and by *Dr. Antoine DePage* and his wife, *Marie DePage,* its founders. Steady progress was made and its nurses were prepared to render skilled services to soldiers of the Belgian, French, and German armies during the first World War.

After several battles had been fought on Belgian soil in which Germany was victorious, hundreds of Allied soldiers were left separated from their regiments. In order to avoid capture and possible death these unfortunate men were compelled to seek shelter in nearby woods and villages. For the avowed purpose of assisting them to escape into neutral Holland, a secret organization of considerable size was formed to which Edith Cavell and Marie DePage gave their support. German forms and stamps were secured and passes forged. Personal guides were provided, and Philippe Baucq, a Belgian lawyer and father, was among these daring men.

As time went on, one after another of the group came under suspicion of the German secret police until thirty five of their number, including Edith Cavell and Philippe Baucq, were apprehended and placed within the walls of St. Gilles prison. At the ensuing trial, two months later, all were found guilty of giving aid to the enemy by assisting in the escape of more than two hundred able-bodied men. The death sentence, "Todes-strafe," for five of the prisoners rang through the somber halls of the jail.

For a reason that has never been clearly understood, Edith Cavell and Philippe Baucq were singled out for immediate execution. At dawn October 12, 1915, they died before a firing squad. The following words of Miss Cavell, uttered to a clergyman as she was leaving her prison cell, are memorable:

"I have nothing to regret. If I had it to do over again, I would do just as I did. Everyone has been most kind to me here in prison and I have been so thankful for these eight weeks of rest. I was very tired and so pressed with the multitude of petty things that life brings that I have not had time for many years for quiet and uninterrupted meditation. It was a welcome rest for me — before the end. I know now that patriotism is not enough; I must have no hatred and no bitterness toward anyone."[1]

Consternation and horror thus came close, not only to nurses of the School of the Rue de la Culture, but to all nurses and all people throughout a bewildered world.

Notwithstanding the loss of its matron, the School of the Rue de la Culture continued building on the foundation that she had established. Dr. Depage, however, suffered another and greater loss. Madame Depage, returning from a trip to the United States, where she had gone to secure funds for carrying on the widely expanded work of the Belgian Red Cross, was among the victims of the ill-fated ship, "Lusitania."

As a tribute to two women who met untimely deaths in their efforts to alleviate human suffering, the *Edith Cavell-Marie DePage School of Nursing* was opened in 1935 as a continuation of the School of the Rue de la Culture in association with the University of Brussels. The school

---

[1]Judson, Helen: Edith Cavell, 1941, p. 281. By permission of The Macmillan Company, New York, publishers.

was generously endowed by both the family of the late Dr. Antoine DePage and the Rockefeller Foundation and receives additional financial assistance from the city of Brussels and the national government of Belgium.

To meet the need for leadership by qualified administrators, instructors, and public health nurses, the University of Belgium instituted, in 1948, a program of two academic years for graduate nurses. So successful has been this school and so high its standing that, through its graduates, its influence has penetrated the neighboring countries of Switzerland, Italy, Greece, Jugoslavia, Lebanon, and Iran.

In 1954 a nurse of the Belgian Army Medical Corps was awarded the signal honor of becoming one of a very few members of a foreign army ever to receive the Bronze Star Medal, a decoration of the U. S. Army. *Captain Marthe Debackere* was cited for her devotion to seriously ill patients in a neurosurgical ward of the Tokyo Army Hospital in Japan, where she was on duty as a United Nations nurse. Her maintenance of smooth and efficient relationships among patients and hospital and government representatives during the Korean Police Action of the UN (1950–1953) gave proof that peoples of all nations can work together even in time of strong emotional bias.

NORTHERN EUROPE

Stories of the development of nursing in the Protestant countries of Northern Europe are similar to those of Protestant Germany. In a region of protracted ice and snow, invigorating climate and energetic people, where the hours of daylight in midsummer lengthen almost to the exclusion of darkness, is one of the most advanced civilizations of Europe. Sweden, Norway, Finland, Denmark, and Iceland have modern nursing schools, nursing practice acts, and national nursing associations. Each has a form of socialized government which sets up uniform standards for nursing schools and employs the greater number of their graduates. While some physicians are engaged in private practice, state medicine is far advanced and physicians are employed by the state in great numbers.

Courses in midwifery are well developed, especially in Sweden, and are offered to young women with no previous preparation for nursing. After completion of a two-year course, graduate midwives visit homes of patients to render a specialized service for which public health nurses are not prepared. In hospitals, the demand is for nurse midwives, and for this service the time required for preparation is four and one-half years.

The Swedish Nurses' Association, in addition to working toward development of nursing to best serve the needs of all the people, takes an active interest in legislation affecting hospital construction and in vocational guidance to interest young people in lines of work requiring long periods of preparation. The association is influential also in matters of general education, movements to counteract alcoholism, and other social issues which have long been supported by *Gerda Hojer,* a Swedish nurse of international reputation. Miss Hojer served as executive secretary and president of the Swedish Nurses' Association, and in 1947 was elected president of the International Council of Nurses. The following year she achieved further distinction when elected to membership in the Swedish parliament.

In the summer of 1948, students enrolled in a postgraduate school sponsored by the Norwegian Nurses' Association, enjoyed an unusual type of instruction. In cooperation with the national associations of Sweden and Denmark, a boat was chartered for the purpose of visiting hospitals, nursing schools, health centers, and public health agencies of their larger cities. For eleven days a program of lectures and field trips was carried on by instructors, doctors, and social workers, the ship waiting in harbor by day and doing most of its traveling by night.

In Norwegian nursing schools, it is said that the psychosomatic approach to illness is stressed with all subjects. Some schools provide special lectures on current world affairs and on social and cultural subjects as well. All students have bicycles and skis and engage in outdoor sports. It is said, too, that in Norway, nurses have ample time to care for their patients!

In addition to their own national associations, Scandinavian nurses have developed a regional organization known as the Association of Northern European Nurses, which meets in convention every four years. Measures encouraging breadth of vision and international understanding have been the outcome of integration of interests. Students of one country often take part of their nursing course in another, and scholarships for advanced study are made available annually. A system instituted by hospitals makes possible an international exchange of their graduates.

ITALY

Italy, a boot-shaped peninsula with its toe reaching to the island of Sicily, juts into the Mediterranean Sea to the west of Greece, its companion peninsula. Rome, capital and largest city, is one of the world's oldest and most historic. This City of Seven Hills, situated on either side of the Tiber River, contains many structures and ruins of antiquity in an excellent state of preservation. Among its ancient temples the Pantheon, erected about 120 A.D. and dedicated to all the gods, is indicative of ancient Rome's tolerant attitude toward the religions of all peoples.

In contrast to ancient structures are modern museums containing priceless literary and art collections as well as modern institutions noted for their excellent educational and cultural facilities. The Appian Way, originally one of the military roads leading to the provinces of the old Roman Empire, is now a modern thoroughfare. Along its borders are to be seen the catacombs, a vast network of subterranean passages, excavated in rock and used as burial chambers by early Christians. During periods of persecution these became places of refuge and religious worship because, under the law, all burial places were granted asylum.

Within the borders of Rome, covering more than a hundred acres on the right bank of the Tiber, is Vatican City, created in 1929 as an independent state to be governed by the Pope. Here are excellent museums and art collections, the papal palace, St. Peter's Church, largest in the world, and the Sistine Chapel, on the walls and ceiling of which are frescoes by world famous artists. Michelangelo's "Last Judgment" completely covers the wall space behind the altar.

Religious orders are in general control of Italian hospitals and nursing with few lay nurses, but large numbers of nurse helpers, employed and directed by nuns. The Italian Red Cross assisted in the introduction of modern methods by establishing Red Cross schools in various parts of the country but it was through the American Red Cross and *Mary Sewall Gardner* that public health nursing came to Italy during the first World War. While a campaign aimed at international tuberculosis control was being carried on, Miss Gardner and fifteen other American public health nurses set sail for Italy where they remained about a year demonstrating methods for controlling the disease through establishment of a public health nursing service. Opposition

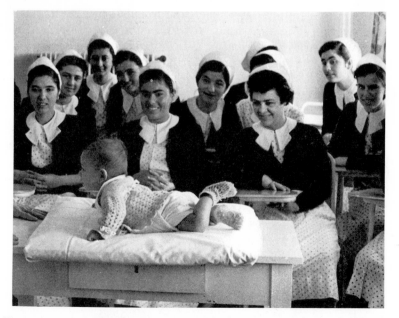

Figure 111. A class in "Mother-Nursing" for student nurses at the Metera Children's Home in Athens. (Courtesy WHO.)

to higher education for nurses and other circumstances proved drawbacks to full acceptance of the plan, which would require time and continued effort to overcome.

Soon after the close of World War II, while Italy was in a greatly impoverished state, the Italian Nurses' Association reorganized, with an executive secretary and an editor of their journal providing volunteer services. Energies were devoted to raising the standard of living of the Italian people through the medium of efficient nursing service. By 1951 there were thirty four nursing schools in Italy, all having established two-year programs and graduating about six hundred nurses annually. While there were as yet no college programs for their graduates, post-graduate courses of seven months in the field of public health were provided. The training of midwives, entirely separate from that of nurses, covers a period of three years. In all schools the poor health of entering students, due to malnutrition associated with privations of war, proved a serious problem in the beginning.

ISRAEL

From Old Testament times Palestine was the home of a Semitic race of people known as Hebrews, Jews, or Israelites. In 63 B.C. their homeland was conquered by the armies of Rome and in 70 A.D. Jerusalem, capital and holy city, was razed by Roman soldiers, leaving the Israelites with no national state for nearly two thousand years. As time went on, great numbers of nomads filtered into Palestine from nearby Arabia, bringing about conflicting claims of rights to territory and other privileges between Jew and Arab and creating antagonisms and perpetual tension.

In the midst of widespread suffering and famine associated with

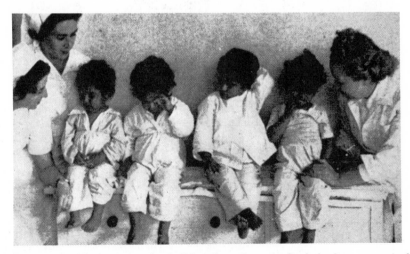

Figure 112. Newcomers to land of Israel receive a medical check-up on arrival at camp. (Cantor, S. L.: Am. J. of Nursing, *51*:162, 1951.)

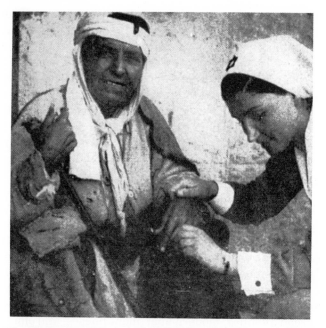

Figure 113. Hadassah public health nurse checking health of resident of old city of Jerusalem. (Courtesy Hadassah.)

World War I, an American Zionist Medical Unit arrived in Palestine to carry on social work of various kinds. This Unit, fully equipped by the *Hadassah Women's Organization,* was made up of registered nurses, doctors, sanitary engineers, and a contingent of the American Red Cross. At that time there were no schools for nurses and the extensive work and influence of this new group were greatly appreciated. In time German deaconesses came to German hospitals, French Sisters of Charity to Catholic hospitals, Scotch missionaries to Scottish hospitals, and British nurses to British mission hospitals. Local Jewish and Arabian girls were trained at the bedside for nursing and midwifery.

In 1922 the League of Nations made Palestine a mandate of Great Britain with the objective of promoting progress through encouragement of immigration. Clashes between Jews and Arabs continued and, in 1948, the General Assembly of the United Nations created an independent Jewish state of *Israel* west of the Jordan River and the Dead Sea, leaving an independent Arab state of *Jordan* to the east. During the first year of Israel's existence, nearly a quarter of a million Jewish immigrants came from many parts of the world, to build permanent homes and aid in its development. The families of these and later arrivals now make up more than one half of the population.

Near Jerusalem and overlooking the Dead Sea the Henrietta Szold School of Nursing, affiliated with the great Rothschild-Hadassah University Hospital and Medical Center, was opened in 1939 by Hadassah, the Women's Zionist Organization of America. Modern in all its aspects, this hospital provides care for Moslem, Jew, and Christian, and affords excellent facilities for teaching purposes. A cosmopolitan atmosphere prevails and students of Polish, German, Latvian, Rumanian, and American, as well as Israeli origin are known to have been in one class.

In 1951 the first Institutions for the Care of Handicapped Immigrants, known as *Malden* and today numbering about fifty, were founded in Israel. These include a large Malden Tuberculosis Hospital at Beer Yaacov, other tuberculosis hospitals, homes for the handicapped and aged, sheltered workshops, rehabilitation centers and, very recently, a nursing school. All patients, and many of the nurses, were immigrants and wanderers from other countries.

Today the city of Jerusalem comprises two sections known as *Old City* and *New City*. Old City, in the heart of Jerusalem, is enclosed by ancient walls and divided into Christian, Jewish, Moslem, and Armenian quarters. In this historic symbol of the Jewish fatherland are locations and structures mentioned in both the Old and the New Testaments. Here also are the Church of the Holy Sepulchre, sacred to Christians, and the Mosque of Omar, sacred to Moslems. New City, now the capital of Israel, was developed during the last century and presents an interesting contrast with broad avenues, modern apartment houses, and office buildings.

AFRICA

Africa, a vast continent comprising many countries, covers sun-seared desert, temperate highlands, dense jungles, magnificent scenery, and seemingly illimitable distances. Its people are of many races and many stages of development, the majority living in isolated areas, each with its own social structure, traditions, and mores which have developed over long, long periods of time. Health workers in many sections find it necessary to teach illiterate, superstitious natives in whose minds evil spirits are still regarded as the cause of all misfortune.

However, this newly stirring continent is awakening to progressive ideas with dramatic speed, but modern methods for control and eradication of infectious disease are still lacking over wide areas. Malnutrition is prevalent among great numbers of its inhabitants and the list of common infections is a long one. Few Africans are free from malaria, and enteric diseases take the lives of thousands of infants and children. Blindness and pain due to trachoma are common in Ethiopia and all of northern Africa, where rows of blind beggars are a common sight in the market places. African sleeping sickness, tuberculosis, smallpox, leprosy, and yaws are causes of distress among great numbers of people, some of whom are afflicted with several diseases at one time.

The first health services were provided by missionaries whose primary purpose was to spread the Christian religion, and there are still far too few medical or nursing schools, or even high schools, to

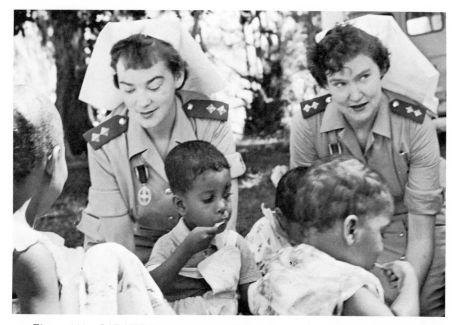

Figure 114. QARANC Lieutenants from East Africa Command at a picnic for young African children. (British Official Photograph: Crown Copyright Reserved. Issued for Britain's Information Services by the Central Office of Information, London.)

provide leaders and trained personnel capable of coping with the situation. However, there are indications that improvement is on the way. Within a five-year period, twenty two African nations achieved independence from colonial rule and are rapidly assuming responsibility for providing educational facilities and medical services for their people. Very recently representatives of thirty four countries held a meeting in Addis Ababa, capital of Ethiopia, and agreed upon a five year program to admit a million children a year to their schools, the high cost to be borne by the countries themselves but help would be sought also from other sources.

In contrast to newly developing areas, noteworthy advances are being made by some nations. Nursing schools of *Nigeria* and *Ghana* are so far advanced as to make it possible for their graduates to register and practice in England. The southern part of Africa and that around the Nile Delta have well established schools, hospitals, health centers, and public health services for rural districts. Graduates of some nursing schools of the *Union of South Africa* are eligible for registration and exchange visits in European and North American countries. It was in what is now Cape of Good Hope Province that need for legal control of nursing practice was first publicly recognized by enactment of a medical and pharmacy law in 1891 which included registration of nurses among its provisions.

As Africa awakens to possibilities of a better way of life, it is being

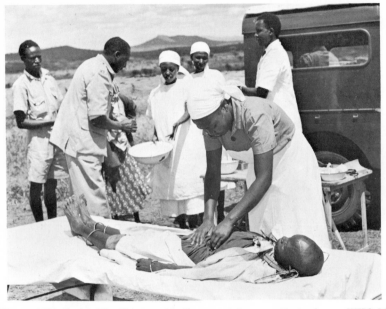

Figure 115. Sarah Wanjiku, a midwife, examining a patient when a WHO Mobile Health Unit comes to Kenya, Africa, with equipment provided by UNICEF. (Nursing Times, March 4, 1960. Photograph by Camera Press, Ltd., London.)

assisted in its efforts by the United Nations. A large scale campaign against trachoma is being carried on by the World Health Organization in Morocco and Tunisia. In 1953 seventeen teams of ophthalmologists and nurses arrived in southern Morocco with a caravan of hospitals. Various other WHO projects, originating in Brazzaville, capital of the Congo Republic and site of the WHO Regional Office for Africa south of the Sahara, are being carried on over the continent.

The United Nations International Children's Fund (UNICEF), with the help of African nurses and other interested persons, is working toward reduction of the high infant mortality rate and ensuring healthy babies for Africa. Hospitals are assisted with teaching and demonstration programs, equipment, powdered milk, and medications. The Food and Agricultural Organization (FAO) is cooperating by teaching up-to-date farming methods and the use of modern equipment to greatly increase the food supply and alleviate malnutrition.

Advancement in all areas of living is being promoted by the United Nations Educational, Scientific, and Cultural Organization (UNESCO), which assists countries to develop their own educational systems from kindergarten to a doctorate. Its social science department concentrates on questions of race relations and discrimination between opportunities for men and women. When requested, it sends top level specialists in education and science to work with the natives and teach them modern systems of education, scientific research, and cultural development. The urgency of the present situation was expressed by the head of the British delegation to a general conference of UNESCO, held in Paris:

"In the field of education, we are all poor and some are poorer than others. UNESCO stands for Education in the broadest sense as WHO stands for Health and FAO stands for Agriculture. We have the right and duty to proclaim the urgent needs of education and to press these claims on our own governments and on the whole family of the United Nations."[2]

As the combined efforts of these great social projects penetrate wider and wider areas, opportunity is afforded for the cultural, moral, and spiritual values of civilization to spread with them.

Dr. Albert Schweitzer. An early independent missionary undertaking in what is now Lambaréné, Gabon, which has become world

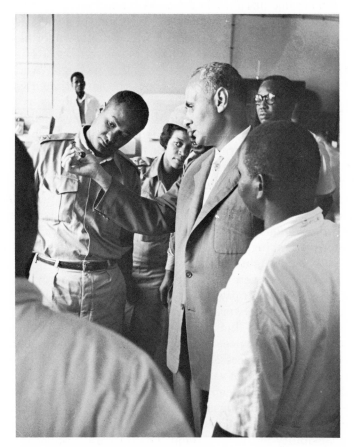

Figure 116. A WHO doctor working with an International Red Cross Medical Team at Bunio, Congo Republic. (Photo courtesy World Health.)

---

[2]UNESCO Courier, Feb. 1961, p. 7.

famous, is that of Dr. Albert Schweitzer, winner of the the 1952 Nobel Prize for World Peace. In the year 1913, in the midst of a mahogany grove on the Ogowe River, Dr. Schweitzer and his wife arrived from Alsace-Lorraine to erect the buildings for a hospital in what has been termed, "the worst climate in the world." No other doctor was to be found for miles around. To the new hospital came at once great numbers of natives suffering from malaria, dysentery, elephantiasis, sleeping sickness, tuberculosis, leprosy, and skin diseases of every description. Conditions requiring surgical procedure were numerous. Patients traveled in canoes or through jungles, sometimes for weeks, arriving with their families and friends, all of whom somehow must be housed and fed.

Dr. Schweitzer had abandoned a career in which he attained fame as a musician, author, and lecturer in order to put into practice his belief that every one has *another job* to do in addition to his art, business, or profession, in serving his fellow men. His study of music began at the age of five, and even as a young man he was well known for his splendid rendition of the compositions of Johann Sebastian Bach. His study of medicine began at the age of thirty in order that he might "work without talking" in his missionary endeavor. About the same time a young lady in whom he was interested entered a school of nursing so as to be prepared to work with him. She became Madame Schweitzer and for many years served as nurse, anesthetist, and general assistant to her husband. Eventually, the state of her health made it necessary for her to return to their home in Alsace-Lorraine.

Dr. Schweitzer's hospital today comprises approximately forty buildings occupying a cleared area of one hundred ten acres. They are well constructed from the standpoint of ventilation and protection from the intense equatorial heat. Conveniences of electricity, refrigeration, modern plumbing, radios, and daily newspapers are lacking. All supplies must be brought in from a distance. Funds to carry on his great humanitarian project were raised through European concert and lecture tours, carried on periodically by Dr. Schweitzer, and through the sale of his writings. Doctors to work with and relieve him during his absence were always difficult to find but nurses of Belgian, Dutch, and French origin gave devoted service, some of them remaining for many years. Now all are finding it necessary to carry on alone since Dr. Schweitzer's death in 1965 at the age of ninety years.

Dr. Schweitzer had a deep conviction that if the lives of fear, disease, and misery of the millions of superstitious and backward African peoples could be observed and understood, civilization would acknowledge its great responsibility for helping them. The core of his philosophy is to be found in his phrase, "reverence for life," which he believed should be the guiding principle for all social, economic, and political systems. His own reverence for life extended to all living things, and he paid the natives for rescuing and bringing to him every creature found in distress. He respected the dignity of all men and recognized his brotherhood with them. All savages were his brothers and sisters. He lived with them and for them. It is fitting that he has been called, "the kindest man in the world," "the greatest living philosopher," and "a little lower than the angels."

REPUBLIC OF INDIA

India, land of origin of two gentle and peaceful religions, Hinduism and Buddhism, is rapidly undergoing social change, but an alarming absence of public health and sanitary measures still exists. Nutritional diseases, malaria, cholera, and leprosy, are prevalent, and it has been estimated that more than two million persons are blind due to preventable or curable causes. The ratio of doctors and nurses to the population remains dangerously low but is increasing with the eagerness of young people to improve the social status and health services of their country. Emphasis is being placed upon the establishment of adequate programs for the preparation of physicians and nurses, especially in the field of pediatrics.

The opening of nursing schools associated with colleges is giving to the profession a higher social and economic status than it had previously known and attracting young people of culture. Among modern schools are the *Vellore Medical College Hospital School of Nursing* and the *College of Nursing of Delhi University* in New Delhi, capital of India. The Vellore School of Nursing, opened in 1902 by *Lillian Hart,* a Canadian, now has a three-year certificate program and a four-year degree program controlled by the nearby University of Madras. Clinical experience for students includes working with well-equipped mobile hospital units which make regular trips into neighboring territory, stopping along the wayside wherever groups of patients have assembled.

The College of Nursing of Delhi University is part of a general movement toward higher education for women which is attracting greater numbers of desirable applicants than can be accommodated. Established in 1946 as a constituent four-year college of the University, it is supported by the central government of India and requires tuition fees corresponding to those of its other colleges.

Clinical experience is obtained at several hospitals and, in addition, students have been working in a nearby village with a Child Welfare Team, supported by WHO and UNICEF, under the direction of a native graduate of the school who obtained advanced public health experience in Toronto, Canada. With these and other promising beginnings the concept of modern nursing and public health practices can be expected to penetrate throughout this great country which today presents an open field for all aspects of health teaching.

Student Nurses' Association of India. In 1929 the Student Nurses' Association of India was established in affiliation with the Trained Nurses' Association of India with the objective of helping nursing to attain professional status and promoting a spirit of understanding and cooperation among students of different schools. Student exhibits are displayed at annual conventions and, in 1952, *Anthony Swami,* a third year student of the Government General Hospital in Madras, received the President of the Republic of India's prize for his exhibit of a model postoperative ward.

CHINA

In China, where women have been expected to marry early and live with their husbands' families on terms of strict obedience and respect toward the older generation, foreign ideas have had to generate many changes. It was within this traditional framework that the early missionaries were required to labor but new impetus was provided by later pioneers. *Nina Gage,* a New York City graduate, while dean of the Hunan-Yale School of Nursing at Changsa and president of the Nurses' Association of China as well as of the International Council of Nurses (1925–1929), was instrumental in bringing about reform. A standard curriculum for nursing schools was developed, laws to provide for accreditation of nursing schools and registration of their graduates were enacted, and conventions of nurses were arranged.

In more recent years many young Chinese, some of them college graduates, were granted the opportunity to study abroad. On their return to China they were equipped to institute the modern methods of foreign lands. Prominent among these were *Elsie Mawfung Chung* who was graduated at Guy's Hospital, London, in 1909, and *Lillian Wu* who came to America and was graduated at the Johns Hopkins School of Nursing, Baltimore. Miss Wu later exerted influence as president of the Nurses' Association of China.

Public health nursing, with all its possibilities for elevation of living standards was inaugurated at Peiping Union Medical College in 1925 and has advanced into many sections, but inevitable setbacks have been experienced. Nevertheless, in spite of many years of civil and international war and great devastation, all fields of Chinese nursing have progressed to a state in which they are able to render invaluable service.

FORMOSA

Formosa, or Taiwan as it is known to the Chinese, is an island about 85 miles off the southern coast of China, its population made up of Chinese, Japanese, and aborigines with the Chinese predominating. Buddhism, Confucianism, and Taoism are all accepted forms of religion and all offer lofty ideals of human thought and conduct. Before World War II nursing schools and those for midwives were managed by doctors at the provincial hospitals, where many patients were cared for by relatives who remained day and night and cooked food at the bedside. Students were admitted at irregular intervals, after completion of eight years of schooling, to a two-year course with no regular classwork.

Formosa was a target for devastating bombing during the war and considerable reconstruction was necessary before hospitals could be re-established. Since the war several modern nursing schools have been founded in Taipeh, capital and chief city. The *National Defense Medical Center School of Nursing* is an integral part of the army and *General Chow Mei-Yo,* a graduate of the school at Peiping Union Medical College, became first dean. The nursing program covers four years with a prerequisite of six months of military training and a requirement of two years of service in army hospitals after graduation.

The *Taiwan University Hospital School of Nursing* has a three-year course. The first director, a Chinese graduate of St. Luke's College of Nursing in Tokyo, has worked toward university status with the assistance of a WHO team of four foreign nurses. The city of Taichung also profited from the services of another WHO team, made up of a Canadian public health nurse, an English nurse midwife, and an American woman obstetrician, who worked toward improved maternal care. All schools of Formosa are greatly in need of teaching and supervisory personnel, textbooks in the Chinese language, and many types of equipment.

In 1952 the Western Pacific Regional Office of the World Health Organization at Manila sponsored a nursing education seminar at Taipeh where twenty nine nurses convened, including the WHO regional nursing advisor and an educational director from the United States. Nurses arrived not only from various parts of Formosa but also from Korea, Japan, China, the Philippines, Malaya, Singapore, North Borneo, New Zealand, Australia, Netherlands, New Guinea, and Vietnam. Tedious and uncomfortable transportation was not permitted to be a drawback. The nurse from Australia traveled eight days by air including necessary stopovers. Another nurse traveled 100 miles by truck and then twelve days by air in order to be present.

JAPAN

The introduction of western methods in Japan by *Linda Richards,* in 1885, has been noted. Under the auspices of the American Board of Missions, she organized at Kyoto the first training school for nurses and guided it through the first five years of its existence. Another major development, founding of the great St. Luke's International Medical Center in Tokyo, was accomplished through the combined efforts of the Protestant Episcopal churches of America and Japan. A school of nursing, established in 1904 in connection with St. Luke's, has become an official college of nursing with a well-planned three-year basic course, and a fourth year for those wishing to specialize in teaching, supervision, or public health nursing.

Japan, like Formosa, sustained serious damage to its hospitals and nursing schools during the second World War, but rapid strides toward reconstruction included founding new schools and the enactment of licensing laws to govern the practice of their graduates. In 1946 the *Red Cross Demonstration School of Nursing* was opened in Tokyo as a model for other schools to follow. The Red Cross Hospital, with which it is associated, is a general hospital of 500 beds maintaining well-equipped classrooms and other adequate teaching facilities. Public health nursing is integrated with other subjects throughout the entire period of study. This school has become a center for refresher courses for nurse administrators, nurse educators, and clinical nursing specialists.

There are now two types or classes of nurses in Japan known as Class A and Class B respectively. Class A nurses correspond to professional nurses of other countries and practice without supervision while Class B nurses correspond to practical or vocational nurses and the law requires that they practice only under direction of a medical practitioner, a dentist, or a Class A nurse.

KOREA

Korea, a peninsula of eastern Asia, is largely mountainous and still in the agricultural stage of development. Little is known of the origin of its people but, because of characteristic features, it is believed that they are a mixture of Mongolian races. Many forms of religion are practiced, including animism, ancestor worship, Buddhism, and Confucianism. Christianity was introduced about 1882 with the arrival of European missionaries. Since that time modern medicine and nursing have been carried on in various isolated centers.

For thirty five years the Japanese government had control of Korea but lost it at the close of World War II, when it was divided temporarily at the 38th parallel into North and South Korea. For the purpose of gaining control of the entire country, the North Korean army began a drive southward in June, 1950. The Security Council of the United Nations took prompt action, and the Korean Police Action of the United Nations followed.

Almost immediate care for wounded soldiers of all armies was provided through the united effort of countries under the banner of the United Nations. Korean nurses, from both North and South Korea, served with Korean armies. The first contingent of foreign nurses arrived one week after the beginning of hostilities to cope with dust and mud and extremes of temperature as they assisted with a continuous flow of combat casualties. The Red Cross societies of many countries became active. The Danish Red Cross contributed a well-equipped hos-

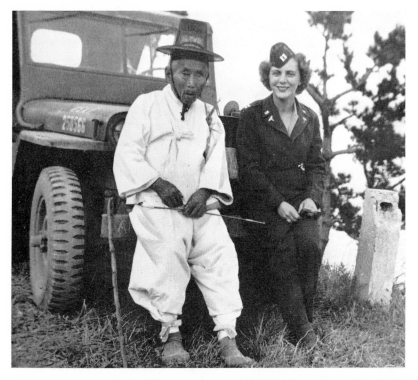

Figure 117. Captain Steele, a Korean patient, and a jeep. (Courtesy of NEWSWEEK.)

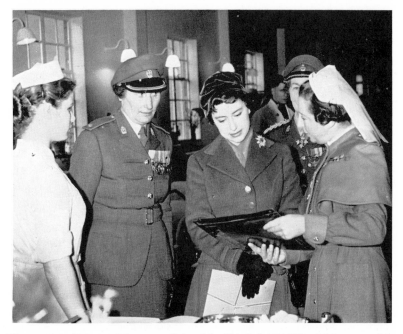

Figure 118. Princess Margaret, Colonel-in-Chief, QARANC, visiting a model ward at the QARANC Preliminary Training School. Work is explained by Major D. Price. (Courtesy Nursing Mirror, April 4, 1958.)

pital ship with a staff of nurses and other personnel. The Swedish Red Cross provided a hospital unit, and the Italian Red Cross sent another whose personnel were all volunteers and prepared to minister solely to the needs of the Korean civilian population.

Nursing Sisters of Queen Alexandra's Royal Army Nursing Corps came from England with equipment for a field hospital. Mobile Army Surgical Hospital (MASH) Units for front line duty were supplied by the United States, and one by Norway. These were so designed as to be capable of moving by jeep and truck closer to the front lines than the field or evacuation hospital. Any available barn, schoolhouse, or church was taken over or, when necessary, tents were rapidly set up and equipped. A staff of doctors, nurses, anesthetists, and corpsmen went into action in preoperative shock wards, postoperative wards, and the operating room. Three or four operating tables were in constant use throughout the day and night until treatment had been given to all the wounded.

Great quantities of whole blood or plasma were used to prevent or overcome shock, and penicillin was administered to all with open wounds. Severe chest, abdominal, and extremity injuries were common. To prevent loss of blood and shock, patients were moved as little as possible, litters elevated on blocks often serving as operating tables. By litter, jeep, and helicopter they arrived, to be evacuated as soon as possible in the same manner, or by ambulance or hospital train.

From evacuation hospitals severely wounded American soldiers were taken to U. S. Army hospitals in Japan, where separate institutions

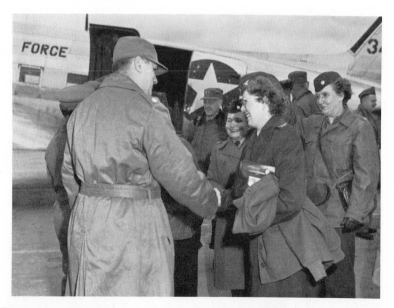

Figure 119. Colonel Mary G. Phillips, Chief of the U.S. Army Nurse Corps, arrives at Seoul, Korea, airfield to begin inspection tour of a mobile army surgical hospital. (From Bulletin of the California State Nurses' Association, May, 1951.)

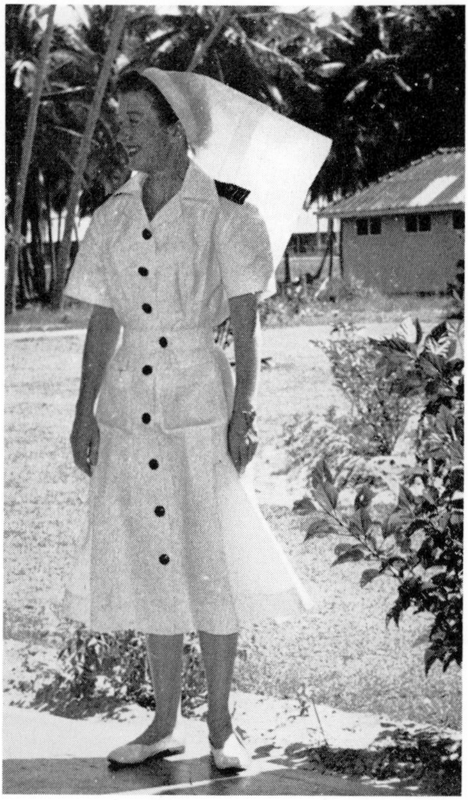

Figure 120. Flight Officer Margaret Maloney, Royal Australian Air Force, outside her quarters at Butterworth, Malaya. (Courtesy Nursing Mirror, March 28, 1958.)

cared for neuro-psychiatric, paraplegic, hepatitis, and frost-bite patients. Here American nurses worked with and taught hospital corpsmen. From Japan, patients unable to return to their regiments were transported by air ambulance or hospital ship to army hospitals in the United States.

In the midst of the conflict nurses from various countries formed what they called a "Little United Nations," in order to become better acquainted. At the first meeting, held in an evacuation hospital, Korean nurses told of Korean nursing service and nursing education and expressed deep appreciation for the assistance their country was receiving. Other speakers from the Netherlands, Sweden, Norway, and the United States told either of nursing in their own countries or of the type of service they were supplying in Korea. A nurse from Thailand explained the similarity between nursing education in her country and that of the United States. A member of the Italian Red Cross Hospital Unit told of their language problem because Korean must first be translated into English and then into Italian, sometimes with startling changes in meaning!

As fighting continued from the north to the south of Korea and the horrors of battle casualties mounted, extreme suffering extended to the

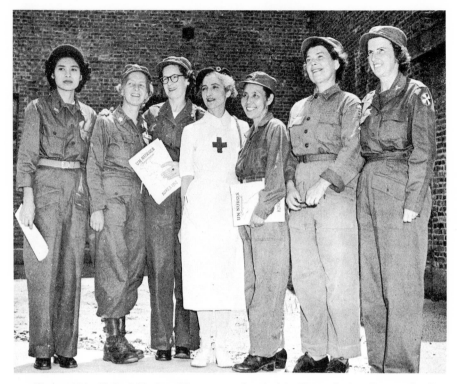

Figure 121. United Nations Nurses at a hospital in Korea during Korean Conflict (1950–1953). (Pamphlet, "The Army Nurse Corps Yesterday and Today" by Mary M. Roberts, Office of Surgeon General, U.S. Army, Washington, D.C. 20402.)

civilian population. Water supplies, purification plants, and health services were disrupted, homes destroyed, civilians injured or killed and little children left without parental or other form of protection, all of which became glaringly apparent when hostilities finally ceased July 27, 1953.

Many countries, working with the United Nations Korean Reconstruction Agency, immediately became active in sending supplies of food, clothing, blankets, and equipment. Boxes of uniforms, shoes, and books were sent to Korean nurses. The American Korean Foundation, working with the United Nations and the Korean Government, provided funds for four Korean nurse leaders to take postgraduate courses in Hawaii and New Zealand and for other Korean graduates to study in Australia, Canada, Hawaii, Japan, and the United States. The American Korean Foundation also opened a Postgraduate School for Nursing in Korea in 1954, and this soon proved more far-reaching in its effectiveness than the plan of sending nurses abroad for advanced study.

References

International Nursing Review. ICN House, 1 Dean Trench Street, London, S.W. 1, England (Some articles are in French, German, and Spanish)

American Journal of Nursing. Official magazine of the ANA. 10 Columbus Circle, New York, New York 10019

Nursing Outlook. Official magazine of the NLN. 10 Columbus Circle, New York, New York 10019

The Canadian Nurse. Published in English and French. 1522 Sherbrooke Street West, Montreal 25, Quebec, Canada

Nursing Times. Journal for the RCN and NCN of the UK. Macmillan & Co., publishers, St. Martin's Street, London, W.C. 2, England

Américas. Pan American Union, 19th St. and Constitution Ave., Washington, D.C. 20006

World Health. The Magazine of the World Health Organization. Columbia University Press, International Documents Service. 2960 Broadway, New York 10027

UN Monthly Chronicle. Columbia University Press, International Documents Service. 2960 Broadway, New York 10027

Index

Abbesses
famous, 81
Radegunde of Poitiers, 82
St. Clare or Clarissa, 103
St. Hildegarde, 114–115
Accreditation of hospitals, 316–317
of nursing schools, 316, 330
Addams, Jane, 237–238
Aeneid, 48
Affiliation, first, 228, 267
Africa, nursing in, 412
Age
Dark, 77
Golden, of ancient Greece, 45
New Stone, or age of farmers, 18
of chivalry, 109
of coma in medicine, 116
Old Stone, or age of hunters, 15
Agency for International Development (AID), 370
Aikenhead, Mother Mary, 178
Alcott, Louisa M., 219–220, 222
Alexander the Great, 21, 45, 47
Alexandria, city of, 21, 45, 66
Alexandrian Empire, 22
Alexian Brothers, 364
Alumnae associations founded, 248–249
American Association of Industrial Nurses, 315
American Association of Nurse Anesthetists, 315
American College of Physicians, 269, 316
American College of Surgeons, 269
American Hospital Association, 269, 271, 306, 316, 317
Council on Nursing, 271
American Indians, 33
American Journal of Nursing, first copy of 252, 329
American Journal of Nursing Company, 335, 336

American Journal of Practical Nursing, 307
American Korean Foundation, 424
American Medical Association, 268–269, 316
Committee on Costs of Medical Care, 282
Committee on Nursing formed, 269, 354
Committee to Study the Nursing Problem, 309
Department of Nursing formed, 269, 354
founding of, 141
Study of nursing education, 309
American Nurses' Association, 324–330
Committee on Economic and General Welfare, 383
Constituent Associations, 326
Counseling and Placement Service, 326
Economic Security Program of, 383
founding of, 249, 259
Joint Subcommittee on Hospital Accreditation, 317
journals and conventions, 329
membership of, 325
reconstruction of, 314–316
research programs of, 341–344
responsibilities of, 324–329
sections of, 325–326
United Nations relationship, 305, 327
units of, 325–326, 343, 378
American Nurses' Foundation, 336, 344–346
Small Grants Program, 345
American Protestant Hospital Association, 271
American Public Health Association, 277
American Red Cross
during World War I, 260
during World War II, 293
founding of, 222–223
Nursing Service established, 255–256

American Red Cross (Continued)
  Red Cross Student Reserve, 293
  textbook of, 262
  Volunteer Nurses' Aide Corps, 293
American Revolution, 170–171
American Society of Dental Surgeons, 269
American Society of Superintendents of Training Schools, 249, 257
American Zionist Medical Unit, 411
Americas, The, 33–34, 394–401
Ancestor worship in China, 31, 420
Animism, 16, 18, 420
Anna Nery School of Nursing, 399
Anthony, Susan B., 145
Antoinette, Marie, 132, 147
Apollo, 39
Apostles of Jesus, 55
Apprenticeship system
  in guild system, 86
  in medicine, 140–141
  in nursing schools, 86
    criticism of, 268
Arabia, 25, 87
Aristotle, 21, 43
Army nursing, organization of, 221
Army Student Nurse Program, 367
Arnstein, Margaret G., 370
Aryan tribes migrate to India, 28
Asceticism, 112
Asklepios, 39, 42, 43
Asoka, king of India, 29–30
Association of Collegiate Schools of Nursing, 315
Association of Northern European Nurses, 408
Association of Operating Room Nurses, 315
Assyria, 23–24
Aswan Dam, 22
Augustinian nuns, 148, 150, 151, 158–160
Australia, 3–11
Avicenna, 90, 115, 116
Ayur Veda or Veda of Longevity, 29
Aztec Indians, 33, 154, 396

Babylonia (now Iraq), 23–24
Baggally, Olive, 285
Barbarians or "Outsiders," 68
Barber surgeons, 116
Barclay, Miss, 227
Barton, Clara, 146, 221, 222–223
Beard, Dr. Richard Olding, 259
Beck, Frances, 7
Bedford College postgraduate courses, 266, 285
Bedouins, 87
Beecher, Catherine, 145
Beecher, Dame Ethel Hope, 260
Beguines of Belgium, 106–107, 120

Belgium, nursing in, 405
Bellevue Hospital, 169, 223, 248, 263
  graduates of training school, 227–230
Benedictine Rule, 80, 114
Bertheau, Caroline, 190
Bethlehem, 54
Bethlehem Hospital (Bedlam), 179
Bible in Latin Vulgate form, 62, 69
Bickerdyke, Mother Mary Ann, 220–221
"Birth of Reason," 43, 46
Black Death, 110, 111
Black Friars, 103
Blackwell, Dr. Elizabeth, 219, 222
Bolton Bill, 294
Bolton, Frances Payne, 276, 277, 294
Books, sacred
  of China, 31
  of Egypt, 22
  of India, 28
  of Palestine, 26
  of Persia, 28
  of the Moslems, 89
Booth, William, 237
Boston graduates, 231–232
Boston Lunatic Asylum, 183
Botticelli, 131
Brahmanism, 29
Brazzaville, 414
Brewster, Mary, 231
Bridges, Daisy C., 4
British Army Nursing Service, 254
British Journal of Nursing, 252
Broe, Ellen, 7
Brotherhood of man, 25
Brothers Minor, 103
Brothers of Mercy, 363
Brothers of St. John of God, 175, 363
Brown, Esther Lucile, 307–308
Browne, Jean, 280
Buddha, the Enlightened One, 29, 30, 47, 53
Buddhism, rise of, 29, 30, 32, 46, 418
Bull Run, battle of, 218
Bureau of Labor Statistics, 341, 342
Byzantine Empire, 88

Cabot, Dr. Richard, 268
Caduceus, emblem of medical profession, 39
Caesar, Augustus, 22, 48, 53, 68
Caesar, Julius, 22, 47, 48
California, most remote spot on earth, 135
Caliphs, Moslem, 96
Cameron, Dr. G. Stewart, 280
Canada, 132, 158–165, 254
Canadian Government Services, 375–376
Canadian Medical Association, 280
Canadian National Association of Trained Nurses, 251

Canadian Nurse, The, 252, 337, 338
Canadian Nurses' Association, 5, 336–339
  Committee on Nursing Affairs, 338
  national headquarters, 338
  organizational chart, 337
  standing committees, 337–338
  structure changes, 336–337
Canadian Nurses' Foundation, 339
Canadian Society of Superintendents of
  Training Schools, 250–251
Cannon, Ida M., 268
Cape of Good Hope Province, 252, 413
Career opportunities for nurses of Canada,
  375–378
  of the United States, 358–374
Carnegie Foundation, 242, 307
Carnegie Study of Nursing, 307
Carrel, Alexis, 242
Cartier, Jacques, 158
Cassiodorus, 81
Catholic Hospital Association of the U.S.
  and Canada, 271
Catholic social reform, 175–178
Cavell, Edith, English nurse
  at ICN Congress, 251
  executed, 261–262
  in Belgium, 405–406
Celsus, 66, 67
Cervantes, 130
Chadwick, Sir Edwin, sanitarian, 143, 193,
  205
Chaptal, Mlle., 402
Charity Hospital of Berlin, 186
Children's Bureau, U.S. Dept. of Health,
  Education, and Welfare, 369, 374, 388
Chile, nursing schools of, 401
China, ancient, 31
China, nursing in, 418
Chiron, strongest centaur, 39
Chivalry, 109, 143–144
Christian churches, 60
Christian religion, 53–65, 67, 69, 78,
  97
Christians, persecution of, 60
Chung, Elsie Mawfung, 418
Church of Holy Sepulchre, 412
Cicero, Roman writer, 49
Civil Service Commission of U.S., 374
  of Canada, 375
Civil War, American, 217–222
  army nursing of, 221
  volunteer nursing of, 219
Civilization, beginnings of, 15
Clamageran, Alice, 10
Clarissa, or Saint Clare, 103–104
Cleopatra, 21
College of Nursing of Delhi University,
  417
College of Philadelphia, 141
Columbus, Christopher, 33, 109, 154, 155,
  394

Commission on Health Needs of the Nation, 310
Commission on Hospital Accreditation,
  316–317
Committee for Study of Nursing Education, 274–275
Committees, medical
  on the costs of medical care, 282, 283
  to study the nursing problem, 309
Committees, nursing
  for the improvement of nursing service,
    309, 349
  on distribution of nursing service, 279
  on grading of nursing schools, 277, 279,
    281
  on the function of nursing, 308
  on practice, 344, 361
Commonwealth Fund, 277
Confucianism, 31
Confucius, 31, 32, 46, 47, 53, 418
Constantine the Great, 61
Constantinople, 91, 96, 108
  breadline of, 64
  fall of, 116
Contracts of employment, 381
Cortez, Hernando, 154, 157, 394, 396
  establishes first hospital in New World,
    156
Council of Trent, 134
Cowley Brothers, nursing fraternity, 190
Creelman, Lyle, of Canada, 4
Crimes versus torts, 382–383
Crusades, 95–99, 142
  gains and losses of, 107
  hospitals of, 97–98
  social changes of, 107–108
Curie, Pierre and Marie, 241

Damascus, Christians of, 56
Dancing mania or St. Vitus' dance, 111
Danish Red Cross, 420
Dark Ages or Early Middle Ages, 77–93
Dark Period of Nursing, 147, 211
Darrack, Dr. William, 277
Daughters of the American Revolution,
  253
da Vinci, Leonardo, 130–131
Day, Philip E., 364–366
Deaconess Order
  early, 58–60, 63
  modern, founded, 184–191
Debackere, Captain Marthe, 407
Deborah, first nurse in history, 26
de Bullion, Madame, 162
Definition of nursing, 343
Delano, Jane, 230, 262
  death of, 263
de la Peltrie, Mme, 158, 159, 162
DePage, Dr. Antoine, 405–406

DePage, Marie, 405, 406
Diakonia, 63
Dickens, Charles, 183–184
Disciples of Jesus, 55–56
Dissection, not permitted, 20, 116
District nursing, 212–213
Divination, 24
Dix, Dorothea Lynde, 146, 212, 222
    organization of army nursing, 221
    reform in care of mentally ill, 182–183
Dock, Lavinia L., 229, 234, 250
Dominican Order, 102, 113, 116, 155
Drake, Sir Francis, 129
Dravidian inhabitants of India, 28
Duchesse d'Aiguillon, 158
Dunant, Henri, 214–216, 222
Dutch West India Company, 169

Early Christian Era, 53
"Ebers' Papyrus," 20
Ecole Florence Nightingale of Bordeaux, 402
Economic security program for nurses, 341, 383–384
"Economic Status of Registered Professional Nurses," 341
Edith Cavell-Marie dePage School of Nursing, 406
Educational Funds, 385–389
Egypt, ancient, 18–22, 26
Ehrlich, Paul, 241
El Salvador, nursing in, 398
Elster, Ruth, of Germany, 11
Embalming, 20
English graduates, 232
Epidauros, Temple of Asklepios, 42–43
Epidemics, 65, 65, 110–111, 140, 142, 179, 412, 416
    bubonic plague, 65, 110–111
    cholera, 165
    influenza pandemic, 263
    leprosy, 101
    malaria, 68, 412, 416
    measles, 140, 156–158
    of Canada, 158, 160
    of New World, 156
    plague, 65, 110
    smallpox, 156–157
    typhus fever, 110, 214, 263
    yellow fever, 140, 165
Erasmus, 130
Escuela Nacional de Enfermeras, 398
    Linda Richards Library of, 399
Establishment for Gentlewomen during Illness, Florence Nightingale superintendent of, 195
Ethiopia, 413
Eurich, Alvin C., 351
Eustochium, daughter of Paula, 63

Fabiola, 62, 92
Factory Act, first, 179
Facts about Nursing, 329
Fallopio, Gabriele, 137
Far East, 28
Feminism, 144–146
Fenwick, Mrs. Bedford
    at St. Bartholomew's Hospital, 232
    at World's Fair in Chicago, 249
    founder of ICN, 250
    founder of Royal British Nurses' Association, 248
    meets Isabel Hampton Robb, 249
    proposes memorial to Florence Nightingale, 259
Fertile Crescent, 23–27
Feudalism, 78, 83–85, 92, 97
Film Service, ANA–NLN, 330
"First Position Paper," 327
Fisher, Alice, 227
Flexner, Abraham, studies medical schools, 242
Fliedner, Caroline Bertheau, 190
Fliedner, Friederike, 184–189
Fliedner, Pastor Theodor, founds modern Order of Deaconesses, 184–191, 403–404
Florence Nightingale Education Division of the ICN, 7, 285–286
Florence Nightingale International Foundation, 7, 284–286
Florence Nightingale Memorial Committees, 285
Foreign Service Nurses, employed by U.S. State Dept., 371
Formosa (Taiwan), nursing in, 418
France, nursing in, 401
Franciscan Order, 102, 103, 120, 155, 157, 363
Franklin, Benjamin, 170
Freedman's Hospital, in Washington, D.C., 374
French and Indian War, 132, 163
Fry, Elizabeth Gurney, 145, 180–181, 183, 190
    meets Pastor Fliedner, 185, 186
Fulbright Scholarships, 390
Fuller, Samuel, 167
Funds for advanced education, 385–390

Gage, Nina, 418
Gainsborough, Sir Thomas, 131
Galen, 66, 67, 89, 90, 91, 115
Gamp, Sairey, 184
Gardner, Mary Sewall, 409
Gaul devastated, 69
General Federation of Women's Clubs, 247
German Nurses Federation, 11
German Prison Association, 185
Germany, nursing in, 403–405

Ghana, nursing schools of, 413
Ginzberg Report, 308, 339
Girard, Alice, 5
Goldmark, Josephine, 275
Good Samaritan, story of, 55
Good Samaritan Hospital, Portland, Oregon, 230
Goodrich, Annie W.
  at Yale School of Nursing, 276
  dean of Army School of Nursing, 262
  gave special lectures at Teachers College, 257
Grading of Nursing Schools, 277–279
Gray, Carolyn E., dean of Western Reserve School of Nursing, 277
Gray Friars, 103
Greece, ancient, 39–46
  "Birth of Reason" in, 43
  care of the sick, 40
  temples of, 41–43
  women of, 46
  xenodochia of, 40
Grellet, Stephen, 180–181
Grenfell, Sir Wilfred T., 238–239
Guilds, 78, 185–186
  of barber surgeons, 116, 137
Gunn, Jean I., 280
Guy's Hospital, London, 418

Hadassah Women's Organization, 411
Hagen, Elizabeth P., 339
Hamilton, Dr. Anna, 401
Hammurabi, King of Babylonia, 23, 24
Hart, Lillian, 417
Harvey, William, 138
Hebrew prophets, 53
Hebrews of Palestine, 25–27
Helen, Sister, of England, 225
Henderson, Virginia, 7, 349, 350
Henrietta Szold School of Nursing, 411
Henry II of England, 122
Henry VIII of England, destroyed monasteries, 147
Henry Street Settlement, 231
Herbert, Sir Sidney, 143, 196, 205, 206
Hill-Burton Act, 310
Hinduism, 28
Hippocrates, 22, 43, 44, 50, 91, 137
Hojer, Gerda, 408
Holmes, Oliver Wendell, 141–142
Homer, author of "The Iliad" and "The Odyssey," 39
Horace, Roman poet, 48
Horus, son of Isis and Osiris, 19
Hospitals
  first of New World, 168–170
  growth of, 117
    in America, 172
  Jesus of Nazareth (formerly Immaculate Conception), 156, 396

Hospitals (Continued)
  La Scala, 112–113
  of Bagdad and Cordova, 90
  of Heilige Geist, 117
  Order of St. John at Valleta, 118–119
  St. John of Jerusalem, 98
  St. Mary Magdalene, 98, 120
  St. Mary of the Teuton, 98
  Santa Fe (Holy Faith), 156
  Santo Spirito of Rome, 92, 117
  three famous, of England, 118
    Bethlehem, 118
    St. Bartholomew's, 118, 169
    St. Thomas in London, 118, 169, 208, 211
Hospitals and Missions of the Americas, 155–157
Hôtel Dieu (House of God), 117, 118
  of Lyons, 92
  of Montreal, 162, 163
  of Paris, 92, 150
  of Quebec, 158, 160, 163
Howard, John, 180
Howe, Julia Ward, 145, 193
Hunan-Yale School of Nursing, 418
Hunayn, an oculist and Moslem translator of Hippocrates and Galen, 90
Hygeia, goddess of health, 39

Iatrion, of ancient Greece, 40
Iliad and Odyssey, 39
Imhotep, priest physician of Egypt, 19
Immortality, belief in, 20
Inca Indians, 33, 154
India, ancient, 28–31
  Buddhism of, 29
  Hinduism of, 28–29
  King Asoka of, 29–30
  medicine of, 30
  nursing in Republic of, 417
  sanitation of, 205
  women of, 30–31
Indians of the Americas, 33, 154, 159, 396
Industrial Nursing, 296–297
Industrial Revolution, 132–133
  women of, 146
Infanticide, 101
Infirmarian, nurse of Benedictine Rule, 80
Influenza pandemic of 1918, 263
Institute of Nursing Sisters, 190
Institute of Research and Service, 339, 340
Interim Classification of Nursing Schools, 310
International Council of Nurses, 3–11, 250, 285–286
  board of directors, 6
  booklet on Nursing Ethics, 7
  booklet on "ICN Basic Principles of Nursing Care," 7
  Code of Ethics, 7

International Council of Nurses (Continued)
  Exchange of Privileges for Nurses Program, 8
  first officers of, 250
  Grand Council, 6, 7, 8
  International Student Nurses' Unit, 9
  Journals and Congresses, 8, 286
  relationship with the United Nations, 305
International Hospital Association, 286
Inventories of Registered Nurses, 342
Isis, Mother Earth, 18
Islam, 86–91
Israel, nursing in, 410
Italian Nurses' Association, 910
Italy, nursing in, 408

Jahoda, Marie, 4–5
Jamestown, settlement of, 166, 167
Janus, temple of, 47
Japan, nursing in, 419
Jenkins, Helen Hartley, 258, 277
Jenner, Edward, 138
Jerusalem
  ancient city of, 88
  modern city of, 412
  seized by Seljuk Turks, 96
Jesuit Order, 134, 155, 158, 159, 162
  "Relations" of, 155, 162
Jesus of Nazareth, 54–55, 60, 92
John, King of England, 108
  signing of Magna Charta, 108
Johns, Ethel, 278
Johns Hopkins Medical School established, 242
Johns Hopkins School of Nurses, 257, 418
Joint Commission on Accreditation of Hospitals, 316
Joint Commission on Distribution of Nursing Service, 279
Jones, Agnes, 213, 214
Jordan, independent Arab state, 411
Journal of Practical Nursing, 306
Journal of the American Medical Association, 268, 269
Journals, first nursing, 252
Judaism, 87
Juno, Roman goddess and woman's patroness, 47
Jupiter, 47

Kaiserswerth Deaconess Institution, 184–190, 403
Kaiserswerth-on-the-Rhine, 404
Karll, Sister Agnes, 251, 404
Karma, Wheel of, 29
Kellogg Foundation, 317, 339, 341
King's Evil (scrofula), 138–139

King's Touch (for cure of scrofula), 138–139
Kircher, Athanasius, and the microscope, 138
Knighthood, education for, 95
Knights Hospitallers, or Military Nursing Orders, 97–99
Koch, Dr. Robert, 241
Koran, sacred book of Moslems, 89
Korea, nursing in, 420
Korean Police Action of the U.N., 366, 407, 420

Labor unions and professional organizations, difference between, 252
Lancet Commission of England, 281
La Scala Hospital, 112–113
Late Middle Ages, 120–122
Latin America, nursing in, 394–401
Latins of ancient Rome, 46
Lazarettos, 92, 98
League of Nations, 266, 267, 411
League of Red Cross Societies, 266, 285
  Nursing Division of, 285
Lees, Florence, 213
Legal status of employed persons, 381
Leone, Lucile Petry, 311
Leprosarium, national, of Carville, La., 369
Leprosy, 82, 92, 101, 120
Licensing of Nurses, 281–282
  interstate licensure, 380
Life insurance and retirement income, 384
Lister, Lord Joseph, 241
"Little United Nations," 423
Livingstone, Nora, 230
Livy, Roman writer, 49
Long, Dr. Crawford, 142
Longfellow, Henry Wadsworth, 201
Louis XIV, 132
Louis XVI, 132
Louisiana, settlement of, 165
Loveridge, Emily L., 230
Loyola, Ignatius, founder of a teaching order, 134
"Lunatics' Tower" in Vienna, 179
Luther, Martin, 130, 133–134

Macdonald, Nursing Sister Margaret, 261
Mack Training School, 227
MacMurchy, Dr. Helen, 252
Magic, black and white, 17
Magna Charta, 108, 132
Malaria in city of Rome, 68
Malden institutions for handicapped, 412
Mance, Jeanne, 162–163
Manual of Charity Hospital of Berlin, 186

Marcella, 62, 78, 92
Marco Polo, 109
Marriage Mart of Canada, 164–165
Marriage Mart of Jamestown, 166
Mars, Roman god of war, 47
Massachusetts General Hospital, 225, 233, 248, 268
Mather, Cotton, 167
Maxwell, Anna Caroline, 232
    at camp hospital of Georgia, 254
Maya Indians, 33, 154, 396
Mayflower, 166, 167
McGee, Dr. Anita Newcomb, 253, 255
McIsaac, Isabel, 262
McLaughlin, L. Margaret, 311
McManus, Prof. R. Louise, 308
Mecca, holy city of Moslems, 87, 88, 89
Medes and Persians, 27
Medical missionaries, 238–239
Medical social service, 268
Medicine
    advances in, 141, 291
    Age of Coma in, 116
    apprenticeship system of, 140
    broader aims in, 268–271
    Byzantine, 115
    early Christian, 65, 66
    enters a revolutionary period, 240
    enters the university, 148
    in ancient China, 32
    in ancient Egypt, 18–20
    in ancient India, 30
    in Babylonia, 24
    in colonial America, 139–142
    in Greece, 42–44
    in Palestine, 26
    in Rome, 49–50, 65–66
    monastic, 114
    of Early Middle Ages, 91
    of Islam (Moslem), 89–90, 115–116
    of Late Middle Ages, 113–116
    of Renaissance, 137
    primitive, 17
    revolution in practice, 240–242
    withdraws from monasteries, 148
Medicine and Nursing, 500–1000 A.D., 91–92
Medicine men (or shaman), 17, 33, 154
Mediterranean Sea, 18
Mediterranean World, 39
Mei-Yo, General Chow, of Formosa, 419
Melbourne, Australia, ICN at, 3
Memorial
    Florence Nightingale International Foundation, 284–285
    to American nurses of World War I, 402–403
    to Florence Nightingale proposed, 259
Men nurses
    Brotherhood of Mexico City, 156
    Brothers of St. John of God, 175, 363

Men nurses (Continued)
    in Belgium, 405
    military nurses or Knights Hospitallers, 97–99
    opportunities for, 363–366
Mendicant Orders, 102, 120
Mental hospitals
    Bethlehem (Bedlam), 118
    Dorothea Lynde Dix and, 182–183
    Linda Richards and, 232–233
    "Lunatic Asylum" at Kaiserswerth, 187
Mental illness
    early care for patients with, 149
    in colonial America, 169
    reform in care for patients with, 182–183
Merryweather, Miss, 212
Merton, Robert, 351
Mesopotamia, 23
Mexico, nursing in, 396–397
Michelangelo, 130
Middle Ages, Early, 77–93
    Late, 94–126
Midwifery, 407
Military nursing, 295–296, 366–367
Military Nursing Orders or Knights Hospitallers, 97–99
    Hospitaller Sisters, 98
    Knights Hospitallers of St. John of Jerusalem, 98
    Knights of St. Lazarus, 98, 101
    Teutonic Knights Hospitallers, 98
Military rank for nurses first granted by Canadian government, 254, 375
Mills School of Male Nurses, 363
Milton, John, 130
Minna, ex-prisoner at Kaiserswerth, 185
Missions in New Spain, 155
Mobile Army Surgical Hospital (MASH) Units, 422
Modern nursing founded, 208–212
Mohammed, founder of Islam, 87–90
Monasteries
    activities of, 80–81
    Benedictine Rule of, 80
    Buddhist, 30
    decline of, 100
    first Christian, 62, 69, 78–83
    loss of interest in, 95
    nursing of, 121
    of Cluny, 96
    of Monte Cassino, 79
    plan of, 79, 80
    preservation of knowledge in, 81
    women of, 81–83
Money, Miss, 227
Monks and nuns, nurses of the Middle Ages, 92
Montag, Mildred, 340
Montcalm, French hero, 163
Monte Cassino, 79

Montezuma, Aztec ruler, 154–156, 396
Montreal General Hospital, 230
Montreal, settlement of, 161
More, Sir Thomas, 130
Mores or customs, primitive, 15
Morocco, 414
Morton, Dr. W. T. G., 269
Mosaic Law, 25
Moses, 25, 26
Moslem Empire, spread of, 22
    weakened, 96
Moslems, 22, 88, 89, 90, 96, 98, 156, 412
Motherhouse system, of Germany, 404
    of Kaiserswerth, 189
Muhlenberg, Reverend, 173
Murdock Report, 309
Mythology, replacing animism, 18

Napoleonic wars, 145
National Association of Brazilian Grad-
    uate Nurses, 399
National Association for Practical Nurse
    Education and Service, 306
National Association of Colored Graduate
    Nurses, 249
National Association of Trained Nurses of
    France, 11, 402
National Committee for the Improvement
    of Nursing Service, 309
National Defense Medical Center School
    of Nursing, on Formosa, 344, 419
National Federation of Licensed Practical
    Nurses, 307
National Health Conference, 284
National Health Surveys, 283–284
National Institutes of Health, USPHS,
    312, 345
National League for Nursing, 330–333
    Constituent Leagues, 331
    Council on Research in Nursing, 347
    Departments and Divisions of, 330–331
    founding of, 315
    membership of, 330–332
    Research and Studies Service of, 346
    research programs of, 346
    special committees of, 332
National Mental Health Act of 1946, 318
National Nursing Council for War Service,
    307, 341, 392, 393
National Student Nurses' Association,
    333–335
Naval Medical School of Bethesda, Mary-
    land, 367
New Amsterdam, becomes New York, 169
New England, 135, 136
    settlement of, 165–170, 178
New England Hospital for Women and
    Children, 223–224
New France, 135–136, 157–158

New Spain, 135–136, 154–157, 178
New York Hospital founded, 170
New York Hospital Training School, grad-
    uates of, 230–231
New York State Charities Aid Associa-
    tion, 223
New York State, nurse practice act of
    1938, 281
New Zealand, 6
New Zealand Registered Nurses' Associa-
    tion, 6
Newgate Prison, 180–181
Nigeria, nursing schools of, 413
Nightingale, Florence, 191–214
    appearance of, 199
    as world consultant, 206
    at Alexandria, 195
    at Kaiserswerth, 195
    birthplace of, 192
    Crimean War service, 196–203
    death of, 259
    early life of, 191–195
    first position, 195–196
    friend of Sir Sidney Herbert and Mrs.
        Herbert, 194, 206
    Julia Ward Howe and Dr. Howe, 193
    honored by Queen Victoria, 203
    memorial to, proposed, 259
    postwar activities, 203–206
    presented with Nightingale Fund, 203
    promotes army sanitation, 204
    promotes district nursing, 212
    promotes hospital and nursing reform,
        204, 225
    promotes sanitation in India, 205
    promotes workhouse infirmary reform,
        213–214
    romance of, 194
    with nuns in Rome, 194
    with Sisters of Charity in Paris and
        Alexandria, 195
    writings of, 204–205
Nightingale Fund, 203, 208–209, 210
Nightingale School of Nursing
    certified nurses of, 210
    founding of, 208–212
    probationary training of, 210
    rules and regulations of, 209
    social grades of students, 209
Nightingale System, basic principles of,
    209, 225–227
    spread of, 223, 227
    to Australia, 227
    to South America, 399
Northern Europe, nursing in, 407–408
Norwegian Nurses' Association, 408
Nurse Draft Bill of World War II, 297–298
Nurse Practice Acts, revision of, 281
Nurse Society of Philadelphia, 171
Nurse, the new, of 1860–1900, 239–240
Nurse Training Act of 1964, 353

Nurses' Association of China, 418
Nurses' Educational Funds, Inc., 386
"Nurses for a Growing Nation," 346
Nursing
　becomes a separate occupation, 121
　decline of, 121, 147
　definition of, 343
　little distinction between medicine and,
　　91
　men in, during Middle Ages, 97–99
　　today, 363–366
　military, 366
　shortage, during World War I, 262–263
　　following World War II, 305–306
　studies of, 307–309
　women lose control of, 148
Nursing methods exposed, 183
Nursing Outlook, journal of NLN, 316, 332
Nursing Reform, nonsectarian, 208
"Nursing Schools Today and Tomorrow,"
　final report of Grading Committee, 279
Nursing Times, journal of Royal College
　of Nursing, 265
Nutting, Mary Adelaide, 229
　develops first school for graduate nurses,
　257–258

Occupational health nursing, 362
Octavius, successor to Julius Caesar, 22
Ohlson, Agnes, 4, 11
Opportunities, career, for senior students,
　358
Orders
　Beguines, 106, 107, 120
　Deaconess, early, 58, 60, 63
　　modern, 184–191
　Dominican, 102, 113, 116, 155
　early Christian, of women, 58–60
　Franciscans, 102–103, 120, 155
　Jesuits, 134, 155, 162
　　"Relations" of, 155, 162
　mendicant, rise of, 102
　military nursing or Knights Hospital-
　　lers, 97–99
　of Mercy, Catholic, 173, 196
　　Protestant, 190, 197
　　Russian, 196, 201
　of St. John at Valetta, 118–119
　of St. John of Jerusalem, 118
　of St. Ursula, 134, 158–161, 164–165
　of Santo Spirito, 117
　of Sisters of Charity, 176–178
　of Tertiaries of St. Francis, 104–105
　Secular, rise of, 104–107
　Sisterhoods of English Church, 190–191
　Sisters of Mercy, Catholic, 173, 196
　　Protestant, 190, 197
　　Russian, 196, 201
　Widows and Virgins, 59, 60, 69

Organization of American States, 395
Organizations, medical
　American College of Physicians, 269
　American College of Surgeons, 269
　American Medical Association, 268–269,
　　277, 354
　American Society of Dental Surgeons,
　　269
Organizations, nursing
　Alumnae associations, 248
　American Association of Industrial
　　Nurses, 315
　American Association of Nurse Anes-
　　thetists, 315
　American Nurses Association, 259, 315,
　　324–330
　American Society of Superintendents of
　　Training Schools, 249, 257–258
　　became National League of Nursing
　　　Education, 259
　Association of Collegiate Schools of
　　Nursing, 315
　Association of Northern European
　　Nurses, 408
　Association of O. R. Nurses, 315
　Canadian National Association of
　　Trained Nurses, became the Cana-
　　dian Nurses' Association, 260
　Canadian Society of Superintendents of
　　Training Schools, 250, 251
　early changes in, 259
　German Nurses' Association, 11, 250
　International Council of Nurses, 3–11,
　　250, 286, 305
　Italian Nurses' Association, 410
　Matrons' Council of Great Britain and
　　Ireland, 248, 250
　National Association for Practical Nurse
　　Education and Service, 306, 380
　National Association of Colored Gradu-
　　ate Nurses, 249, 315
　National Association of Graduate
　　Nurses of France, 402
　National Council of Nurses of Great
　　Britain and Northern Ireland, 248,
　　250
　National Federation of Licensed Prac-
　　tical Nurses, 307
　National League for Nursing, 315, 316,
　　330–333
　National League of Nursing Education,
　　259, 277, 306, 315
　National Organization for Public Health
　　Nursing, 259, 315
　National Student Nurses' Association,
　　333–335, 386
　Navy Nurse Corps Candidate Program,
　　367
　Norwegian Nurses' Association, 408
　Nurse Society of Philadelphia, 171–
　　172

Organizations, nursing *(Continued)*
    Nurses' Associated Alumni of the United
        States, 249, 250
        became the American Nurses' Associ-
            ation, 259
    Nurses' Association of China, 418
    Royal British Nurses' Association, 248
    Royal College of Nursing, 263–265
    Student Nurses' Association of England,
        263–265
    Swedish Nurses' Association, 407
Osborn, Lucy, 227
Osiris, husband of Isis, 19
Osler, Sir William, 379

Palestine, 23, 25, 54, 55, 410–411
Palmer, Sophia, 249, 252
Pan American Health Organization, 311,
    395, 400
Pan American Sanitary Bureau, 395
Pan American Union, 395
Panacea, healer of all ills, 39
Pantheon, temple of Rome, 408
Papyri, 20, 31
Paracelsus, 137
Paré, Ambroise, 137
Parthenon, temple of Athens, 41
Partnership for Progress, initiated by
    AHA, 317
Passavant, Reverend William, 173, 189
Pasteur Institute founded, 241
Pasteur, Louis, 205, 240–241, 401
Paula, 63, 78, 92
Pavlova, Grand Duchess of Russia, 201
Peace Corps, 371–372
Peiping Union Medical College, 418, 419
Pelton, Garnet, 268
Pennsylvania Hospital, founded, 170
    school of nursing for men, 364
People-to-People Health Foundation, 374
Pergamum, birthplace of Galen, 66
Permanent Army Medical Corps Nursing
    Service of Canada, 261
Persia (now Iran), 27
Peru, 154
Peter, the Apostle, 57
Pfefferkorn, Blanche, 278
Pharaohs, of Egypt, 19, 20, 21
Philadelphia Dispensary, 171
Philadelphia General Hospital (formerly
    Blockley Hospital), 169, 227
Philip of Macedonia, 45
Phoebe, a Greek lady, 57, 58
Pilgrimages to Palestine, 94–95
Pinel, Philippe, 138
Plagues, Great, of Late Middle Ages, 110–
    113
    of third century, 65
Plato, 43

Poor Clares or Clarissas, 104
Pope, Georgina F., 254, 261
Pope Innocent III, 117
Pope Urban II, 96
Postwar developments following World
    War II, 298
Practical nurses, 306–307
Preliminary courses, first in Scotland, 233
    first in the United States, 233
        at Johns Hopkins Hospital, 233
        at Simmons College, 233
Priest physicians, 17, 19, 20, 26
Prig, Betsy, 183–184
Primitive man, 15
Princess Margaret, 265
Princess Mary's Royal Air Force Nursing
    Service, 260
Prisons, conditions in, 149–150, 179
    reform of, 180–181, 185
Procurement and Assignment Service of
    World War II, 293
Professional Credentials and Personnel
    Service of ANA, 329
Professional Liability Insurance, 379–380,
    384
Protestant nursing sisterhoods, 190
Protestant Sisterhood of All Saints, 225
Protestant Social Reform, 178–184
Provincial associations, of Canada, 338
    of Manitoba and Ontario, 251
Psychiatry, rise of, 318
Psychosomatic medicine, 318
Public health nursing, 361
Public Workhouse and House of Correc-
    tion, 169
Pueblo Indians, 154
Pyramids of Egypt, 20

Quebec, founding of, 158–161
Queen Alexandra's Royal Army Nursing
    Corps, 255, 260, 422
Queen Alexandra's Royal Naval Nursing
    Service, 260
Queen Elizabeth I, 132, 143, 165
Queen Elizabeth II, 265
Queen Elizabeth, the Queen Mother, 265
Queen Isabella of Spain, 122, 154
Queen Mary of Scotland, 143
Queen Victoria, 142, 146, 203, 376–377

Radegunde of Poitiers, 82, 122
Raphael, 131
Rathbone, William, 182, 212–214
Raymond Rich Associates, 314
Reconstruction following World War I, 265
Red Cross Demonstration School of Nurs-
    ing in Tokyo, 420

Red Cross enrollment changes, 307
Red Cross Hospitals
  of France, 401
  of Germany, 404
  of Mexico City, 398
  of Tokyo, 420
Red Cross Societies
  birth of, 214
  flag of, 217
  founded in the United States, 222, 223
  International Committee of, 216
  of Denmark, 420
  of France, 403
  of Germany, 404
  of Italy, 409, 422
  of Japan, 420
  ready to assist armies, 253
  Treaty of Geneva, 216
Reform in nursing
  Catholic, 176–178
  in the United States, 223
  in workhouse infirmaries, 213
  nonsectarian, 208, 225–227
  Pre-Nightingale, 223
  Protestant, at Kaiserswerth, 184–207
Reformation or Protestant Revolt, 133, 148
Reforms, Social, 175–183, 236–239
Registration of Nurses, 247–248
  and licensing, 281–282
  first laws enacted, 252–253
  spread of, 252–253
Rehabilitation
  expansion of services, 319
  first Rehabilitation Act, 265
  following World War I, 265
  following World War II, 319
  vocational, 265–266
  Workman's Compensation Board Reha-
    bilitation Center of Malton, Ontario,
    Canada, 319–320
Reichardt, Gertrud, 186
Reincarnation, 29
"Relations" of the Jesuits, 155, 162, 189,
  190
Rembrandt, 131
Renaissance, 129–153
  classical revival of, 130–131
  decline in nursing of, 147
  industrial revolution of, 132
  medicine of, 137
  political revolution of, 131
  women of, 143–147
Republic of India, nursing in, 417
Republic of Sudan, 22
Research programs
  associate degree, 340–341
  expansion of, 339
  Institute of Research and Service, 339
  of American Nurses' Foundation, 344–
    346
  of ANA, 341–344

Research programs (Continued)
  of NLN, 346–347
  of USPHS, 348–350
  of Yale University, 349–350
Responsibilities of nurses, moral and legal,
  379
Revision of Nurse Practice Acts, 281–282
Revolution
  American, 132, 170–171
  French, 132, 147
  Industrial, 132–133
    women of, 146
  Latin American, 132
  political, 131–132
Reynolds, Sir Joshua, 131
Rhazes of Persia, 90
Richards, Linda, 223–224
  first trained nurse in America, 224, 232
  Linda Richards Library, 399
  work in Japan, 419
Richelieu, Cardinal, of France, 158
Robb, Isabel Hampton, 249, 257, 258
  at Illinois Training School, 228
  at Johns Hopkins Training School, 228
  books of, 229, 234
  inaugurates affiliations, 228
Roberts, Mary M., 252, 308, 350
Robinson, Mary, 212
Rockefeller Foundation, 274–275, 277,
  281, 339, 345, 407
Rockefeller Institute for Medical Research,
  242
Rockefeller, John D., 242
Rogers, Linda L., 231
Roman Empire
  extent of, 53, 68
  fall of, 68–70
  ladies of, 81–83
Roman matrons, 61–63
Rome, ancient, 46–51
  army hospitals of, 50
  dispensaries of, 50
  Greece under control of, 45
  medicine and nursing in, 49
  Palestine under rule of, 25
  sanitation of, 49–50
  temples of, 47
  women of, 50–51, 57
Romulus and Remus, 47
Rothschild-Hadassah University Hospital,
  411
Royal Australian Air Force band, 3, 10
Royal Australian Nursing Federation, 3
Royal British Nurses' Association, 248
Royal Canadian Army Medical Corps
  Nursing Service, 254
Royal Children's Orthopedic Hospital of
  Frankston, Australia, 10
Royal College of Nursing and National
  Council of Nurses of the United King-
  dom, 265

Rubens, 131
Rule, of St. Augustine, 98
  of St. Benedict of Nursia, 79–81
Russell, Dr. Kathleen, 280

St. Augustine, 98
St. Bartholomew's Hospital, founding of, 118
St. Basil of Caesarea, 64, 65, 92
St. Benedict of Nursia, rule of, 79–81
St. Catherine of Siena, 111–113, 122
St. Clare, or Clarissa, 103–104
St. Dominic, 102, 113, 116
St. Elizabeth of Hungary, 105–106, 122
St. Elizabeth's Hospital, Washington, D.C., 374
St. Francis of Assisi, 102–105, 108, 116, 120, 122
  Mendicant Order of, 103
  mission in honor of, 157
  Second Order of, 103–104
  Third Order of, 104–105, 120
St. Hildegard, 114–115
St. Jerome, 62, 69, 78, 91
St. Louise de Marillac, 176, 177, 401
St. Luke, "the beloved physician," 57
St. Luke's International Medical Center, Tokyo, 419
St. Mungo's Medical College, Scotland, 233
St. Paul (Saul), 56–58, 59
  attitude toward women, 57
St. Peter, first bishop of Rome, 57
St. Peter's Cathedral, 409
St. Radegunde, 82, 122
St. Thomas' Hospital, 208–212
  founding of, 118
  Nightingale School founded at, 208–212
St. Ursula, Order of (see Ursuline nuns)
St. Vincent de Paul, 175–178, 187, 401
Saladin, Moslem conqueror of Jerusalem, 107
Salerno, in Italy, first medical school at, 92, 115, 116
Salvation Army, 237
Sanitary Commission of Civil War, 217–218
Sanitation
  era of, 142–143
  of English army, during Crimean War, 204
  of Hebrews, 26
  of India, 205
  of Romans, 49
"Santo Filomena," poem by Longfellow, 201
Santo Spirito Hospital of Rome, 92, 117
Saul of Tarsus (St. Paul), 56–58
School Data Survey of 1949, 309
School nursing founded in the United States, 231

School of the Rue de la Culture, Belgium, 405
Schools, medical
  attempts at reform of, 242
  development of, in America, 141, 172
  established in Mexico City, 136
  grading of, 242
  Johns Hopkins founded, 242
  of aviation medicine, 367
  Salerno, Italy, first to be founded, 92, 115, 116
Schools, nursing
  apprenticeship system in the U.S., 225–227
  Carnegie study of, and Brown report, 307
  curriculum for, first, 259
  early American, 225
  early endowed, 209, 276
  first modern, 208–212
  grading of, 277–279
  Interim Classification of, 310
  national accreditation of, 316
  Nightingale reform in the U.S., 225
  prevailing methods, early, 234–235
  Rockefeller Survey of, 274–277
  school data survey of, 309
  system of apprenticeship in the U.S., 225–227
Schweitzer, Dr. Albert, 415–417
Scott, Jessie M., 314
Seaman, Dr. Valentine, first to lecture to nurses, 170
Seljuk Turks, seize Jerusalem, 96
Semitic Tribes from Arabia, 25
Semmelweis, Ignaz, of Vienna, 142
Senior students, opportunities for, 367
Serra, Father Junipero, Franciscan friar, 157
Seton, Mother Elizabeth, 173, 178
Settlement houses, 237
Sewall, Judge Samuel, 167
Shakespeare, William, 130
Shattuck, Lemuel, 143
Shaw, Clara Weeks, 231, 234
Shean, Marion, 310
Simpson, Sir James, 142
Sister Helen, 225
Sisters of Charity, Order of
  founding of, 176–178
  instruction by St. Louise de Marillac, 176–178
  introduced into America by Mother Elizabeth Seton, 173, 178
  introduced into Ireland by Mother Mary Aikenhead, 178
  service during Crimean War, 178
  uniform dress of, 177
Sisters of Mercy, Catholic Order of, in Pittsburgh, 173, 196
  Protestant Order of, 190, 197
  Russian, 196, 201

Sisters of St. John's House, 190, 197
Sisters of St. Lazarus, 120
Sisters of St. Mary Magdalene, 120
Sistine Chapel of the Vatican, 131, 409
Slaves, great physicians as, 47, 65, 66
  Greek scholars as, 47
Smith, Captain John, 166
Snively, Mary Agnes, 229, 250, 251
Social agencies, development of, 208–242
Social problems, of England, 178–180
  of Middle Ages, 99–101
Social reform, 175–184
Social Security Act of 1935, 283
Social Security protection by ANA, 384
Social Service established, 175
Society of St. Joseph de la Flèche, 162–163
Socio-economic studies of nursing, 341–342
Socrates, 43
Solferino, battle of, 214–216
Soranus of Ephesus, 66
South American republics, nursing in, 399–401
S. S. Hope, 372
Stanton, Elizabeth Cady, 145
State Boards of Medical Examiners established, 242
Stewart, Isabel Maitland, comes to Teachers' College, 258
  gratitude due to, 350
  honored by chair in nursing research, 339
Stewart, Isla, 232, 248
Stone Age, 15, 18
Stowe, Harriet Beecher, 145
Strong, Mrs. Rebecca, of Scotland, 233, 257, 267
Structure changes in organized nursing, 314–316
Student meetings at Melbourne, Australia, 8–10
Student Nurses' Association
  of England, 263–264
  of India, 417
  of the U.S., 333–335
Studies of F.S. & Q., 342–344, 345
Studies of Nursing, Three, 307–309
Surgeon General's Consultant Group, 350–354
  President Kennedy's message to Congress, 350–351
  publishes Toward Quality in Nursing, 351
  recommendations of, 352–353
"Survey and Assessment of Research in Nursing," 349
Survey of medical practice, 282–283
"Survey of Nursing Education in Canada" by Professor George Weir, 281
Surveys of nursing
  by AMA, 309
  by Carnegie Foundation, 307

Surveys of nursing (Continued)
  by Grading Committee, 277–279
  by Rockefeller Foundation, 274–278
  by Teachers College, 308–309
  in Canada and England, 280–281
Surveys of nursing and medicine, 274–288
Swami, Anthony, 418
Sweating sickness, 111
Swedish Nurses' Association, 407, 408
Sydenham, Thomas, 138, 240

Taiwan University Hospital School of Nursing, 419
Taoism, 418
Tarsus, Saul of (St. Paul), 56
Teachers College, Columbia University, 268
  first graduate courses at, 257, 268
  study of nursing, 308
Temples
  of Asklepios, 42–43
  of Egypt, 19–20
  of Epidauros, 42
  of Greece, 41–42
  of Karnak, 19
  of Luxor, 19
  of Rome, 47
Textbooks for nurses, first, 233–234
Thirty Years War (1618–1648), 134
Tiber River, 47, 65
Tithing, Hebrew system of, 27
Titian of Venice, 131
Today's Health, an AMA publication, 268–269
Toltec Indians, 33, 154, 396
Toronto General Hospital, 229
Torts versus crimes, 382–383
"Toward Quality in Nursing – Needs and Goals," 351
Toynbee Hall, 237
Trained Nurses Association of India, 417
Traineeship Awards of USPHS, 336, 353, 386–388
Treaty of Geneva, 216
Trends in nursing (1893 to 1920), 267–268
  Modern, 323–357
Tuke, William, 138
Tunisia, 414
Turkestan, invaders from, 96

Uniform dress
  adoption of, in America, 235–236
  lack of, in early convents, 82–83
  lineage of the cap, 236
  of Civil War, 221
  of Crimean War, 202
  of Dominican Order, 103
  of Franciscan Order, 103

Uniform dress *(Continued)*
  of Kaiserswerth deaconesses, 188–189
  of Knights Hospitallers, 99
  of monasteries of Late Middle Ages, 122
  of New France, 164
Uniforms, first in the United States, 235–236
Union of South Africa, 413
United Arab Republic, 22
United Nations, 300–305
  Economic and Social Council (ECOSOC), 301, 302, 305
    Specialized Agencies of, 302–305
      FAO, 302, 414
      ILO, 302, 305
      UNESCO, 22, 302, 414–415
      WHO, 4, 303–305, 414, 417, 419
  General Assembly, 300
  International Court of Justice, 301
  Korean Police Action, 420
  Korean Reconstruction Agency, 424
  Secretariat, 305
  Security Council, 301
  Trusteeship Council, 301
  UNICEF, a special body, 302, 304, 305, 414, 417
UNRRA, 299–300
U.S. Army Nurse Corps established, 255
U.S. Army School of Nursing organized, 262
U.S. Cadet Nurse Corps, 293–295
U.S. Civil Service Commission, 374
U.S. Department of Health, Education, and Welfare, PHS, 283, 311–314
U.S. Department of Labor, 341
U.S. Exchange Visitor Program, 378
  ANA a sponsor, 378
U.S. Government Services, 366–369
U.S. Marine Hospital and Public Health Service, 311
U.S. Marine Hospital Service, 311
U.S. Navy Nurse Corps established, 255
U.S. Public Health Service, Dept. of HEW
  associated with Pan American Health Organization and WHO, 311
  Division of Nursing, 313
  five Bureaus share responsibilities, 312–314
  history of, 311
  national health surveys by, 283–284
  National Institutes of Health, 312
  national inventory of registered nurses, 293
  National Library of Medicine, 312
  nursing opportunities with, 364, 369
  nursing research programs, 348–349
  Professional Nurse Traineeship Awards, 386–388
  Public Health Reports, official USPHS journal, 312
  Student Training and Extern Program, 369

U.S. Veterans Administration, 265, 368
Universidad Nacional del Litoral of Argentina, 400
Universities
  Columbia, 257–259
  Dartmouth, 141
  Harvard, 141
  Heidelberg, 405
  New York, 364
  of Belgium, 407
  of Bologna, Italy, 116, 139
  of British Columbia, 280
  of Cambridge, England, 116
  of Delhi, India, 417
  of Madras, India, 417
  of Mexico, 397
  of Minnesota, 259
  of Montpelier, France, 116
  of Oxford, England, 116
  of Paris, 116
  of Pennsylvania, 141
  of Salerno, Italy, 92, 116
  of Texas, 257
  rise of, 116
  Western Reserve, 276
  Yale, 141, 276, 405
University of Pennsylvania Hospital, 230
Upanishads, sacred, of India, 28, 31
Urban II, Pope at Rome, 96
Ursuline nuns
  convent of, in Quebec, 158–161
  first instructors of nurses on American continent, 161
  founding of order, 134
  in New Orleans, 165
  with Marriage Mart from France, 164–165

van Dyck, 131
van Leeuwenhoek, Anton, 138
van Rensselaer, Euphemia, 235
Vassar Training Camp of World War I, 262
Vatican City, 409
Vedas, sacred, of India, 28, 31
Veils, 82, 83
Velasquez, 131
Vellore Medical College Hospital School of Nursing, 417
Versailles, marvel of, 132
Vesalius, Andreas, 137
Victoria, queen of England, 142, 146, 376, 377
Victorian Order of Nurses for Canada, 376–378
Virgil, 48
Virginia, settlement of, 166
Voluntary Aid Detachment (V.A.D.) of World War I, 260
von Behring, Emil, 241
von Lersner, Olga, 405

Wald, Lillian D.
  inaugurates public health nursing in the
    U.S., 231
  inaugurates school nursing in the U.S.,
    231
  instructor at Teachers College, New
    York, 258
  represents nurses at Cannes Conference,
    266
Waldron, Martha M., 224
Walter Reed Army Research Institute, 367
War
  American Civil, Sanitary Commission
    of, 217–218
    volunteer nursing in, 219–221
  American Revolution, 132, 168, 170–171
  Franco-Prussian, 222
  French and Indian (Seven Years' War),
    163
  Napoleonic, 132, 145
  South African (Boer War), 254
  Spanish American, 253–254, 255
  Thirty Years', 134
  World War I, 260–263
  World War II, 291–298
    postwar problems, 298
Wardroper, Mrs. Sarah Elizabeth, 208, 211
Warrington, Dr. Joseph, 172
Weir, Prof. George, 280–281
Wellington, Duke of, 132
Western Pacific Regional Office of the
  WHO, 419
Whitman, Walt, 221
Willard, Emma C., 145
Willard, Frances E., 145
Wilson, President Woodrow, 266
Winslow, C. E. A., 275
Winslow-Goldmark Report, 276
Witchcraft, belief in, 167–168
Woman's Hospital of Philadelphia, 224
Women
  barbarian, 69
  early Christian Orders of, 58–60
  following the Civil War, 247
  in monasteries, 81–83
  of American Indian tribes, 34, 155
  of American Revolution, 170
  of ancient Babylonia, 24
  of ancient China, 32

Women (Continued)
  of ancient Egypt, 20
  of ancient Greece, 46
  of ancient India, 30
  of ancient Rome, 50–51, 57
  of Late Middle Ages, 109
  of Palestine, 26
  of the Renaissance, 143, 147
  pioneers in America, 163–165
  under feudalism, 84–85
  under Islam, 90–91
Women's Zionist Organization of America,
  411
Workhouses
  of England, 179, 183
  Workhouse and House of Correction in
    New York, 169
  Workhouse Infirmary of Liverpool, re-
    form of, 213
World Federation for Mental Health, 286,
  318
  ICN and ANA members of, 318
World Health Conferences, 305
World Health Organization, 4, 303–305,
  398, 400, 417, 419
  Expert Committee on Nursing, 302, 305
  Fellowships for foreign study, 389
  six regional offices of, 305, 311, 385
World's Fair of Chicago, 249
Wu, Lillian, 418

Xenodochia, Christian, 63–64, 69
  of ancient Palestine, 27, 40
  of Late Middle Ages, 97
  of St. Basil of Caesarea in Asia Minor,
    64
Xenodochion of the ancient Greeks, 40

Yale Index, 350
Yale's Study of Studies, 349
Y.M.C.A. and Y.W.C.A., 238

Zendavesta, 28
Zoroaster, 28